Mental Health in Bangladesh

S. M. Yasir Arafat
Editor

# Mental Health in Bangladesh

## From Bench to Community

Springer

*Editor*
S. M. Yasir Arafat
Department of Psychiatry
Bangladesh Specialized Hospital Limited
Dhaka, Bangladesh

ISBN 978-981-97-0609-9 ISBN 978-981-97-0610-5 (eBook)
https://doi.org/10.1007/978-981-97-0610-5



This Springer imprint is published by the registered company Springer Nature Singapore Pte Ltd.
The registered company address is: 152 Beach Road, #21-01/04 Gateway East, Singapore 189721, Singapore

Paper in this product is recyclable.

*This book is dedicated to our forefathers of Bangladesh Psychiatry*
*Prof. Dr. A. K. M. Nazimuddowla Chowdhury*
*Prof. Dr. Hidayetul Islam*

# Foreword by Hidayetul Islam

Mental health is an integral component of health. Unfortunately, and historically, this fundamental aspect has been neglected in Bangladesh and its nearby regions. There are several challenges in this way like inadequate resources and research, poor health and mental health literacy, and high stigma attached to mental disorders. As a discipline, psychiatry gets little attention in the undergraduate medical curriculum in Bangladesh.

The evolution of psychiatry started in 1957 through the establishment of Pabna Mental Hospital in Bangladesh during the Pakistan period. After the liberation, along with the overall medical science, psychiatry has marched forward. The establishment of the National Institute of Mental Health (NIMH), Dhaka is another milestone in Bangladesh psychiatry. Over the decades, the mental health services have been expanding in the country. However, Bangladesh lags far behind regarding the local evidence, research, and books on almost all aspects of mental health.

*Mental Health in Bangladesh: From Bench to Community* was an immediate necessity in Bangladesh. I am delighted to see this first book on Psychiatry accumulating local evidence and expertise on the global platform. It is a historical milestone in Bangladesh psychiatry. The book is the first of its kind and unique as it highlights what we have and what we need to do.

Despite the limited number of evidence, the book covers the important aspects of mental health in Bangladesh. It mentions both personal and services development historical aspects of Bangladesh, the evolution of psychotropics in the Bangladesh market, epidemiology of psychiatric disorders, child psychiatry, substance abuse, and psychosexual disorders. The editor sheds light on neglected, however, domains of psychiatry like forensic psychiatry, community psychiatry, geriatric psychiatry, suicide prevention, and public mental health. It includes some emerging aspects of psychiatry like climate change, technology and mental health, and the mental health of vulnerable populations.

This book certainly fills an important gap and contributes to existing knowledge in mental health in Bangladesh. It will be useful for students and faculties working in mental health in Bangladesh. I believe this book will inspire many more to delve into mental health research which will pull Bangladesh Psychiatry to the next level. I hope it will serve as a useful resource for all of us.

Dhaka, Bangladesh Prof. Dr. Hidayetul Islam

# Foreword by Anwara Begum

This is the first comprehensive book on psychiatry in Bangladesh based on limited local evidence and expertise. In addition to all other chapters, it is the first book published on the history of psychiatry in Bangladesh. It contains personal history, the history of mental health services development, and historical aspects of the treatment of psychiatric disorders in Bangladesh. Through this book, all psychiatrists, doctors, and common people will know about the historical evolution of psychiatry in Bangladesh. It is a daunting task. The editor, authors, and publisher put in immense effort and worked tirelessly to make it happen. I appreciate the efforts and wish you all the best and I hope this book will inspire many more.

Dhaka, Bangladesh | Prof. Dr. Anwara Begum

# Preface

Bangladesh is a densely populated country in South Asia with about 170 million population. It has had significant economic growth over the last decades and recently it has improved from low-income to lower middle-income country. Currently, Bangladesh is facing a double burden of communicable and non-communicable diseases where about 60% of the burden has been incurred by non-communicable illness. Mental disorders are one of the top fifth burdens of non-communicable disease in the country after heart diseases, diabetes mellitus, chronic respiratory diseases, and cancer. The prevalence of psychiatric disorders in Bangladesh is 18.7%. However, the country has an extreme dearth of budgetary allocation and other resources to cope with the burden of psychiatric disorders. The treatment gap for psychiatric disorders is more than 90% with inadequate and inequitable distribution of manpower. Psychiatrists are posted only at tertiary care level of health services in Bangladesh. Due to the existing high stigma and low literacy, people visit nonmedical persons like traditional healers and religious leaders. As there is no insurance coverage for mental illness, the out-of-pocket expense is more than 70%. There is an extreme dearth of research in the country. I did not find any book on mental health in Bangladesh neither in English nor in vernacular language (i.e., Bangla). Therefore, a comprehensive book on mental health in Bangladesh based on existing evidence and expertise was an immediate necessity.

I tried to provide a comprehensive overview of mental health from academics to door step with the limited existing literature and expertise. In the first chapter, I include the prominent persons in the establishment of psychiatry in Bangladesh considering the historical perspective. Subsequently, the epidemiology and burden of mental health disorders in Bangladesh have been discussed. The chapter includes the prevalence of different psychiatric disorders and their impact on people, society, and the country. Next, I mention historical development and the current status of mental health services delivery in Bangladesh. The chapter includes the existing mental health service delivery structure in different levels of health services, human resources in mental health services, help-seeking behavior for mental health care in Bangladesh, current status, and potential challenges to accessing mental health care in the country. Thereafter, I organized the pharmacological and psychosocial management of psychiatric disorders in Bangladesh. The chapters indicate the gaps in advanced interventions like neuro-modulation in Bangladesh. I incorporated a chapter on child and adolescent mental health in Bangladesh. It encompasses the epidemiology and burden of child psychiatric disorders and the current status of service delivery in this area. In the next chapter, I include issues related to substance abuse and mental health in Bangladesh. The chapter discusses the current status of substance use disorder and available services for substance abuse patients in regard to medical management and rehabilitation. Then I include community psychiatry, forensic psychiatry, sexual medicine, suicide and suicide prevention in Bangladesh. I shed light on education and research aspects of mental health in the following chapter. It emphasizes the psychiatry curriculum in undergraduate medical schools and postgraduate courses. It also discusses the psychiatry journals in Bangladesh. I place a chapter discussing research conducted on common mental disorders in Bangladesh. It highlights potential research gaps in the county. Subsequently, I shed light on emerging aspects of mental health like public mental health aspects, climate change and its impact on mental health in Bangladesh, technology-based interventions for mental health support, mental health of vulnerable populations, geriatric psychiatry status and services, and NGOs working in mental health in Bangladesh. Throughout the process, I was careful to reduce overlaps and repetitions of contents among the chapters. However, there are minimal overlaps to make the chapters stand alone.

Psychiatry is a neglected branch of Medicine in Bangladesh. Academically, it has also been under-addressed and under-researched. This book is the first of its kind to address multiple domains of mental health in Bangladesh. It identifies research gaps and gives recommendations for improving mental health services in Bangladesh. The book could serve as a useful resource for students, faculties, researchers, policymakers, public health specialists, mental health professionals as well as non-governmental and voluntary organizations, and advocacy groups interested in mental health in Bangladesh.

Dhaka, Bangladesh S. M. Yasir Arafat

**Acknowledgements** I am grateful to Ms. Hasina Akter, Dr. Towhidul Islam, Dr. Sujita Kumar Kar, and Dr. A. M. Fariduzzaman for their support in different phase of preparing the book.

# Contents

# About the Editor

**Dr. S. M. Yasir Arafat** is currently working as an Associate Consultant of Psychiatry at Bangladesh Specialized Hospital Ltd. (BSHL), Dhaka, Bangladesh. He is affiliated with Dnet as an honorary Research Fellow and Biomedical Research Foundation, Bangladesh as Senior Research Fellow. He was affiliated with the University of Bristol, UK as Visiting Senior Research Associate (August 2021–2023). He completed MD in Psychiatry from Bangabandhu Sheikh Mujib Medical University, Dhaka and MBBS from the Dhaka Medical College, Dhaka, Bangladesh. He also did an MPH in Health Economics and MBA in Marketing. He has (co)authored more than 350 peer-reviewed articles and book chapters, and (co)edited several books with Springer. He has been included in the global 2% researcher list in 2021, 2022, and 2023. He is acting as editorial member in more than 10 leading journals in mental health published by Frontiers, Wiley, Springer, and Taylor and Francis. His research focused on mental health, suicidal behavior, psychometrics, panic buying, and psychosexual disorders.

# List of Figures

# List of Tables

# Chapter 1
# Prominent Figures in Psychiatry in Bangladesh

**Nafia Farzana Chowdhury, A. M. Fariduzzaman, and S. M. Yasir Arafat**

**Abstract** The current status of psychiatry in Bangladesh is the summation of all efforts since its commencement in 1957 at *Pabna Mental Hospital* during the Pakistan period. It is the collective effort of all individuals. However, for historical purposes, we mention the prominent persons of psychiatry in Bangladesh considering their extraordinary contribution to the mental health of the country. We mention the personal history of Professor Dr. AKM Nazimuddowla Chowdhury who is the first psychiatrist in the country, Professor Dr. Hidayetul Islam who played a fundamental role in the establishment of the *National Institute of Mental Health*, Dhaka, Professor Dr. Anwara Begum who is the first female psychiatrist in the country, Dr. Shamim Matin Chowdhury who is the first Child and Adolescent psychiatrist, Professor Dr. Syed Kamaluddin Ahmed for his contribution to research and regional services delivery of mental health, Prof. Dr. Abul Hasnat Mohammad Firoz who contributed to raising awareness and fought against stigma among community people, and Professor Mohammad SI Mullick who contributed to the establishment of Child and Adolescents Psychiatry in the country. We hope this is the beginning of historical contributions for inspiration of future leaders and hopefully, this section will be enriched in the future editions of the book.

**Keywords** Bangladesh · Prominent figures · Bangladesh psychiatry · Mental health · Psychiatric services · Human resource

N. F. Chowdhury
Department of Psychiatry, Bangabandhu Sheikh Mujib Medical University, Dhaka, Bangladesh

A. M. Fariduzzaman
Department of Psychiatry, Chandpur Medical College and Hospital, Chandpur, Bangladesh

S. M. Y. Arafat (✉)
Department of Psychiatry, Bangladesh Specialized Hospital Limited, Dhaka, Bangladesh
e-mail: arafatdmc62@gmail.com



S. M. Y. Arafat (ed.), *Mental Health in Bangladesh*,
https://doi.org/10.1007/978-981-97-0610-5_1

## 1.1 Introduction

The People's Republic of Bangladesh is located in South Asia. It is surrounded by the Indian border in its North, East, and West and the Bay of Bengal in the South. It has an area of 147,570 km$^2$ and according to the latest *Population and Housing Census* 2022, its total population (adjusted) is about 170 million (Bangladesh Bureau of Statistics, 2023). Mental health services are relatively newer in the region as no mental hospital was found before 1957. The first mental health hospital setup was reveled about six and half decades ago (in 1957) in Pabna (a district town 175 km from the capital, Dhaka), the *Pabna Mental Hospital* (PMH). The development of mental health services has been discussed in Chap. 3 of this book (Arafat, 2024). Mental health services were introduced at *Dhaka Medical College* (DMC) in 1974. In 1975, the Department of Psychiatry was started at the *Institute of Postgraduate Medicine and Research* (IPGMR) (now *Bangabandhu Sheikh Mujib Medical University*, BSMMU). In 1981, the *National Institute of Mental Health* (NIMH) was started (For details see Arafat, 2019, 2024; Arafat et al., 2024).

Mental health as an entity and Psychiatry as a discipline has been under developed due to an extreme stigma and low literacy in the region, specially in Bangladesh. Our forefathers of psychiatry had to fight to overcome the stigma and misconceptions related to the causation and treatment of mental disorders. With their strong determination and resilience, they nudged to establish infrastructure, mental health care services, academic curriculum, and developed human resources to provide inclusive mental health care services for the entire country.

The current status of psychiatry in Bangladesh is the summation of all efforts of all individuals. Our pioneer psychiatrists are our trendsetters, and teachers to us and for the whole nation for providing mental health services. Nevertheless, many of the young mental health professionals of Bangladesh do not know the contributions of early leaders and evolution of psychiatry in the country. With the demise of our seniors, we may lose some important information forever. Hence, for historical purposes, we mention some prominent persons of psychiatry in Bangladesh considering their extraordinary contribution to psychiatry in Bangladesh (Box 1.1). We considered our seniors who have already died and/or retired from regular job. We collected the information by interviewing the family members of those who died already and interviewing the leaders who are alive. In a country like Bangladesh, it is challenging to classify with perfect precision due to inadequate research and lack of scientific culture. However, we intend to prioritize the historical assimilation of extra-ordinary personal efforts that created additional momentums for psychiatry in Bangladesh. We hope in future the list will be enriched by new additions in future editions of this book or upcoming many other articles, chapters, and books.

**Box 1.1: Prominent figures in Bangladesh Psychiatry and their remarkable contributions**

1. Professor Dr. A K M Nazimuddowla Chowdhury- The first psychiatrist

2. Professor Dr. Hidayetul Islam- Establishment of the NIMH
3. Professor Dr. Anwara Begum- The first female psychiatrist
4. Dr. Shamim Matin Chowdhury- The first Child and Adolescent psychiatrist
5. Professor Dr. Syed Kamaluddin Ahmed- Research and contribution in regional mental health services delivery
6. Professor Dr. Abul Hasnat Mohammad Firoz- Raising awareness
7. Professor Dr. Mohammad SI Mullick- Establishment of Child and Adolescent Psychiatry

### *1.1.1 Professor Dr. A K M Nazimuddowla Chowdhury*

Professor Dr. Nazimuddowla Chowdhury was born on 30 September 1929 in the Northern part (Gaibandha district) of Bangladesh. He completed his Bachelor of Medicine, and Bachelor of Surgery (MBBS) degree from DMC in 1954. After completing his medical graduation Dr. Chowdhury went to the United Kingdom (UK) to pursue his post-graduation degree in Pediatrics. Upon reaching there, he met a Bangladeshi family who were close to him and were going through mental trauma. This family and their situation changed his mind and at that time he realized that Bangladesh didn't have any mental health services. The people and the physicians of Bangladesh were not aware of this discipline at all. He discussed his insightful concern with his guide there and changed his subject of post-graduation from Pediatrics to Psychiatry. He completed a Diploma in Psychological Medicine (DPM) in 1958, came back to Bangladesh, and joined PMH in 1960. While working in PMH, Dr. Chowdhury used to take classes on a regular basis at DMC to introduce psychiatry and raise awareness among undergraduate medical students. In 1971, Dr. Chowdhury left PMH and joined IPGMR (now BSMMU). In 1975 Dr. Chowdhury started the Department of Psychiatry at IPGMR at that time with the help of Minister Mosharraf Hossein. He started DPM in IPGMR in 1975. He was awarded honorary Fellowships from the Royal College of Physicians, London, UK (FRCPsych) and Bangladesh college of Physician and Surgeons (FCPS in 1989). Prof. Chowdhury was the Founder, Director and Chief Consultant, of Central Drug Addiction Cure Centre, Tejgaon, Dhaka and he retired in 1989. During that time, he worked tirelessly to ensure the center was well equipped and well stuffed with the mission to provide comprehensive service. Prof. Chowdhury was awarded two Gold Medals for his enormous contribution in the field of Psychiatry; *Ibrahim Memorial Gold Medal* was awarded by the *Association of Physicians of Bangladesh* in 2000 and gold medal for medical education on *World Mental Health Day* by *National Forum of Psychiatrist* in 2002. Prof. Chowdhury used to do private practice at Samorita Hospital till 2012. He died of multi-organ failure on 25 September 2014 at Samorita Hospital. He is the first psychiatrist in Bangladesh and is considered as the father of Psychiatry in the country. His contribution to the field of Psychiatry is profound and unforgettable.

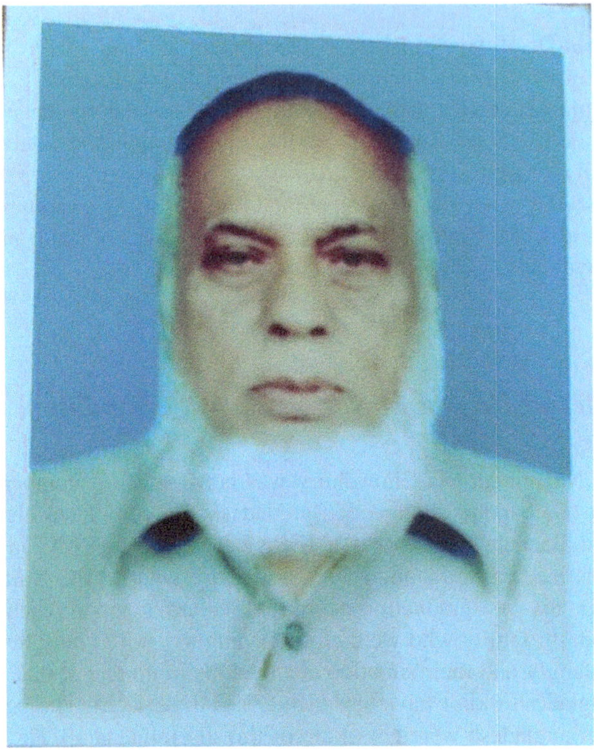

**Fig. 1.1** Professor Dr. A K M Nazimuddowla Chowdhury. *Source* Authors

He is the source of inspiration of mental health services in Bangladesh. We present his single photo in Fig. 1.1. (We collected the information from his daughter Dr. Ferdouse Ara Chowdhury by NFC.)

### *1.1.2 Professor Dr. Hidayetul Islam*

Professor Hidayetul Islam was born in 24 September 1934 in south-central part of Bangladesh (Faridpur District). Dr. Islam Completed his MBBS from DMC in 1960. During the early days of his career, Dr. Islam thought to persue his career in Medicine that eventually turned to Psychiatry. After Professor AKM Nazimuddoula Chowdhury, Dr. Islam along with his colleague (Dr. Khalilur Rahman) went to the UK with a scholarship to complete his DPM in 1962. He did training in different hospitals in the UK namely, *Hammersmith Hospital*, *Wittington Hospital*, *Westminster Hospital*, *Maudsley Hospital*. After completing his DPM degree he worked in different hospitals of the UK from 1964 to 1969 in different positions. Dr. Islam came back to Bangladesh in 1969 and initially joined the *Mymensingh Medical*

*College Hospital* for a few months. After that he joined PMH in 1970 and started his work with Professor AKM Nazimuddoula Chowdhury. During the liberation war of Bangladesh, Dr. Islam was in-charge of the PMH when he supported many freedom fighters. He arrange to provide mental health services to 156 freedom fighters and few rape victims. While working in Pabna he also used to give lectures in *Sylhet Medical College* and *Chattogram (Chittagong) Medical College* (CMC).

Dr. Islam left PMH in 1977 and after some bureaucratic delay he joined Suhrawardy Hospital in 1978. He started *Organization of Training in Mental Health* (OTMH) in 1978 as a development project and which later was included in revenues in 1981. This project turned into NIMH in 1992 and Dr. Islam was the prime person worked for the establishment of it. After having a conflict with the authority of Suhrawardy Hospital about space required for psychiatric work Dr. Islam shifted OTMH to Mitford Sir Salimullah Medical College Hospital (SSMCH) in 1983. While working in Mitford Hospital he used to hold four posts, Director of SSMCH, Professor Department of Psychiatry, Project Director of World Health Organization (WHO) mental health program Bangladesh and elected member of Bangladesh Medical Research Council (BMRC) and Bangladesh Medical and Dental Council (BMDC). Dr. Islam retired in 1993 as professor of Psychiatry and the director of NIMH. He was awarded "Leadership Award" for his outstanding contribution in the field of Psychiatry in his country in the second world congress of behavioural science Washington DC in 1997. We present his single photo in Fig. 1.2. (We collected the information from Professor Hidayetul Islam by SMYA.)

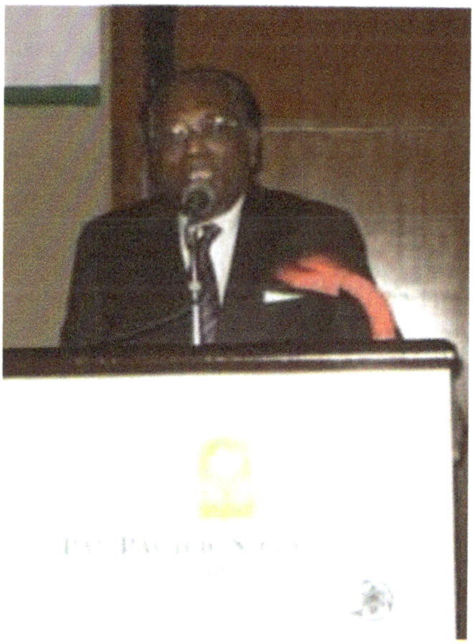

**Fig. 1.2** Professor Dr. Hidayetul Islam. *Source* Authors

### *1.1.3 Professor Dr. Anwara Begum*

Professor Dr. Anwara Begum has been widely acclaimed as one of the pioneers in the field of psychiatry in Bangladesh. She was born on 05 November 1940 in Jashore (Jessore) situated in the south-western part of the country. After completing her MBBS from DMC in 1965, she joined the Army Medical College of Pakistan in January 1967. Her career took an unexpected turn during the liberation war of Bangladesh in 1971 when she was posted as a flight lieutenant of air force at Tejgaon, Dhaka. Serving from 1971 to 1974, she witnessed the horrors of war and its toll on mental health.

Dr. Anwara Begum went to the UK to pursue her postgraduate studies in Gynaecology. While she was undergoing training, she saw the sufferings and management of psychiatric patients that turned her career to Psychiatry. During her time there, she underwent training at various hospitals and became the first female psychiatrist from Bangladesh to obtain an MRCpsych degree. In 1982, she returned to Bangladesh and joined DMC as an Associate Professor in the Department of Psychiatry. From 1982 to 1985, she also worked in the Central Drug Addiction Treatment Center, Tejgaon. She was promoted as professor of psychiatry in 1988, and was posted to the PMH. In 1994, Professor Anwara Begum joined the NIMH as a professor of psychiatry and the Director of the institute. Her service time at NIMH was marked by her tireless efforts to expand and enhance the services provided by the institute. She played a crucial role in acquiring the land of NIMH and introducing psychology specially, clinical psychology along with psychiatry, ensuring a comprehensive approach to mental health care. In recognition of her efforts and dedication to the development of mental health services in Bangladesh, she was awarded an honorary FCPS from the Bangladesh college of Physician and Surgeons (BCPS). After retirement, Professor Anwara Begum continues to serve as a consultant in BIRDEM General Hospital and shares her wealth of knowledge and experience with the next generation of doctors.

In addition to her contributions to psychiatry, she has also made significant contributions to Bangla literature. Her novels, short stories, and children's books are written with insightful portrayal of human psychology. In 2010, she received the Bangla Academy Literary Award, followed by Annanya Shahitya Puroshkar, Shishu Academy Puroshkar, and Ekushey Padak in 2019 for her remarkable literary contributions. Professor Anwara Begum's life and achievements stand as a testament to her unwavering dedication to the field of psychiatry and her tireless efforts to improve mental health services in Bangladesh. Her substantial contributions have undoubtedly left an indelible mark on the landscape of psychiatry and literature in the country. We present her single photo in Fig. 1.3. (We collected the information from Professor Dr. Anowara Begum by AMF).

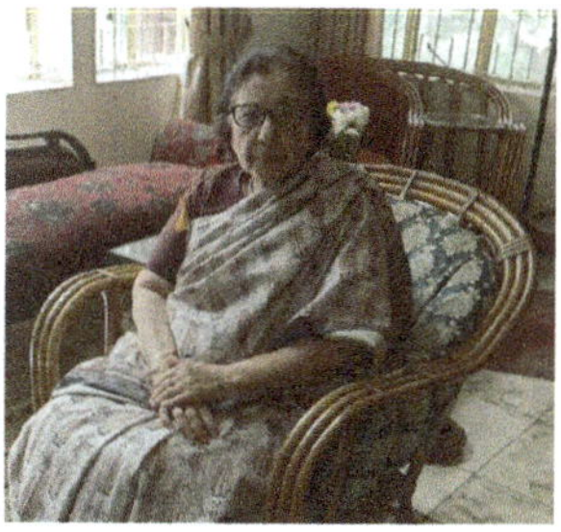

**Fig. 1.3** Prof. Dr. Anwara Begum. *Source* Authors

### *1.1.4 Dr. Shamim Matin Chowdhury*

Dr. Shamim Matin Chowdhury was born on 11 June 1950 in Dhaka, the capital city of the country. After graduating from DMC in 1976, she began her career as a lecturer of Pharmacology at DMC and later at Sir Salimullah Medical College. During her internship, her interest in psychiatry sparked, leading her to pursue post-graduation in the field. She completed her Membership of the College of Bangladesh and Surgeons (MCPS) in Psychiatry from BCPS in July 1987. She became the first psychiatrist in Bangladesh to achieve a Diploma in Child and Adolescent Psychiatry (DCAP) from the prestigious Institute of Psychiatry and Maudsley Institute of Child Health in the UK in 1990. She worked at Tejgaon the Central Drug Addiction Treatment Center from 1991 to 1997 when she was promoted to assistant professor. Dr. Shamim became the director in charge of the Tejgaon Drug Addiction Center from 1997 to 1999. In 1999, she became the director of Tejgaon Drug Addiction Center and served till 2002. She worked as a treatment consultant at the United Nations International Drug Control Program (UNDCP) which was renamed as United Nations Office on Drugs and Crime (UNODC) in 2022 and UNODC. She contributed to preparing a training manual for UNDCP during her tenure. In 2004, Dr. Shamim made the decision to take early retirement from PMH to establish her own practice as a child psychiatrist. She further expanded her impact by founding a school for special children called "Beautiful Mind" a center for autistic and mentally challenged children. The school provides meaningful care and education for 200 children with special needs. At that time there was no such organization for special children having psychiatric comorbidity and Autism. She felt a desperate need for some kind of institution to help these children and families. Dr. Shamim also joined Special Olympics in 1994 and she is the current Chairperson of Special Olympics Bangladesh and the Chairperson of Asia Pacific Advisory Council of Special Olympics. This Olympics represents the children who are mentally challenged and also suffering from Autism. Besides being a psychiatrist she wanted to train these special children in sports as well.

Dr. Shamim Matin Chowdhury worked in several institutes namely IPGMR, NIMH, and PMH. She published research papers regarding drug abuse, self-harm, patterns of referral in the psychiatry outpatient department, clinical patterns of Dhat syndrome, and risk behavior among drug abusers in the spread of HIV in Bangladesh.

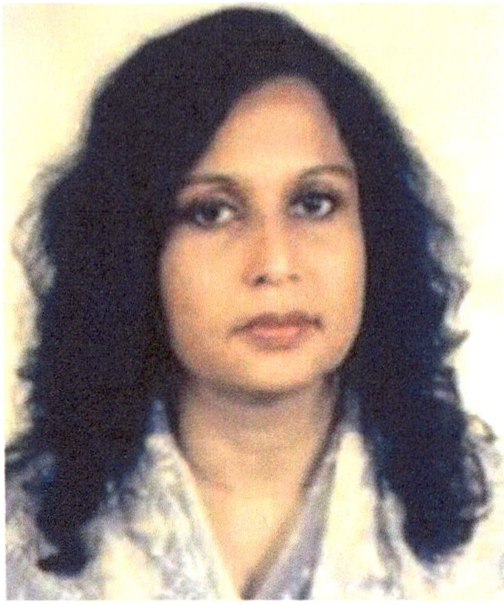

**Fig. 1.4** Shamim Matin Chowdhury. *Source* Authors

She attended several international conferences and availed several trainings on drug abuse.

Dr. Shamim Matin Chowdhury's dedication and expertise have made a significant difference in the lives of countless children who are mentally challenged and suffering in Bangladesh. She believes God has been kind to give all kinds of opportunities to psychiatrists to help and serve people who have psychiatric illnesses both adults and children and who are related to psychiatry must help these special groups of people with heart's content. We present her single photo in Fig. 1.4. (We collected the information from Dr. Shamim Matin Chowdhury by NFC).

### *1.1.5 Professor Dr. Syed Kamaluddin Ahmed*

Professor Dr. Syed Kamaluddin Ahmed was born in 19 March 1953 at South-eastern part of Bangladesh Chattogram (Chittagong), the port city. He completed his MBBS from CMC in 1978 and a Fellowship, *Fellow of College of Physicians and Surgeons* (FCPS) in Psychiatry from *Bangladesh College of Physicians and Surgeons* (BCPS) in July 1982. Then, he obtained fellowship training from several international institutions namely the *National Institute of Mental Health and Neurosciences* (NIMHANS), India, *University of Colombo*, Sri Lanka and the *WHO Collaborating Centre for Research in Mental Health* at *McGill University*, Canada. In 2005, he was awarded a Fellowship, *Fellow of the Royal College of Physicians of Edinburgh* (FRCPE) from the *Royal College of Physicians of Edinburgh* in 2005 (Royal College of Physicians of Edinburgh, 2023).

Dr. Ahmed started his career by joining the Government health services and worked there for about 18 years. He joined the Department of Psychiatry of the

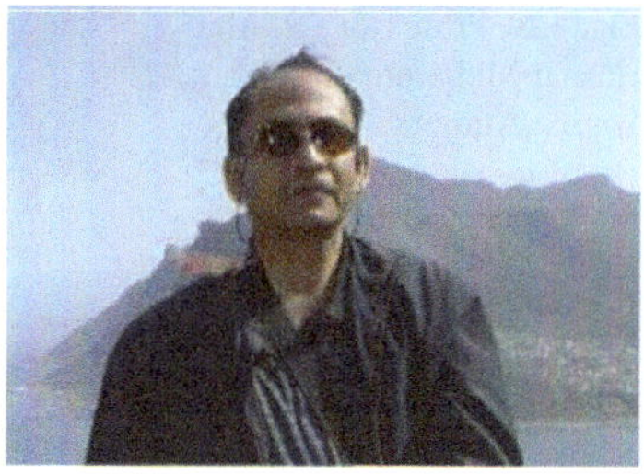

**Fig. 1.5** Professor Dr. Syed Kamaluddin Ahmed. *Source* Authors

IPGMR in 1984 as a faculty member. He was promoted as an associate professor in 1989 and he continued his work at IPGMR till 1993. Then, he joined at the Tejgaon Drug Addiction Center as the Chief Consultant and Director where he worked till 1996. Later on, Prof. Ahmed joined the UNDCP and the *United Nations Development Programme* (UNDP) as 'drug demand reduction' and 'behavior change' consultant. In 1988, Dr Ahmed played a leading role in a UNDCP program of drug demand reduction in the Maldives.

Dr Ahmed's conducted research on biological aspects of psychiatry, behavioral intervention and substance abuse. He (co)authored more than 40 articles and he conducted the first epidemiological survey of drug abuse as one of the leading investigators funded by the WHO. Dr Ahmed had expertise in medical ethnography and he conducted a landmark study on distribution of buprenorphine use in Bangladesh. Dr Ahmed performed validation of the *Present State Examination* (PSE) in Bangla, which has been widely used in further research.

Prof. Ahmed acted as a member of editorial board of several academic journals. He acted as the Editor-in-Chief of the *Journal of the Bangladesh College of Physicians and Surgeons* and the *Journal of Medical Science and Research.* He was an international advisory board member of the *International Journal of Addiction Sciences.*

Dr Ahmed was well known for his uncompromising professionalism, honesty, ethics, and integrity. Prof. Ahmed died on 21 December, 2011 from gastric cancer at the age of 58 years. At that time, he was working as a Professor of Psychiatry at the *Holy Family Red Crescent Medical College,* Dhaka. We present his single photo in Fig. 1.5. (We collected the information from already available sources by NFC).

### *1.1.6 Professor Dr. Abul Hasnat Mohammad Firoz*

Professor Dr. Abul Hasnat Mohammad Firoz was born on 15 December 1956 at the Northern part of Bangladesh (Rangpur District). He completed MBBS from DMC in 1982 and perused a fellowship (FCPS in Psychiatry) from BCPS in 1988. After that, he was posted in Tejgaon Central Drug Addiction Treatment Center in 1988 as Residential Medical Officer (RMO). In 1996 he was appointed as head of the Department of Psychiatry of DMC. He was an active member of more than twenty

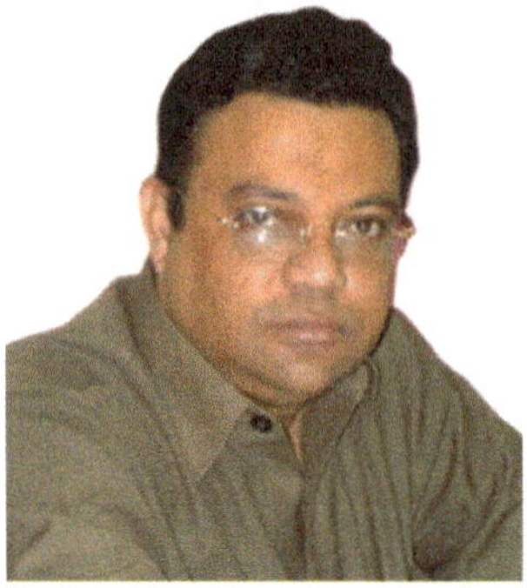

**Fig. 1.6** Professor Dr. Abul Hasnat Mohammad Firoz. *Source* Authors

international organizations. In the year 2001 he received a membership (MRCP) and a fellowship (FRCP) from *Royal College of Physicians and Surgeons*, UK. In 2002 he was appointed as professor and Director of NIMH, Dhaka. In the same year he was selected as a member of National Narcotics Control Board and National AIDS (Technical) Committee of Bangladesh. He Passed away at the age of 55 years on 5 June 2012 in Dhaka.

In his initial days every month on a Friday he used to organize a discussion meeting on mental health issues. He used to gather twenty five people from Madrssa, Islamic Mowlana, and university students to make them understand about mental illness and how these illnesses can be treated. This was his own way of making awareness among general populations. To encourage people and make these discussions successful he provided them with lunch packet and a certificate. This was a great step by him to spread awareness about mental health and create an understanding about it. He published many leaflets and booklets and distributed different places of Bangladesh to raise awareness among general people about mental illness and treatment. Dr. Firoz was founder editor of "Monthly Monojagot" which was the first ever published magazine on mental health in Bangla. The magazine was distributed and got popularity in the whole country. We present his single photo in Fig. 1.6. (We collected the information from his wife Dr. Ferdous Ara Chowdhury.)

### *1.1.7 Professor MSI Mullick*

Professor Mohammad S I Mullick is a leading general psychiatrist and child & adolescent psychiatrist in Bangladesh. He was born at Khulna on 31 March 1956. He graduated from Sher-E-Bangla Medical College, Barisal in 1983 and joined Government Health Services as an Assistant Surgeon, Sher-E-Bangla Medical College Hospital, Barisal in the same year. He had a dream to be a psychiatrist when he was a medical student influenced by his own inherent inquisitiveness about 'mind' and chose psychiatry at the first chance. Later, he selected child psychiatry enhanced by getting an aligned opportunity of British scholarship on this specialty and became a child and adolescent psychiatrist. He obtained FCPS in Psychiatry from BCPS in 1991. He got a diploma in child and adolescent psychiatry from King's College London in 1997. After that, he obtained MRCPsych and then FRCPsych from the Royal College of Psychiatrists, UK, in 2004 and 2011 respectively. He did a PhD in child and adolescent psychiatry from the University of Dhaka in 2007.

He started his teaching career as an Assistant Professor in the Department of Psychiatry, IPGMR, Dhaka, in 1995 and continued as Associate Professor of Psychiatry, Associate Professor of Child and Adolescent Psychiatry, and then Professor of Child and Adolescent Psychiatry at BSMMU till his retirement in 2022. He held the post of Chairman, of the Department of Psychiatry, BSMMU, from 2009–2015.

In his long 28 years of teaching life, Professor Mullick set an example of devotion in teaching and training in psychiatry. He drafted a curriculum for FCPS Psychiatry when he was Secretary of the Faculty of Psychiatry, BCPS that was adopted and published in 2000. Subsequently, he came up with updating and developing the curriculum of MD Psychiatry non-residency and residency programs of BSMMU that were approved in 2003 and 2013 respectively. Further, he worked on the curriculum for the MD residency program in child and adolescent psychiatry that was implemented by BSMMU in 2015. He headed the committee for drafting the curriculum of FCPS Child and Adolescent Psychiatry accepted in 2022. Still, he is contributing to psychiatry education as the Chairman, the Faculty of Psychiatry, BCPS.

The development of child and adolescent psychiatry in Bangladesh was his long-cherished dream. As the founding head of the Child and Adolescent Psychiatry Division, Department of Psychiatry, BSMMU, Professor Mullick set up a Child Mental Health Clinic at BSMMU in 1998 that was the first formal Child and Adolescent Mental Health Services (CAMHS) in Bangladesh. Subsequently, he expanded high-quality CAMHS and arranged child and adolescent psychiatry training for mental health professionals. Through his constant effort and persuasion, the MD residency program on child and adolescent psychiatry was started from 2015 at the University which is certainly a great milestone in child and adolescent mental health in Bangladesh. Afterward, he worked with the concerned team for the FCPS course in child and adolescent psychiatry that was started in BCPS in early 2022.

During his job as Assistant Registrar in the then Institute of Mental Health and Research from 1988–1995, Professor Mullick served and coordinated continued training on mental health for GPs, nurses, and health workers. He provided all-out assistance in the planning, approval, and implementation of the project for the establishment of the NIMH, Dhaka.

As a devoted researcher, Professor Mullick is always meticulous with his research work. He conducted the first child psychiatric epidemiological study in Bangladesh in 2005, and the first prevalence study of psychiatric disorders among preschool children in the country in 2018. His other remarkable work includes establishing validity and reliability of the Bangla version of reputed screening and structured measures of child psychopathology and developing a stress scale with adult & adolescent versions. He wrote some guiding articles on developing Mental Health Services including CAMHS in Bangladesh and low and middle-income countries (LMICs). He wrote

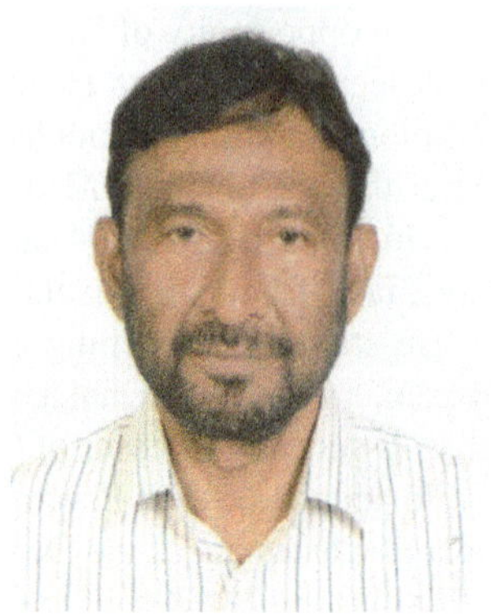

**Fig. 1.7** Prof. Dr. MSI Mullick. *Source* Authors

a unique book on case-based learning exercises for the residents and trainees in psychiatry.

Professor Mullick is diligently involved with the advocacy groups. As a committed member, he created momentum for the Bangladesh Association of Psychiatrists by drafting the constitution and initiating the relevant organizational activities. He was Secretary of Scientific Affairs of the Association for 6-years. He is on the editorial board of the Association's Journal from its first issue. He convened and founded the Bangladesh Association for Child and Adolescent Mental Health (BACAMH) in 2008. He worked hard to expand and create the firm base of the Association and hold office as Secretary General and then President.

Professor Mullick is one of the most influential psychiatric consultants in Bangladesh. He is a strong exponent of evidence-based and value-based practice for patients. He will be remembered for his singular role in establishing child and adolescent psychiatry in Bangladesh. We present his single photo in Fig. 1.7. (We collected the information from Prof. MSI Mullick).

### *1.1.8 Others*

Some other important names should be mentioned here to reveal the historical aspects. We obtained the information from personal communication with several senior psychiatrists of the country. Dr. Mohammad Hossain Ganguly, the civil surgeon of that time established the PMH at at *Sitlai House* (an abandoned land lord's house). Dr. Nosin was the first physician worked in PMH before joining of Professor Nazimuddowla Chowdhury. He was trained in Ranchi Mental Hospital and UK. Dr. Farhana Haque was the first female psychiatrist worked at DMC in Bangladesh before the independence. She was an Urdu speaking psychiatrist.

## 1.2 Conclusion

We mention some prominent personal contributions to Psychiatry in Bangladesh which may not reflect all the events. It is important to mention that the current status of psychiatry in the country is the collective progress of all efforts from every corner of the country and every personal effort. We consider the chapter as an initial effort of acknowledging the contributions of our forefathers for the inspiration of future leaders. We hope this list will be enriched in due course of time.

## References

Arafat, S. M. Y. (2019). History of psychiatry in Bangladesh. *Asian Journal of Psychiatry, 46*, 11–12. https://doi.org/10.1016/j.ajp.2019.09.024

Arafat, S. M. Y. (2024). Mental health services in Bangladesh. In S. M. Y. Arafat (Ed.), *Mental health in Bangladesh: From bench to community*. Springer Nature. https://doi.org/10.1007/978-981-97-0610-5_3

Arafat, S. M. Y, Giasuddin, N. A., & Mazumder, A. H. (2024). Access to mental health care in Bangladesh—Current status, potential challenges, and ways out. In S. M. Y. Arafat, & S. K. Kar (Eds.), *Access to mental health care in South Asia—Current status, potential challenges, and ways out*. Springer Nature. https://doi.org/10.1007/978-981-99-9153-2_3

Bangladesh Bureau of Statistics. (2023). *Population. Population and Housing Census 2022*. Retrieved December 12, 2023, from https://bbs.gov.bd/site/page/47856ad0-7e1c-4aab-bd78-892733bc06eb/Population-&-Housing

Royal College of Physicians of Edinburgh (2023). Dr Syed Kamaluddin Ahmed FRCP Edin. Retrieved September 19, 2023 from https://www.rcpe.ac.uk/obituary/dr-syed-kamaluddin-ahmed-frcp-edin

# Chapter 2
# Epidemiology and Burden of Mental Disorders in Bangladesh

**Atiqul Haq Mazumder**

**Abstract** This chapter explores the epidemiology and burden of mental disorders in Bangladesh. It synthesizes the literature on the prevalence, risk factors, and impact of mental disorders in various segments of the population. The chapter reveals that mental disorders are common in Bangladesh, affecting about one-fifth of adults and one-eighth of children and adolescents. The most frequent disorders are depression and anxiety disorders. Women and urban dwellers are more vulnerable to mental illness. The COVID-19 pandemic has also worsened the mental health of young people. It discusses the legislative and strategic initiatives taken by the government and other actors to cope mental health burden. It concludes that a comprehensive understanding of the psychiatric burden and its implications in Bangladesh is still missing.

**Keywords** Mental disorders · Epidemiology · Bangladesh · Burden · Psychiatric disorders

## 2.1 Introduction

Epidemiology of mental health involves investigating the frequency, spread, root causes, and effects of mental disorders within specific populations (Burger & Neeleman, 2007). Mental disorders, as defined by the World Health Organization (WHO) in 2023, are severe disruptions in a person's thinking, emotional control, or behavior. These disturbances typically cause distress or hinder the individual's ability to function in significant aspects of life (WHO, 2023a). Mental disorders can be classified into different categories based on their symptoms, causes, and course. The most widely used classification systems are the *International Classification of Diseases* 11th Revision (ICD-11) and the *Diagnostic and Statistical Manual of Mental Disorders* 5th Edition Text Revision (DSM-5-TR) (MSD Manuals, 2022). Diagnosis of mental disorders involves assessing the presence and severity of the symptoms, as

A. H. Mazumder (✉)
Ministry of Health and Family Welfare, Government of Bangladesh, Dhaka, Bangladesh
e-mail: Atiqul.Mazumder@oulu.fi



S. M. Y. Arafat (ed.), *Mental Health in Bangladesh*,
https://doi.org/10.1007/978-981-97-0610-5_2

well as ruling out other possible causes or conditions. Diagnosis can be done by trained mental health professionals using standardized criteria and tools, such as interviews, questionnaires, or tests (World Health Organization, 2023b). Diagnosis can help to identify the appropriate treatment and support options for people with mental disorders. Epidemiology of mental health is crucial to comprehend the trends, triggers, and consequences of mental disorders, and to create potent strategies and regulations for their prevention and treatment.

## 2.2 Prevalence of Mental Disorders Among Adults

### *2.2.1 Findings from Empirical Studies*

I present a comparison of the prevalence of mental disorders among adults in Table 2.1. The earliest study conducted in an urban setting in 1975, shows that mental health had been a significant issue in Bangladesh for many decades (Chowdhury et al., 1975). Out of 652 interviewed cases, 31.4% had only psychogenic conditions, 45% had only organic diseases, and 14.8% reported symptoms of both psychogenic and organic features which suggests a high prevalence of mental health issues, underlining the importance of ongoing research and improved mental health services in the country.

Later in 1978 another urban setting study shows that nearly one third of patients were found to be dealing with a mental health problem (Alam, 1978). This high prevalence underscores the necessity of integrating mental health services into primary healthcare settings. It also highlights the importance of training general practitioners to recognize and manage mental health conditions, given their significant role in providing healthcare in urban settings.

In 1981, community-based rural study in Bangladesh reveals a lower prevalence of psychiatric disorders (3.4%) compared to the urban setting previously mentioned (Chowdhury et al., 1981). Additionally, it identifies 2.9% of the population as having both psychiatric and physical disorders. Psychiatric diseases were more prevalent in females than in males. Depression and anxiety were noted to be the most common conditions. These differences might be attributed to numerous factors, including variations in lifestyle, environmental factors, access to healthcare services, and the stigma associated with mental health in different settings. This information emphasizes the need for localized and context-specific mental health strategies and interventions.

An additional study in 2001 provides valuable insight into the prevalence of mental disorders among 415 women of 18–65 years of ages in a rural setting in Bangladesh (Ara et al., 2001). With 16.4% of the women in the study having a mental disorder and depression being the most common at 8.9%, it suggests that depression is a significant concern among women in these areas. It also highlights the need for increased awareness, screening, and treatment services specifically tailored for

**Table 2.1** Prevalence of mental disorders among adults in different studies in Bangladesh

| Study | Year | Setting | Age range (years) | n (sample size) | Prevalence of behavioral/ psychiatric disorders | Most common conditions | Gender difference | Implications |
|---|---|---|---|---|---|---|---|---|
| Chowdhury et al. | 1975 | Urban | ≥13 | 652 | 46.2% of outpatients | Psychogenic conditions | Not specified | High prevalence of mental health issues in urban settings |
| Alam | 1978 | Urban | All | 1,764 | 29% of patients | Not specified | Not specified | Need for integrating mental health services into primary healthcare settings |
| Chowdhury et al. | 1981 | Rural | All | 1,181 | 6.5% of population | Depression and anxiety | Females suffered more than males | Lower prevalence of psychiatric disorders might be due to inclusion of children less likely to suffer from mental disorders |
| Ara et al. | 2001 | Rural | 18–65 | 415 (Women) | 16.4% of women | Depression (8.9%) | Not applicable | Emphasizes the importance of enhancing awareness, screening, and treatment services specifically for women in rural areas |

(continued)

Table 2.1 (continued)

| Study | Year | Setting | Age range (years) | n (sample size) | Prevalence of behavioral/ psychiatric disorders | Most common conditions | Gender difference | Implications |
|---|---|---|---|---|---|---|---|---|
| Islam et al. | 2003 | Urban | ≥18 | 1,145 | 28% of participants | Not specified | Females suffered more than males | Higher prevalence of mental disorders might be due to inclusion of older people more likely to suffer from mental disorders |
| Karim et al. | 2006 | Rural and Urban | ≥18 | 327 | 12.2% of participants | Neurotic disorders (7%) | Females suffered more than males | The diversity of psychiatric disorders in the population, as shown by prevalence rates, emphasizes the multitude of mental health challenges people face |

(continued)

**Table 2.1** (continued)

| Study | Year | Setting | Age range (years) | n (sample size) | Prevalence of behavioral/ psychiatric disorders | Most common conditions | Gender difference | Implications |
|---|---|---|---|---|---|---|---|---|
| Hossain et al. | 2007 | Rural | 18–60 | 766 | 16.5% of participants | Depressive disorders (8%) | Nearly same for both genders | In rural areas, mental health services should focus on depressive and anxiety disorders due to their high prevalence |

(continued)

**Table 2.1** (continued)

| Study | Year | Setting | Age range (years) | n (sample size) | Prevalence of behavioral/ psychiatric disorders | Most common conditions | Gender difference | Implications |
|---|---|---|---|---|---|---|---|---|
| NIMH, B and WHO | 2007 | Rural and Urban | ≥18 | 13,080 | 16.1% of population | Neurotic disorders (8.4%) | Females suffered more than males | Higher levels of awareness, care, and attitudes towards mental illness may be attributed to nationwide mental health programs and the influential role of the expanding media |
| MOH&FW | 2021 | Rural and Urban | ≥18–99 | 7,270 | 18.7% of population | Depressive disorders (6.7%) | Females suffered more than males | The similar rates of mental health disorders in both rural and urban environments suggest that these issues are common concerns needing attention in various regions |

*Source* Author

women in rural settings. These findings can help shape public health initiatives and policies to better address the mental health needs of this population.

An urban community-based study in 2003 found a much higher prevalence of psychiatric disorders, with 28% of 1,145 participants aged 18 years and above, diagnosed by a psychiatrist (Islam et al., 2003). This significant difference from the rural study could be due to various factors, including environmental stressors, lifestyle differences, or increased access to diagnostic services in urban areas. These findings further emphasize on the need for effective mental health policies to cater to different communities within the country. The same study reported higher prevalence of mental disorders among women and persons with higher socioeconomic status. This observation suggests that gender and socioeconomic status play a role in the prevalence of psychiatric disorders in Bangladesh. Women and people from higher socioeconomic classes being more likely to have a psychiatric disorder could be due to a variety of reasons. For instance, women may be more likely to seek help and therefore be diagnosed, or they may face different stressors related to societal roles. As for higher socioeconomic classes, it could be due to more access to diagnostic services, or different types of stress related to their lifestyle. These insights can help guide targeted mental health policies and interventions. A recent study on mental healthcare-seeking behavior of women in Bangladesh finds about one-third women to be reluctant to seek mental healthcare (Koly et al., 2022). Conclusions of this study underlines the importance of a comprehensive and community-centered approach to improving mental healthcare for women in Bangladesh. By raising awareness about mental health issues, eliminating stigma, and designing culturally sensitive and evidence-based interventions, more women may feel comfortable seeking help. Multisectoral collaborations can also ensure a more holistic approach. This includes involving not just the health sector, but also education, social services, and other sectors that can contribute to a supportive environment for mental health. This approach could lead to better mental health outcomes and greater healthcare coverage for women in Bangladesh.

The 2006 study (Karim et al., 2006) among 327 adult population again highlights the prevalence of psychiatric disorders to be higher in females than males in a suburban setting in Bangladesh. The prevalence rates of 13.9% in females and 10.2% in males show a notable gender difference. Neurotic disorders, which include conditions like anxiety disorders, obsessive–compulsive disorder, and panic disorders, have a prevalence of 7.0 per 1000 population. Major depressive disorder is a health condition, as marked by enduring emotions of sorrow and a consistent disinterest in engaging in activities, has a prevalence of 4.0 per 1000 population. Lastly, psychotic disorders, which include conditions like schizophrenia that involve distorted perceptions of reality, have a prevalence of 1.2 per 1000 population, according to this study. These prevalence rates provide a breakdown of specific types of psychiatric disorders in the population. These rates highlight the variety of mental health issues faced by the population and underline the need for a range of mental health services to cater to these different conditions.

Additionally, the study's finding that psychiatric morbidity is higher among the middle and lower socio-economic classes contradicts a previous finding that suggested higher prevalence in higher socio-economic classes. This discrepancy could be due to differences in study settings or methodologies, or it could suggest that individuals across all socio-economic classes are vulnerable to mental health issues, but the types or causes of these issues might vary.

These findings underline the need for a nuanced understanding of mental health prevalence and its determinants in different sub-populations, and highlight the need for tailored interventions that can cater to these different groups.

A rural community-based study in Bangladesh among 766 adults aged 18–60 years provides valuable insights into the prevalence and types of psychiatric disorders in the country's rural areas (Hosain et al., 2007). The prevalence of psychiatric disorders was determined to be 16.5%, which is a substantial figure. Depressive disorders were the most common type of psychiatric disorder, affecting 8% of the population, or about half of those suffering from any psychiatric disorder. Anxiety disorders also had a significant prevalence, affecting 5% of the population, or about a third of psychiatric disorder sufferers. Prevalence rates were same for both genders. Males suffered more from depressive disorders and females suffered more from anxiety disorders.

These findings suggest that mental health services in rural areas of Bangladesh should prioritize interventions for depressive and anxiety disorders. Additionally, given the overall high prevalence of psychiatric disorders, there is a clear need for accessible, affordable, and effective mental health services in these areas.

A systematic review dated back in 2014 provides a range for the prevalence of psychiatric disorders in both adults and children in Bangladesh (Hossain et al., 2014). For adults, the prevalence ranges from 6.5 to 31.0%, and for children, it's between 13.4 and 22.9%. These figures highlight a significant portion of both adult and child populations in Bangladesh are affected by psychiatric disorders. It underlines the need for effective mental health programs and interventions to support these individuals and reduce the overall burden of mental disorders in the country. The same review study also recognized three major tools to diagnose and assess mental disorders within the Bangladeshi population; The *Self Reporting Questionnaire* (SRQ), *General Health Questionnaire* (GHQ), and the *Structured Clinical Interview for Diagnostic and Statistical Manual of Mental Disorders* (SCID). These are all reputable tools used globally for diagnosing mental health conditions. They provide a standardized way to measure and understand mental disorders.

### *2.2.2 The First National Mental Health Survey on in Bangladesh (2003–2005)*

Indeed, the first national survey carried out from 2003 to 2005 in Bangladesh highlights the substantial impact of mental disorders within the nation (NIMH, B and WHO, 2007). This survey has been critical in providing an initial understanding of the prevalence and types of mental disorders in the population. It has also offered insights into the demographic and socioeconomic factors associated with these conditions. These findings would then guide the development of national mental health strategies and policies, and inform the prioritization of resources. It's important for such surveys to be conducted periodically to monitor trends and evaluate the effectiveness of interventions.

This comprehensive report provides an in-depth look into the prevalence of mental disorders within a population of 13,080 people in Bangladesh. The overall prevalence of mental disorders was 16.05%, with a higher occurrence in women than in men (19.0 vs. 12.9%).

The analysis of individual disorders shows that neurotic disorders are the most common (8.4%), followed by a major depressive disorder (4.6%), and then psychotic disorders (1.1%). Among neurotic disorders, generalized anxiety disorder was fairly common (2.9%). The study also points to a significant relationship between mental illness and socioeconomic deprivation, indicating that poorer individuals may be more prone to mental health issues. Interestingly, while there was a high level of awareness about mental illness and a generally good attitude towards those with mental health conditions, many respondents held misconceptions about the causes of mental illness, with more than half believing in supernatural causation. Despite these misconceptions, a high percentage (85%) expressed a willingness to treat mental health conditions using modern psychiatric methods. These findings highlight the importance of continued education and awareness campaigns to dispel myths about mental health. It also underscores the need for accessible and affordable mental health services, especially for those in lower socioeconomic brackets.

### 2.2.3 *Prevalence of Mental Disorders Among Children and Adolescents*

There are variations of prevalence of mental disorders among children in Bangladesh among the studies (Table 2.2). The earliest report on mental health among urban primary school children in Bangladesh provides important insights into the prevalence of behavioral disorders in this population (Rabbani & Hossain, 1999). The finding that 13.4% of children had some type of behavioral disorder is notable and suggests a need for early mental health interventions and support in schools. The gender difference is also striking, with boys being twice as likely as girls to be affected by behavioral disorders (20.4 vs. 9.9%). This could be due to a range of factors, including biological differences, societal expectations, or differences in the way boys and girls express and cope with emotional distress.

Data from this study also indicates the prevalence of specific types of behavioral disorders among children. Emotional disorders, which can include conditions like anxiety and depression, were found in 3.2% of the children. Conduct disorders, which are characterized by antisocial behavior such as theft, aggression, or vandalism, were the most common, affecting 8.9% of the children. Lastly, undifferentiated disorders,

**Table 2.2** Prevalence of mental disorders among children and adolescents in different studies in Bangladesh

| Study | Year | Setting | Age range (years) | n (sample size) | Prevalence of behavioral/ psychiatric disorders | Most common conditions | Gender difference | Implications |
|---|---|---|---|---|---|---|---|---|
| Rabbani and Hossain | 1999 | Urban primary school | | 1,288 | 13.4% of children | Conduct disorders (8.9%) | Boys twice as likely as girls (20.4 vs. 9.9%) | Need for early mental health interventions and support in schools |
| Mullick and Goodman | 2001 | Psychiatric clinic, Community | | 161 | Not specified | Not specified | Not specified | Validated and used DAWBA and SDQ tools for assessing child and adolescent psychiatric disorders |
| Jahan et al | 2004 | Urban slum | 10–16 | 210 | 22.9% of children | Not specified | Girls slightly more likely than boys (25.5 vs. 20.0%) | Need for targeted mental health interventions for children living in disadvantaged conditions |
| Mullick and Goodman | 2005 | Urban, Rural and Urban Slum | 5–10 | 922 | 15.2% of children 19.5% in urban slum | Post-traumatic stress disorder in children in urban slum | Not specified | Higher prevalence of obsessive–compulsive disorder than in previous studies |
| Khan et al | 2009 | Rural | 2–9 | 453 | 14.6% of children suffering by behavioral problems | Enuresis (9%) | Not specified | Holistic assessment and qualitative questioning important to differentiate 'developmental' problems from 'behaviour' problems |

(continued)

**Table 2.2** (continued)

| Study | Year | Setting | Age range (years) | n (sample size) | Prevalence of behavioral/psychiatric disorders | Most common conditions | Gender difference | Implications |
|---|---|---|---|---|---|---|---|---|
| Rabbani et al | 2009 | Urban and Rural | 5–17 | 3,564 | 18.4% of children | Enuresis (3%) | Boys slightly more likely than girls (19.2 vs. 17.5%) | It's crucial to establish community-based child mental health services and school mental health services |

(continued)

**Table 2.2** (continued)

| Study | Year | Setting | Age range (years) | n (sample size) | Prevalence of behavioral/ psychiatric disorders | Most common conditions | Gender difference | Implications |
|---|---|---|---|---|---|---|---|---|
| Mullick and Islam | 2020 | Urban | 3–4 | 160 | 11.9% of preschool children | Conduct disorders (5.6%) | Girls having more emotional disorder and boys having more behavioral disorder | Critical in implementing appropriate screening methods and subsequent handling of these conditions |
| MOH&FW | 2021 | Rural and Urban | 7–17 | 2,163 | 12.6% of population | Neurodevelopmental disorders (NDDs) (5.1%) followed by Anxiety Disorders (4.7%) | Boys suffered more than girls | The increased prevalence in boys versus girls, in urban settings over rural areas, and the most frequent diagnosis of neurodevelopmental disorders provide essential information that can guide the formulation of mental health policies and interventions for children and adolescents |

*Source* Author

which are characterized by symptoms that do not clearly fit into any specific category, were found in 1.2% of the children. These findings highlight the range of mental health issues that can affect children, and underscore the importance of early detection and intervention. By identifying and addressing these issues early on, it's possible to prevent long-term negative impacts on a child's development, academic performance, and overall well-being. They also highlight the importance of providing mental health support to children from a young age, and of taking gender differences into account when designing these interventions. They also underscore the need for further research to understand the causes of these gender differences and to develop effective strategies to address them.

A study in 2004 among socially disadvantaged children living in urban slums in Bangladesh reveals a higher prevalence of psychiatric disorders compared to the general population (Jahan et al., 2004). It was found that 22.9% of these children had some form of psychiatric disorder. Interestingly, the gender disparity observed in the general population was reversed in this study, with a slightly lower prevalence of psychiatric disorders in boys (20.0%) compared to girls (25.5%). This could potentially be attributed to the additional stresses and challenges faced by girls in disadvantaged settings, but further research would be needed to confirm this. This study underscores the need for targeted mental health interventions for children living in disadvantaged conditions, who are at a higher risk of psychiatric disorders. It also highlights the importance of considering gender-specific factors when developing these interventions.

Mullick and Goodman validated the *Development and Well-Being Assessment* (DAWBA) and used the *Strengths and Difficulties Questionnaire* (SDQ) tools in 261 Bangladeshi children aged 4–16 focusing on a comprehensive evaluation of the mental health of children of this country (Mullick & Goodman, 2001). The DAWBA is a suite of surveys, interviews, and scoring methods created to establish ICD-10 and DSM-IV diagnoses for individuals aged 2–17 years. It's a reliable tool for assessing psychiatric disorders in children and adolescents, making it particularly beneficial for research studies centering on mental health in these younger demographics. Conversely, the SDQ is a concise behavioral assessment questionnaire for 4–16 year olds. It comprises five sections that assess emotional symptoms, behavioral issues, hyperactivity/inattention, problems with peer relationships, and pro-social behavior. The usage of these tools enables an in-depth comprehension of the mental health scenario among children and adolescents in Bangladesh. Moreover, it ensures the collected data is uniform and can be compared with data from other regions or countries that use the same tools.

A 2005 study in Bangladesh offers important insights into the prevalence of mental disorders in children of the age group 5–10 in different settings across the country (Mullick & Goodman, 2005). The prevalence of mental disorders was determined to be 15.2%, with the highest prevalence observed in urban slum regions at 19.5%. The study also found that the estimated prevalence of any diagnosis according to the ICD-10 was 15%, which falls within the 95% confidence interval of 11–21%. One notable finding was that the prevalence of obsessive–compulsive disorder was found to be greater than what earlier studies had reported. This suggests that this particular disorder may be more common in the population than previously thought, or that diagnostic practices have improved to better identify this condition.

Furthermore, children residing in slum areas were considerably more prone to serious behavioral issues, and slightly more likely to suffer from post-traumatic stress disorder. This underlines the impact of social conditions and environmental factors on mental health, particularly in vulnerable populations such as children living in slums. Overall, these findings highlight the need for comprehensive mental health services that are accessible and tailored to the needs of different population groups in Bangladesh.

Another more recent study (Khan et al., 2009) among children indicates a significant prevalence of behavioral problems among children in rural Bangladesh, as reported by their parents. The finding that 14.6% of children are affected suggests that behavioral problems are a common issue in this population. Nocturnal endures is the most common (9.3%) behavioral problem followed by pica, aggression and others. Parental reports can be a valuable source of information in studies of this kind, as parents often have a detailed understanding of their child's behavior in various contexts. However, it's also important to note that these reports can be influenced by a variety of factors, including the parents' own mental health and their understanding and interpretation of their child's behavior. Regardless, this high prevalence rate underscores the need for accessible mental health services for children in rural areas of Bangladesh. Early intervention can help address behavioral problems before they become more severe or lead to other issues, such as academic difficulties or social problems. The study also underscores the need for comprehensive assessments of children and the use of qualitative questioning to distinguish 'developmental' issues from 'behavioral' ones.

A recent quantitative, cross-sectional, and descriptive study (Mullick and Islam, 2020) among 3–4 year old preschool children in an urban setting included 86 boys and 74 girls. The overall predicted prevalence of psychiatric disorder was 11.9%, with 4.4% being emotional disorder, 5.6% being conduct disorder, and 1.9% being hyperactivity. The prevalence of predictive psychiatric disorders was roughly the same for both 3 and 4 year olds. Girls were more prone to emotional disorders, while boys exhibited more behavioral disorders. There was a high rate of comorbidity, with significant overlap among the types of psychiatric disorders. This research corroborates previous discoveries of mental health issues in preschool-aged children, which could be critical in implementing appropriate screening methods and subsequent handling of these conditions.

### 2.2.4 *Mental Disorders, Mental Retardation, Epilepsy and Substance Abuse in Children: Survey Report 2009*

This community based descriptive cross sectional study was conducted in Dhaka division, Bangladesh between July and December 2009, reported that a significant proportion of surveyed children aged 5 to 17 years were suffering from various mental health issues (Rabbani et al, 2009). The study found that the prevalence for mental disorders, mental retardation (MR), epilepsy, and substance-related disorders (SRD) were respectively found to be 18.4%, 3.8%, 2.0%, and 0.8%. 19.2% males and 17.5% females had mental disorders. The most common mental disorders included enuresis (3%), somatoform pain disorder (1.9%), communication disorder (1.6%), obsessive–compulsive disorder (1.3%) and generalized anxiety disorders (1.3%), among others. Children aged 5 to 11 years had a higher prevalence of epilepsy and MR, while children aged 12 and above experienced more mental disorders and substance abuse. The study also found a significant association between child mental disorders, MR and SRD, and factors such as rural residence, low father's education, family history of psychiatric illness, history of head injury in perinatal period, and prolonged psychiatric illness of parents. The findings suggest a need for improved child mental health services in Bangladesh. The Reporting Questionnaire for Children (RQC) for child and adolescent mental disorders, Structured screening questionnaire for substance abuse for population among 10–17 years, Screening questionnaire for epilepsy and Screening questionnaire for psychotic disorders were implemented in this study. The survey report recommended for training skilled professionals in child and adolescent mental health, implementing community-based mental health services with a primary health care approach, expanding school mental health services, revising high school curriculum to cover mental health and substance abuse, promoting public education campaigns on child mental health, and continuing research support from national and international organizations.

### 2.2.5 Mental Health Status of Adolescents in Post-Covid Era

The COVID-19 pandemic has presented unique challenges and strains for youth globally. According to the web search results, there are some studies that have explored the mental health status of adolescents in Bangladesh during the pandemic, as well as the associated risk factors. Here are some key findings from these studies:

A cross-sectional study carried out on 322 adolescents (aged 12–19) from various urban and semi-urban regions in Bangladesh from January 22 to February 3, 2021, revealed that 67.08% of them were experiencing different levels of depression, 49.38% had anxiety, and 40.68% had stress according to the *Depression Anxiety Stress Scale*-21 (DASS-21) (Afrin et al., 2022). The study also pinpointed several factors that significantly correlated with mental health burdens. These factors included age, gender, education level, mother's profession, total monthly income, participation in sports, performing household chores, leaving the house, watching television, using the internet, attending online classes, altering eating habits, and communication with friends.

A different cross-sectional study carried out on 672 individuals from Bangladesh, aged between 15 and 65 years, from April 15 to May 10, 2020, estimated the prevalence of loneliness, depression, anxiety, and sleep disturbance at 71%, 38%, 64%, and 73%, respectively (Das et al., 2021). Factors like being female, unemployment, being a student, obesity, and living without family were identified as significant contributors to poor mental health during the COVID-19 crisis. The study also found noteworthy correlations among the different mental health issues measured.

A systematic review and meta-analysis of nine studies carried out on the Bangladeshi population during the COVID-19 pandemic revealed that the combined prevalence of depression, anxiety, and stress was 37.9%, 41.9%, and 34.7% respectively (Hosen et al., 2021). Factors associated with mental health issues included gender, age, area of residence, family size, monthly family income, educational level, marital status, physical activity, smoking, alcohol consumption, fear of COVID-19, presence of chronic illness, unemployment status, and exposure to COVID-19-related news and social media.

These studies imply that the COVID-19 pandemic has had a significant negative effect on the mental health of adolescents and other age groups in Bangladesh. They underscore the necessity for psychological assessments and counselling through both online and offline platforms to enhance the deteriorating mental health states of the impacted population. Additionally, these studies stress the criticality of increasing awareness and knowledge about mental health concerns among the general public, healthcare professionals, and policy makers.

## 2.2.6 *National Mental Health Survey 2019*

### 2.2.6.1 Prevalence of Mental Disorders in Adults

1. Prevalence of Mental Disorders: The survey revealed that 18.7% of the adult population (18 years and older) in Bangladesh were experiencing mental disorders, with a 95% confidence interval of 17.4–20%. This represented an increase from the earlier national survey conducted in 2003–2005, which reported a prevalence of 16.1% (Ministry of Health and Family Welfare, 2021).
2. Gender and Age Differences: The rates of mental disorders varied by gender and age. Females had a higher prevalence of 21.5%, compared to males at 15.7%. Additionally, individuals aged 60 years and above had the highest prevalence, with 28.1%.
3. Common Mental Disorders: The most common mental disorder among adults was depression, with a prevalence of 6.7%, followed by anxiety disorders at 4.7%. Other notable diagnoses included somatic symptom disorder (2.3%), psychoses (1%), obsessive–compulsive disorder (OCD, 0.6%), and bipolar disorder (0.5%).
4. Rural and Urban Prevalence: The survey found that the prevalence of psychiatric disorders was nearly equal in rural and urban settings, indicating that mental health issues are not limited to any specific geographic area.

#### 2.2.6.2 Prevalence of Mental Disorders in Children and Adolescents

1. Prevalence of Mental Disorders: Among children and adolescents (7–17 years), the prevalence of psychiatric disorders was 12.6%.
2. Gender Differences: Boys had a slightly higher prevalence (13.7%) compared to girls (11.5%).
3. Common Mental Disorders: The most common diagnosis among this age group was neurodevelopment disorder (NDD, 5.1%), followed by anxiety disorders (4.7%), disruptive disorders (1.7%), and depression (0.4%).
4. Rural and Urban Prevalence: The occurrence was more pronounced in rural children (12.9%) compared to their urban counterparts (11.5%).

These findings underscore the importance of addressing mental health concerns in the population, particularly among specific demographics like females, the elderly, and children and adolescents. It also suggests the need for targeted mental health interventions and support in Bangladesh.

The prevalence of psychiatric disorders in Bangladesh has been increased by more than 2% from the initial study conducted in 2003–2005. This could be due to a multitude of factors such as increased awareness, improved diagnostic procedures, or societal and environmental changes. It's important to note that the prevalence of psychiatric disorders can vary over time due to various factors, such as changes in diagnostic criteria, accessibility of mental health services, and societal attitudes. It's also notable that the data shows some differences in prevalence based on age, gender, and location. It's crucial that these findings are used to inform mental health interventions and support systems in the country. The gender disparity and higher prevalence in the elderly also underline the need for targeted mental health interventions. The most common disorders being depression and anxiety aligns with global trends. The nearly equal prevalence of psychiatric disorders in rural and urban settings indicates that mental health issues are a widespread concern that requires attention across different areas. For the younger population (7–17 years), the higher prevalence in boys and the most common diagnosis being neurodevelopment disorders provides valuable insights to shape child and adolescent mental health policies and interventions. This information can contribute to developing targeted approaches to support the mental well-being of children and adolescents in Bangladesh.

## 2.3 Burden of Mental Illness in Bangladesh

Bangladesh is grappling with a dual burden of diseases, encompassing both communicable and non-communicable illnesses. Around 60% of the disease burden is due to non-communicable diseases (Ahmed, 2018). Among the non-communicable diseases, mental illness was noted as one of the top fifth burdensome condition in Bangladesh (Ahmed, 2018). While mental health plays a vital role in leading a healthy and productive life, mental disorders often lack sufficient research focus and are not treated as a serious public health concern in countries like Bangladesh. The occurrence of mental disorders is extremely high and increasing among various demographic groups in Bangladesh (Arafat et al., 2024). A lack of public mental health facilities, scarcity of skilled mental health professionals, insufficient financial resource distribution, inadequately stewarded mental health policies and stigma contribute to making current mental healthcare significantly inadequate in Bangladesh (Arafat et al., 2024; World Health Organization, 2020). Bangladesh allocates 0.5% of its overall health budget to mental health, and the annual mental health spending per individual is 0.1 USD (WHO, 2022). Over 70% of health sector expenses in Bangladesh are out-of-pocket costs (World Bank, 2023). It is reasonable to assume a similar situation likely exists within the country's mental health care sector. There is a low level of awareness and knowledge about mental health issues among the general public, health professionals, and policy makers (Arafat et al., 2024; Hossain et al., 2014). Many people have negative attitudes and stigma towards people with mental disorders, and often resort to traditional or religious healers instead of seeking professional help (Faruk & Rosenbaum, 2023). People with mental disorders may face different forms of stigma, such as self-stigma, public stigma, professional stigma, and institutional stigma.

## 2.4 Coping Initiatives

### *2.4.1 The Mental Health Act (MHA) of 2018*

The Mental Health Act of 2018 is the commendable steps taken by the government of Bangladesh to improve the situation of mental health in the country (Hossain et al., 2019). The Mental Health Act 2018 replaced the 105-year-old Lunacy Act, 1912. However, there are still many challenges and gaps that need to be addressed, such as increasing the mental health budget, expanding the community-based services, training more mental health professionals, integrating mental health into primary care, raising public awareness and reducing stigma (The Borgen Project, 2021). There is a provision in Mental Health Act of 2018 that can potentially penalize medical practitioners for providing false certificates of mental illness in Bangladesh (Hossain et al., 2019). This provision might deter the already limited number of psychiatrists in the country from diagnosing and treating ambiguous cases out of fear of punishment. In this situation, it would be beneficial to have clearer guidelines or definitions surrounding what constitutes a "false certificate" and to ensure that there are sufficient protections and resources for mental health professionals. This could include increased training, legal protections, and better access to resources and support.

### 2.4.2 The National Mental Health Strategic Plan 2020

The National Mental Health Strategic Plan 2020–2030 represents a significant commitment by the government of Bangladesh to improve mental health across the country (Government of The People's Republic of Bangladesh, 2022). This ten-year plan, implemented through a series of 5-year action plans, likely outlines a comprehensive strategy to boost mental health services, raise awareness, reduce stigma, and provide support to individuals with mental health conditions. Though the plan's precise elements are not outlined here, a typical strategic plan would usually involve aspects such as enhancing mental health services and incorporating mental health care into primary healthcare environments, training healthcare providers, improving mental health research, and promoting mental well-being in schools and workplaces. The implementation of this strategic plan will be an important step towards improving mental health outcomes in Bangladesh and ensuring that individuals with mental health conditions receive the care and support they need.

### 2.4.3 Bangladesh National Mental Health Policy (NMHP) 2022

The NMHP 2022 is a landmark document that reflects the commitment of the Government of Bangladesh to strengthen national mental health services (National Mental Health Strategic Plan, 2020–2030). It is based on the principles of human rights, equity, accessibility, quality and community participation. It also aligns with the global mental health agenda and the Sustainable Development Goals.

Some of the key features of the NMHP 2022 are:

- It provides a comprehensive definition of mental health that includes emotional, psychological and social well-being, as well as resilience and positive coping skills.
- It recognizes the diversity of mental health needs and challenges across different age groups, genders, regions, cultures and contexts.
- It identifies six priority areas for action: promotion and prevention, service delivery, human resources, advocacy and awareness, research and monitoring, and governance and financing.
- It proposes a range of strategies and interventions to address each priority area, such as integrating mental health into primary care, developing a national mental health workforce plan, establishing a national mental health authority, allocating at least 5% of the health budget to mental health, and conducting regular surveys and evaluations.
- It highlights the importance of including individuals with personal experiences of mental health conditions, their families and caregivers, civil society organizations, professional associations, academic institutions, and other stakeholders in the design, execution, and assessment of mental health policies and programs.

The NMHP 2022 is a visionary document that sets the direction for transforming the mental health system and services in Bangladesh. However, it also faces some challenges and gaps that need to be addressed. For example:

- The NMHP 2022 is not yet fully operationalized and implemented. There is a need for a detailed action plan with clear roles and responsibilities, timelines, indicators and budgets for each strategy and intervention.
- The NMHP 2022 does not adequately address some of the emerging issues and trends in mental health, such as gender-based violence, substance misuse, suicide prevention, digital mental health and climate change.
- The NMHP 2022 does not explicitly state the method for ensuring the quality and standards of mental health services and safeguarding the rights and dignity of individuals with mental health conditions. There is a need for a robust regulatory framework, accreditation system, quality improvement mechanism and good governance system.
- The NMHP 2022 does not reflect the voices and perspectives of all segments of the population, especially those who are marginalized and vulnerable. There is a need for more inclusive and participatory processes to ensure that the policy is responsive to the needs and preferences of all people.

### *2.4.4 The Persons with Disabilities Rights and Protection Act 2013*

The Rights and Protection of Persons with Disabilities Act of 2013 recognizes the rights of people with autism, intellectual disability, hyperactivity, mental disabilities like schizophrenia, clinical depression, bipolar disorder, traumatic stress, post-traumatic stress, anxiety or phobic disorders (International Labor Organization, 2014). It covers various aspects of disability rights, such as recognition, education, employment, health care, social security, accessibility, and protection from discrimination and abuse4. However, this Act does not explicitly address the rights of people with mental diseases that do not qualify as a mental disability. Therefore, a separate legislation may be needed to safeguard the rights of this group of people, such as:

- The right to access quality mental health care and treatment without discrimination or stigma.
- The right to be involved in decisions regarding their own mental health and well-being.
- The right to receive quality mental health care and treatment without facing discrimination or stigma.
- The right to participate in decision-making about their own mental health and well-being.
- The right to privacy and confidentiality regarding their mental health information.
- The right to protection from harm, exploitation, violence, and neglect.

– The right to advocacy and support from peers, family members, and civil society organizations.

## 2.5 Ways Forward

There is a requirement for further research and data to investigate the epidemiology and impact of mental disorders in Bangladesh. The major challenges and limitations of the existing studies are underreporting, underdiagnosis, small sample size and poor study design (Arafat, 2024; Arafat et al., 2024; Hasan et al., 2021). These factors can affect the validity and reliability of the findings and limit the generalizability and applicability of the results. Therefore, it is important to conduct more large-scale, well-designed epidemiological studies and clinical trials that can address these issues and provide more accurate and comprehensive data on the prevalence, determinants, impact and treatment of mental disorders in Bangladesh.

Some of the possible ways to enhance the quality and scope of mental health research in Bangladesh are:

– Developing a national mental health research agenda that identifies the priority areas, questions and methods for mental health research in Bangladesh. This can be done through a consultative process involving researchers, policymakers, practitioners, service users, funders and other stakeholders (Hasan et al., 2021)
– Strengthening the capacity and infrastructure for mental health research in Bangladesh, including training and mentoring researchers, establishing research networks and collaborations, improving data collection and management systems, ensuring ethical standards and oversight, and securing adequate funding and resources (Arafat et al., 2022; Kemp et al., 2022).
– Applying rigorous and innovative research methods and designs that can capture the complexity and diversity of mental health issues in Bangladesh, such as mixed methods, longitudinal studies, randomized controlled trials, implementation research, participatory research and digital technologies (Barksdale et al., 2022).
– Disseminating and translating the research findings into policy and practice, through effective communication strategies, stakeholder engagement, evidence synthesis and reviews, policy briefs and recommendations, advocacy and awareness campaigns, and scaling up of effective interventions (Jayaweera et al., 2019).

## 2.6 Conclusions

The epidemiology and burden of psychiatric disorder are yet to be explored precisely in Bangladesh. There is an increase of prevalence of disorders based on the national mental health surveys. However, there are variations in the estimates among the empirical studies and national mental health surveys when we compare the distribution of disorders. These are complex and interrelated issues that require a holistic and multi-sectoral approach to address them.

## References


Afrin, S., Nasrullah, S. M., Dalal, K., Tasnim, Z., Benzadid, M. S., Humayra, F., Said-Ur-Rahman, K. M., & Hawlader, M. D. H. (2022). Mental health status of adolescents in-home quarantine: A multi-region, cross-sectional study during COVID-19 pandemic in Bangladesh. *BMC Psychology, 10*(1), 116. https://doi.org/10.1186/s40359-022-00819-3

Ahmed. (2018). Non-communicable diseases and their prevention: A global, regional and Bangladesh perspective. *National Bulletin of Public Health (NBPH), 1*(3), 2–4.

Alam, M. N. (1978). Psychiatric morbidity in general practice. *Bangladesh Medical Research Council Bulletin, 4*(1), 38–42.

Ara, N., Hossain, G. M. M., & Islam, M. T. (2001). Women mental health in rural part of Bangladesh. *Bangladesh Journal of Psychiatry, 15*(2), 5–10.

Arafat, S. M. Y, Giasuddin, N. A., Mazumder, A. H. (2024). Access to Mental Health Care in Bangladesh—Current Status, Potential Challenges, and Ways Out. S. M. Y. Arafat, & S. K. Kar (Eds.) *Access to mental health care in South Asia—Current status, potential challenges, and ways out*. Springer Nature Singapore.

Arafat, S. M. Y. (2024). Psychiatric Education and Research System in Bangladesh. S. M. Y. Arafat, (Ed.) Mental health in Bangladesh: From bench to community. Springer Nature Singapore. https://doi.org/10.1007/978-981-97-0610-5_12

Arafat, S. Y., Ali, S. A., Saleem, T., Banerjee, D., Singh, R., Baminiwatta, A., & Shoib, S. (2022). Academic psychiatry journals in South Asian countries: Most from India, none from Afghanistan, Bhutan and the Maldives. *Global Psychiatry Archives, 5*(1), 1–9. https://doi.org/10.52095/gp.2021.4395.1036

Barksdale, C. L., Pérez-Stable, E., & Gordon, J. (2022). Innovative directions to advance mental health disparities research. *The American Journal of Psychiatry, 179*(6), 397–401. https://doi.org/10.1176/appi.ajp.21100972

Burger, H., & Neeleman, J. (2007). A glossary on psychiatric epidemiology. *Journal of Epidemiology and Community Health, 61*(3), 185–189. https://doi.org/10.1136/jech.2003.019430

Chowdhury, A. K., Alam, M. N., & Ali, S. M. (1981). Dasherkandi project studies. Demography, morbidity and mortality in a rural community of Bangladesh. *Bangladesh Medical Research Council bulletin, 7*(1), 22–39.

Chowdhury, A. K., Salim, M., & Sakeb, N. (1975). Some aspects of psychiatric morbidity in the out-patient population of a general hospital. *Bangladesh Medical Research Council Bulletin, 1*(1), 51–59.

Das, R., Hasan, M. R., Daria, S., & Islam, M. R. (2021). Impact of COVID-19 pandemic on mental health among general Bangladeshi population: A cross-sectional study. *British Medical Journal Open, 11*(4), e045727. https://doi.org/10.1136/bmjopen-2020-045727

Faruk, M. O., & Rosenbaum, S. (2023). Mental illness stigma among indigenous communities in Bangladesh: A cross-sectional study. *BMC Psychology, 11*(1), 216. https://doi.org/10.1186/s40359-023-01257-5

Government of The People's Republic of Bangladesh. (2022). National Mental Health Strategic Plan, 2020–2030.

Retrieved 02 May 2023, from https://dghs.gov.bd/sites/default/files/files/dghs.portal.gov.bd/notices/e27171cb_a80b_42d4_99ad_40095adef31b/2022-08-16-08-42-af8622e2c4936593dd45601b84f4920f.pdf

Hasan, M. T., Anwar, T., Christopher, E., Hossain, S., Hossain, M. M., Koly, K. N., Saif-Ur-Rahman, K. M., Ahmed, H. U., Arman, N., & Hossain, S. W. (2021). The current state of mental healthcare in Bangladesh: Part 2—setting priorities. *Bjpsych International, 18*(4), 82–85. https://doi.org/10.1192/bji.2021.42

Hosain, G. M., Chatterjee, N., Ara, N., & Islam, T. (2007). Prevalence, pattern and determinants of mental disorders in rural Bangladesh. *Public Health, 121*(1), 18–24.

Hosen, I., Al-Mamun, F., & Mamun, M. A. (2021). Prevalence and risk factors of the symptoms of depression, anxiety, and stress during the COVID-19 pandemic in Bangladesh: A systematic review and meta-analysis. *Global Mental Health (cambridge, England), 8*, e47. https://doi.org/10.1017/gmh.2021.49

Hossain, M. D., Ahmed, H. U., Chowdhury, W. A., Niessen, L. W., & Alam, D. S. (2014). Mental disorders in Bangladesh: A systematic review. *BMC Psychiatry, 14*, 216. https://doi.org/10.1186/s12888-014-0216-9

Hossain, M. M., Hasan, M. T., Sultana, A., & Faizah, F. (2019). New mental health act in Bangladesh: Unfinished agendas. *The Lancet. Psychiatry, 6*(1), e1. https://doi.org/10.1016/S2215-0366(18)30472-3

International Labor Organization, 2014. The Persons with Disabilities Rights and Protection Act 2013. Retrieved October 30, 2023, from https://www.ilo.org/dyn/natlex/natlex4.detail?p_lang=en&p_isn=95795&p_classification=08

Islam, M. M., Ali, M., Ferroni, P., Underwood, P., & Alam, M. F. (2003). Prevalence of psychiatric disorders in an urban community in Bangladesh. *General Hospital Psychiatry, 25*(5), 353–357. https://doi.org/10.1016/s0163-8343(03)00067-7

Jahan, N. A., Hasan, M. K., & Mohit, M. A. (2004). Prevalence of psychiatric disorders among socially disadvantaged children. *Bangladesh Journal of Psychiatry, 18*(2), 27–40.

Jayaweera, K., Craig, J. M., Zavos, H. M. S., Abeysinghe, N., De Alwis, S., Andras, A., Dissanayake, L., Dziedzic, K., Fernando, B., Glozier, N., Hewamalage, A., Ives, J., Jordan, K. P., Kodituwakku, G., Mallen, C., Rahman, O., Zafar, S., Saxena, A., Rijsdijk, F., Saffery, R., … We would like to acknowledge the other members of the SEARCH Group (2019). Protocol for establishing a child and adolescent twin register for mental health research and capacity building in Sri Lanka and other low and middle-income countries in South Asia. *BMJ open, 9*(10), e029332. https://doi.org/10.1136/bmjopen-2019-029332

Karim, E., Alam, M. F., Rahman, A. H. M., Hussain, A. A. M., Uddin, M. J., & Firoz, A. H. M. (2006). Prevalence of mental illness in the community. *TAJ: Journal of Teachers Association, 19*(1), 18–23.

Kemp, C. G., Concepcion, T., Ahmed, H. U., Anwar, N., Baingana, F., Bennett, I. M., Bruni, A., Chisholm, D., Dawani, H., Erazo, M., Hossain, S. W., January, J., Ladyk-Bryzghalova, A., Momotaz, H., Munongo, E., Oliveira E Souza, R., Sala, G., Schafer, A., Sukhovii, O., Taboada, L., … Collins, P. Y. (2022). Baseline situational analysis in Bangladesh, Jordan, Paraguay, the Philippines, Ukraine, and Zimbabwe for the WHO Special Initiative for Mental Health: Universal Health Coverage for Mental Health. *PloS one, 17*(3), e0265570. https://doi.org/10.1371/journal.pone.0265570

Koly, K. N., Tasnim, Z., Ahmed, S., Saba, J., Mahmood, R., Farin, F. T., Choudhury, S., Ashraf, M. N., Hasan, M. T., Oloniniyi, I., Modasser, R. B., & Reidpath, D. D. (2022). Mental healthcare-seeking behavior of women in Bangladesh: Content analysis of a social media platform. *BMC Psychiatry, 22*(1), 797. https://doi.org/10.1186/s12888-022-04414-z

Khan, N. Z., Ferdous, S., Islam, R., Sultana, A., Durkin, M., & McConachie, H. (2009). Behaviour problems in young children in rural Bangladesh. *Journal of Tropical Pediatrics, 55*(3), 177–182. https://doi.org/10.1093/tropej/fmn108

Ministry of Health and Family Welfare. (2021). National Mental Health Survey 2019. Retrieved October 30, 2023, from http://nimh.gov.bd/wp-content/uploads/2021/11/Mental-Health-Survey-Report.pdf

MSD Manuals 2022. Classification and Diagnosis of Mental Illness. Retrieved October 30, 2023 from https://www.msdmanuals.com/home/mental-health-disorders/overview-of-mental-health-care/classification-and-diagnosis-of-mental-illness

Mullick, M. S., & Goodman, R. (2001). Questionnaire screening for mental health problems in Bangladeshi children: A preliminary study. *Social Psychiatry and Psychiatric Epidemiology, 36*(2), 94–99. https://doi.org/10.1007/s001270050295

Mullick, M. S., & Goodman, R. (2005). The prevalence of psychiatric disorders among 5–10 year olds in rural, urban and slum areas in Bangladesh: An exploratory study. *Social Psychiatry and Psychiatric Epidemiology, 40*(8), 663–671. https://doi.org/10.1007/s00127-005-0939-5

National Institute of Mental Health and Hospital (Bangladesh), WHO Bangladesh: Prevalence, Medical Care, Awareness and Attitude Towards Mental Illness in Bangladesh. In Karim, M. E., Zaman, M. M. 2007:1–27. http://books.google.com.bd/books/about/Prevalence_Medical_Care_Awareness_and_At.html?id=cixINwAACAAJ&redir_esc=y

National Mental Health Strategic Plan, 2020–2030. Retrieved 02 November, 2023, from https://dghs.gov.bd/sites/default/files/files/dghs.portal.gov.bd/notices/e27171cb_a80b_42d4_99ad_40095adef31b/2022-08-16-08-42-af8622e2c4936593dd45601b84f4920f.pdf

Rabbani, M. G., & Hossain, M. M. (1999). Behaviour disorders in urban primary school children in Dhaka, Bangladesh. *Public Health, 113*(5), 233–236. https://doi.org/10.1016/s0033-3506(99)00165-1

Rabbani, M. G., Alam, M. F., Ahmed, H. U., Sarkar, M., Islam, M. S., & Anwar, N. (2009). Prevalence of mental disorders, mental retardation, epilepsy and substance abuse in children, Bangladesh. *Journal of Psychiatry, 23*(1), 11–54.

The Borgen Project 2021. (2022). The State of Mental Health in Bangladesh. Retrieved October 30, 2023, from https://borgenproject.org/mental-health-in-bangladesh/. Government of The People's Republic of Bangladesh.

World Bank. (2023). Out-of-pocket expenditure (% of current health expenditure)—Bangladesh. Retrieved November 09, 2023, from https://data.worldbank.org/indicator/SH.XPD.OOPC.CH.ZS?locations=BD.

World Health Organization. (2023a). Mental disorders. Retrieved October 30, 2023, from https://www.who.int/news-room/fact-sheets/detail/mental-disorders

World Health Organization. (2023b). ICD-11 International Classification of Diseases 11th Revision. Retrieved October 30, 2023, from https://icd.who.int/en

World Health Organization. (2022a.) Mental Health Atlas 2020 Country Profile: Bangladesh. Retrieved November 09, 2023, from https://www.who.int/publications/m/item/mental-health-atlas-bgd-2020-country-profile

World Health Organization (2020). Bangladesh. Special Initiative for Mental Health Situational Assessment. Retrieved October 30, 2023, from https://www.who.int/docs/default-source/mental-health/special-initiative/who-special-initiative-country-report-bangladesh-2020.pdf?sfvrsn=c2122a0e_2

# Chapter 3
# Mental Health Services in Bangladesh

**S. M. Yasir Arafat**

**Abstract** Bangladesh is one of the most densely populated countries in the world with more than 90% of the mental health treatment gap. After abolishing the Dhaka asylum, the *Pabna Mental Hospital* and the *National Institute of Mental Health* are the prominent services set up in the country. There are inadequate and inequitable distributions of human resources. Psychiatric services are focused only at the tertiary care level. There are high stigma, low literacy, inadequate funds and research, a non-existent referral system, lack of insurance facilitates, and huge out-of-pocket expenses in regard to mental health services in Bangladesh. Traditional healers play an important role in the treatment of mental disorders in Bangladesh due to the perceived causative role of supernatural forces in mental disorders. I discuss historical aspects of mental health services development, mental health services delivery system, human resource in mental health services, help-seeking behavior in mental health care, and current challenges and ways out for mental health care in Bangladesh.

**Keywords** Bangladesh · Millstones of psychiatry · Mental health · Psychiatric services · Human resource

## 3.1 Introduction

Bangladesh is a country with an area of 147,570 square kilometers and a population of about 170 million (World Population Review, 2023). Psychiatric services are under-developed in comparison to the demand in the country. The latest nationwide mental health survey revealed that the prevalence of mental disorders is 18.7% among adults and 12.6% among children and adolescents (7–17 years) (Ministry of Health and Family Welfare, 2021). The survey also found that the treatment gap was 91% indicating that 91% of psychiatric patients in Bangladesh are not getting mental health services. This chapter focuses on the developmental milestones of psychiatric services, and current systems of services delivery in Bangladesh. It also mentions

S. M. Y. Arafat (✉)
Department of Psychiatry, Bangladesh Specialized Hospital Limited, Dhaka, Bangladesh
e-mail: arafatdmc62@gmail.com

 
S. M. Y. Arafat (ed.), *Mental Health in Bangladesh*,
https://doi.org/10.1007/978-981-97-0610-5_3

the help-seeking and referral patterns along with potential challenges and ways out in the country.

## 3.2 Historical Developments of Psychiatric Services in Bangladesh

### 3.2.1 Development of Public Service Points

The historical aspects of mental health services were previously published in some articles where it has revealed that the first mental health services establishment was found during the British period in 1815 in Dhaka (for details see Arafat et al., 2020, 2024; Arafat, 2019, 2020; Mullick, 2007; Karim et al., 2006; Rabbani et al., 2016). Subsequently, the *Pabna Mental Hospital* (PMH) and the *National Institute of Mental Health* (NIMH) were established. In this chapter, I mention the development milestones and mental health services in Bangladesh (Box 3.1). During the British period, there were asylums in the Indian subcontinents. There were regional distributions from where patients were admitted in different asylums (Arafat, 2019; Arafat et al., 2024). During the Pakistan period, there were 60 admitted patients in the Ranchi Mental Hospital from East Pakistan and the Government had to make payments for their expenses. Then it was decided to build a hospital in East Pakistan. As a result of this decision, PMH was established and the sixty patients were returned from Ranchi Mental Hospital. The hospital was established by Dr. Mohammad Hossain Ganguly, the civil surgeon of that time.

### 3.2.2 Development of Private Services Points

The development of private services for psychiatric patients was started in the early 1980s in Dhaka. The *Dhaka Monorog Clinic* and *Zaman's Clinic* are the initial setups in Dhaka. Currently, there are lots of private clinics across the country (Arafat et al., 2024).

**Box 3.1. Historical developmental milestones of mental health services in Bangladesh (Arafat et al., 2024; Basu, 2004; Sharma & Varma, 1984).**

1. Before British period
   a. Some asylums in 15th century (1436–1469) during the regime of Mohammad Khilji
   b. There was a mental hospital at *Dhar, Madhya Pradesh*, India and a physician named *Maulana Fazulur Hakim*

2. British period-asylum
   a. Before the British period , no identifiable service establishment
   b. Asylum period
   c. Lunatic asylum at Muralibazar/Murli Bazar (now Bakshibazar) in Dhaka in 1815
   d. It was connected with the central jail
3. Pakistan period-PMH
   a. 1947–1971
   b. Hospital period
   c. Establishment of Pabna Mental Hospital in 1957 at *Sitlai House* by Mohammad Hossain Ganguly
   d. Started with 60 inpatients beds
   e. Currently there are 500 inpatient beds
   f. There was recommendations of building mental health institute
4. Bangladesh period
   4.1 NIMH
   a. After 1971 along with regular health services, *National Institute of Mental Health (NIMH), Dhaka* is a major establishment
   b. Started in February 1981 at Suhrawardy Hospital as *organization in training in mental health*
   c. In 1988 it was shifted to *Sir Salimullah Medical College* with a 50-bed inpatient facility
   d. Then it was shifted to Dhaka Medical College Hospital (DMCH)
   e. In 1992, it was started as NIMH at Sher-e-Bangla Nagor with the facility of 100 inpatients beds and other regular outpatient services
   f. It started at the current location in 2001
   g Currently 400 inpatient beds

4.2 The Central Drug Addiction Treatment Center (CTC)
   a. Established in 1988

4.3 DMCH
   a. Out-patient services were started in 1974

### *3.2.3 Advocacy Groups*

There are a few advocacy groups and societies are working in psychiatry in Bangladesh. Some leading groups are mentioned in Box 3.2.

**Box 3.2. Prominent advocacy groups in mental health services in Bangladesh (Arafat et al., 2020)**

A. Bangladesh Association of Psychiatrists (BAP)
   I. established in 1975
   II. promotion of mental health and advancement of psychiatry in Bangladesh
   III. advancing all mental health as a prime mover in the country

B. Bangladesh Association for child and adolescent mental health (BACAMH)
   I. established in 2008
   II. national organization in child and adolescent psychiatry
   III. promotion of child and adolescent mental health and wellbeing by ensuring training, services, research, advocacy, peer support and collaboration

C. Association of Therapeutic Counselors, Bangladesh (ATCB)
   I. established in 2010
   II. a national, non-profitable organization
   III. advancement of counseling as a profession and to ensure augmented service

### 3.2.4 Development of Legal Frames

The latest Mental Health Act was passed on November 14, 2018, which inactivates the previously enacted Lunacy Act, of 1912 (Mental Health Act, 2018). The *Neurodevelopmental Disability Protection Trust* act was passed in 2013. The *National Mental Health Policy* and the *National Mental Health Strategic Plan 2020–2030* were accepted in 2022. The Bangladesh Rehabilitation Council Act was passed in 2018 (World Health Organization, 2022a).

## 3.3 Mental Health Services Systems in Bangladesh

### *3.3.1 Components of Mental Health Services in Bangladesh*

There are four components of health sector in Bangladesh by which health services are managed and delivered (Fig. 3.1). They are government sector, private sector, nongovernmental organization (NGO) sector, and donor agency driven services (World Health Organization, 2015).

The private sector plays a fundamental role in mental health service delivery in Bangladesh. It covers services of Western medicine as well as alternative medicine (Unani, Ayurvedic, Homeopathic). Services are available in different avenues namely corporate hospitals, private medical college hospitals, diagnostic centers, private chamber and diagnostics complexes, clinics, and hospitals (World Health Organization, 2015).

Consultants and physicians in Bangladesh (both government and non-govt.) practice medicine and perform surgeries in private settings outside their office time. For this practice, several corporate chamber complexes Labaid, Popular, Ibn Sina, Medinova, etc.) have been built in almost all the cities in Bangladesh. Private practice

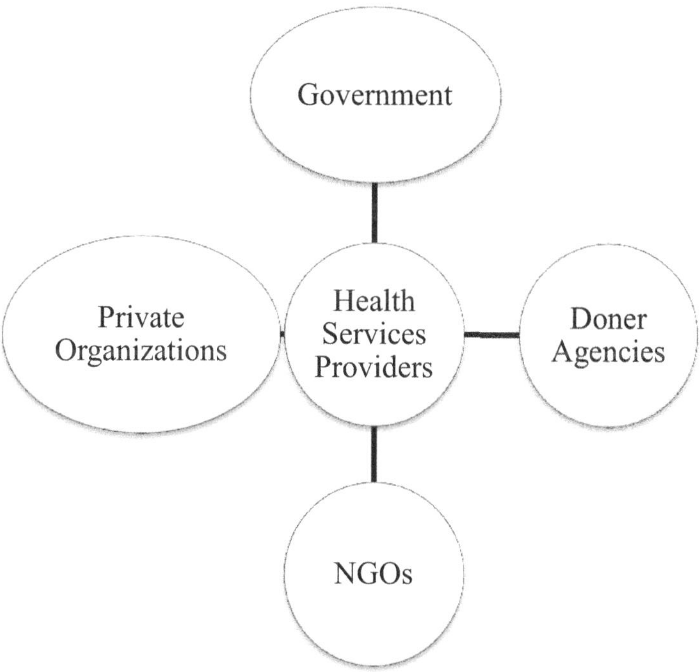


**Fig. 3.1** Components of Health Services Delivery in Bangladesh (Adapted from World Health Organization, 2015)

and the private sector are grossly unregulated and many incidents have been noted that persons practicing as doctors by falsifying the Bangladesh Medical & Dental Council (BMDC) registration. In addition to that psychiatrists visit their nearby cities to consult patients during the weekends (Andalib & Arafat, 2016).

NGOs and donor agencies usually prioritize the deprived and marginalized portion of society as well as the rural areas of the country (World Health Organization, 2015). They played a significant role in mental health and psychosocial support (MHPSS) efforts for refugees and other marginalized people (Kemp et al., 2022).

### *3.3.2 Level of Government Mental Health Services in Bangladesh*

There are three different levels of government health services in Bangladesh i.e. primary level, secondary level, and tertiary level (Fig. 3.2). The primary level care has three services points; (1) community clinic (the end-point of health services), (2) union sub-centers (referral point of community clinic), (3) upazila health complexes. The secondary level of health services is composed of district hospitals and the tertiary level includes medical college hospitals and specialized institutions (Government of The People's Republic of Bangladesh, 2022). According to the current organogram, psychiatrists are only posted in tertiary care level and no post is available at primary and secondary care levels for psychiatrists (Government of The People's Republic of Bangladesh, 2022).

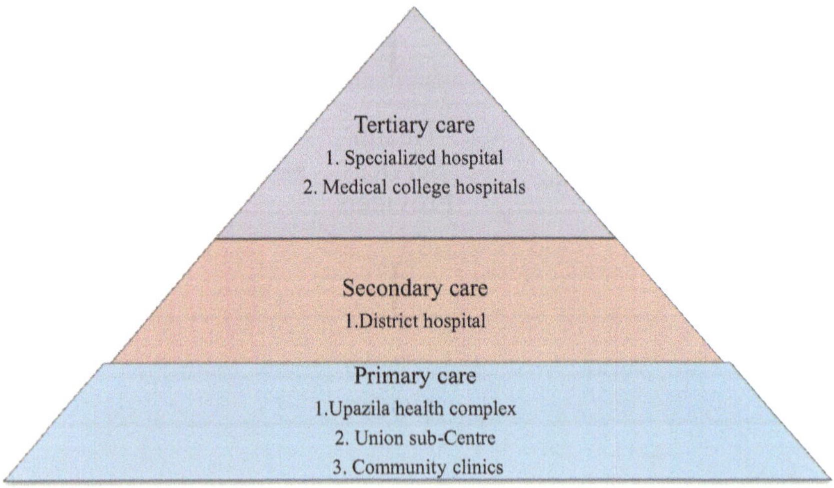


**Fig. 3.2** Level of Health Services in Bangladesh (adapted from Facility Government of the People's Republic of Bangladesh, 2022; Registry, 2023)

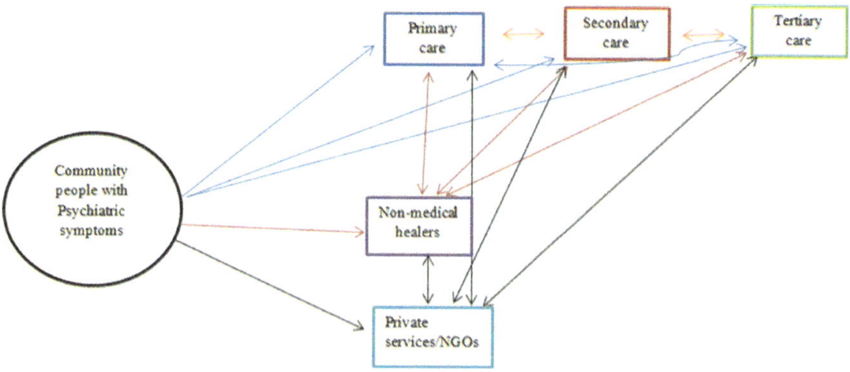


**Fig. 3.3** Help seeking pathways in psychiatric disorder in Bangladesh (Adapted from Arafat et al., 2024)

### *3.3.3 Formal and Informal Services*

Mental health services in Bangladesh are sought both in formal and informal service settings. The formal services are rendered through outpatient consultations, inpatient admissions, residential facilities in hospitals and clinics, and other facilities like rehabilitation services (World Health Organization, 2007). The informal service is rendered by unqualified village doctors, pharmacy men, homeopathic physicians, kobiraj, and religious healers (World Health Organization, 2015). Formal services are well practiced in urban areas whereas informal services are more availed in rural areas (World Health Organization, 2015).

### *3.3.4 Referral System*

The referral system in Bangladesh has no boundaries. The private sector does not have any restrictions to follow. The public sector does not follow any specific pattern. The community people can attend any physician, in any sector (Fig. 3.1), and at any level (primary, secondary, or tertiary; Fig. 3.2) in exchange for a consultation fee (Fig. 3.3). There is no epidemiological catchment area for any specific mental health services point (Arafat et al., 2024; World Health Organization, 2015).

### *3.3.5 Telepsychiatry*

Along with the in-person services telepsychiatry is an emerging treatment mode in Bangladesh psychiatry. With the rapid expansion of smartphone and internet users, telepsychiatry has been expanding day by day. The necessity has been well substantiated by the COVID-19 pandemic even though the services were started in 1999. During the COVID-19 pandemic, telepsychiatry was practiced through Skype, WhatsApp, Messenger, IMO, and FaceTime. In recent days, psychiatrists, especially the younger ones, usually share their WhatsApp numbers with the patients for communication. Telepsychiatry was started at the *National Institute of Mental Health* (NIMH), Dhaka which has been ceased later (Arafat et al., 2024). Psychiatrists in Bangladesh use telepsychiatry services for Bangladeshi expatriates living in different countries of the work (Arafat et al., 2024).

### 3.3.6 Current Psychiatric Services in Bangladesh

Currently, NIMH has 400 inpatient facilities and PMH has 500 inpatient beds. There are 15 beds for forensic inpatient services. The mental health services were started in 1974 in *Dhaka Medical College Hospital* (DMCH) where there are 25 inpatient beds at present (Government of the People's Republic of Bangladesh, 2022; Karim et al., 2006). The *Bangabandhu Sheikh Mujib Medical University* (BSMMU) has 40 inpatient beds. There are about 72 outpatient services attached to a hospital and 62 inpatient services with 195 inpatient beds across the country (World Health Organization, 2022a, 2022b). Among the 37 government medical colleges, inpatient services are available only in ten medical colleges and *Cox's Bazar District Hospital* has an indoor facility (Government of the People's Republic Of Bangladesh, 2022). Among the 63 private medical colleges in the country, psychiatric inpatient services is available in only four medical colleges (*Enam Medical College and Hospital, Z. H. Sikder Women's Medical College, Bangladesh Medical College, and Uttara Adhunik Medical College and Hospital*) with a total of 38 allocated seats (Government Of The People's Republic Of Bangladesh, 2022). *Shishu Bikash Kendra* (SBK) has been started in 34 medical college hospitals (tertiary care level) and one district hospital (secondary care level) aiming to provide comprehensive care for autism spectrum disorders and other neurodevelopmental disorders, including epilepsy (World Health Organization, 2022a).

### 3.3.7 Essential Drugs in Psychiatry in Bangladesh

According to the *National Mental Health Strategic Plan*, 2020–2030, the below mentioned drugs have been considered as national essential medicines for common mental disorders in Bangladesh (Box 3.3; Government of the People's Republic of Bangladesh, 2022).

**Box 3.3. National Essential Medicines for common mental disorders for Bangladesh (adapted from Government of The People's Republic of Bangladesh, 2022)**

1. Anti-depressants-Fluoxetine and Amitriptyline
2. Anti-psychotics—Haloperidol, Risperidone, Chlorpromazine, Fluphenazine
3. Anticholinergics—Biperiden and Trihexyphenidyl
4. Mood stabilizers—Lithium Carbonate, Sodium valproate and valporic acid and Carbamazepine
5. Anti-dementics—Cholinesterase inhibitors (Donepezil and Galantamine) and Memantine

## 3.4 Human Resource in Mental Health Care in Bangladesh

Bangladesh has a scarcity of human resources in mental health. According to a recent WHO report, there are 350 psychiatrists, about 700 mental health nurses, and 656 psychologists in Bangladesh for 170 million populations (World Health Organization, 2022a). It revealed that there are 0.2 psychiatrists, 0.4 psychiatric nurses, and 0.3 psychologists per 100,000 population in the country (World Health Organization, 2022a). A mathematical calculation indicates that one psychiatrist has been allocated for 93,500 psychiatric patients (I considered the prevalence 18.7% and availability of psychiatrists 0.2 per 100,000 populations). We acknowledge that positive mental health and well-being is something outside the treatment of mental disorders. Then the burden is mounting. Additionally, psychiatrists usually live in districts and divisional cities. So, the scarcity is more severe in rural areas of Bangladesh (Government of The People's Republic of Bangladesh, 2022).

## 3.5 Help-Seeking Behavior in to Mental Health Care in Bangladesh

There is a high prevalence of stigma and low status of mental health literacy in Bangladesh. There are several enduring beliefs attributing to the causative and curative role of supernatural power on mental health (Islam & Howard, 1993). One study found that 61% of participants believed in revealed Jinn possession, 50% attributed black magic, and 44% attributed the evil eye to the causation of mental illness (Mullick et al., 2013). Jinn and black magic are two prominent concepts in the causation of mental illness and treatment of it (Selim & Satalkar, 2008; Mulick et al., 2013). Therefore, traditional healers and religious healers deal with a good proportion of psychiatric patients. The second important factor is the non-existence of a referral system and the absence of a catchment area. Therefore, people can consult any caregiver level of the caregiver (Fig. 3.3). The third important factor for consideration is misconceptions about the treatment of psychiatric disorders. People think that psychiatrists only prescribe high doses of sedatives and keep the patients sleeping. Therefore, people are sometimes reluctant to consult psychiatrists. All these conditions are attributed to the high treatment gap and the availing of traditional healers/ informal services.

The traditional healers include unqualified mental health experts such as community health workers, pharmacy men, Palli cikitsak or village doctors, practitioners of alternate medicine, herbalist, "Ojha", "Kabiraz", "Baba", "Pirr", "Sufi", "Fakir", "Huzur", "Samans", and "Homeopathy" (Giasuddin et al., 2015; Nuri et al., 2018; World Health Organization, 2015). Traditional healers include "Ojha", "Kabiraz", "Baba", "Pirr", "Sufi", "Fakir", "Huzur", "Samans", "Homeopathy", "and alternate medicine" (Haque et al., 2018; Giasuddin et al., 2015; Nuri et al., 2018).

One study revealed that 84% of patients with mental illness visited other service points before reaching a mental health expert, 44% attended general physicians, 22% visited religious healers, and 12% visited polli cikisak (Giasuddin et al., 2012). Another study identified that 30% of patients with mental illness visited non-medical caregivers and 42.5% attended non-psychiatric physicians as their primary contact point (Nuri et al., 2018). One earlier study found that more than one-quarter of patients (26.3%) visited traditional and religious healers along with herbalists (Islam et al., 2001). The latest national mental health survey identified that 30% of children with psychiatric disorders consulted traditional healers as the first point of service (Ministry of Health and Family Welfare, 2021). From the available evidence, it has been extrapolated that about 25–50% of psychiatric patients visited informal services.

## 3.6 Potential Challenges and Ways Out

Mental health services have expanded remarkably in Bangladesh since its independence. However, there are ways ahead to move. There are multiple challenges and some recommendations to improve the status quo. These are discussed by Arafat et al., in 2024 and mentioned in Table 3.1.

## 3.7 Conclusions

Like other developing countries, Bangladesh has inadequate mental health services to deal with the current burden of psychiatric illness. Proper attention is needed to revamp the sectors for mental health patients which could mitigate future demands. The shortage and inequitable distribution of mental health professionals is a common challenge in the country. Both short- and long-term strategies are warranted to produce psychiatrists with standard quality and adequate quantity in Bangladesh.

**Table 3.1** Potential challenges and ways out for mental health services in Bangladesh (Adapted from Arafat et al., 2024; World Health Organization, 2022b)

| Potential challenges | Ways Out |
|---|---|
| 1. High treatment gap- more than 90% | 1. Augmented research and funding |
| 2. Unregulated help seeking pattern- no functional referral system and catchment area | 2. Expansion of services and creating awareness |
| 3. Poor fund and research- <0.5 of the total health budget, 10 Taka for mental health in a year, only 35 peer reviewed articles were published on mental health in 2020 | 3. Functioning referral system |
| 4. Inadequate and inequitable manpower | 4. Country-wide distribution of mental health professionals |
| 5. Huge out of pocket expense->70% | 5. Human resources development |
| 6. Poor mental health literacy | 6. Health insurance |
| 7. Lower-Middle income status and income disparity | 7. Awareness creation targeting the mental health literacy |
| 8. High stigma | 8. Dedicated programs for non-medical responders |
| 9. Non-judicious prescribing (poly pharmacy) | 9. Good governance |
| | 10. Availability of psychotropic medications |
| | 11. Involvement of the clients and their family in the service delivery process |
| | 12. Inter-sectoral collaboration |
| | 13. Protection of human rights |
| | 14. Disaster preparedness |
| | 15. Clinical audits |

## References


Andalib, A., & Arafat, S. Y. (2016). Practicing pattern of physicians in Bangladesh. *International Journal of Perceptions in Public Health, 1*(1), 9–13.

Arafat, S. M. Y, Giasuddin, N. A., Mazumder, A. H. (2024). Access to mental health care in Bangladesh—current status, potential challenges, and ways out. S. M. Y. Arafat, S. K. Kar (Eds.) Access to mental health care in South Asia—Current status, potential challenges, and ways out. Springer Nature. https://doi.org/10.1007/978-981-99-9153-2_3

Arafat, S. M. Y., Mullick, M. S. I., & Islam, H. (2020). Development of psychiatric services in Bangladesh. *Asian Journal of Psychiatry, 47*, 101870. https://doi.org/10.1016/j.ajp.2019.101870

Arafat, S. M. Y. (2020). The current status of psychiatric education in Bangladesh. *Asian Journal of Psychiatry, 52*, 102108. https://doi.org/10.1016/j.ajp.2020.102108

Arafat, S. M. Y. (2019). History of psychiatry in Bangladesh. *Asian Journal of Psychiatry, 46*, 11–12. https://doi.org/10.1016/j.ajp.2019.09.024

Basu, A. R. (2004). A new knowledge of madness-nineteenth century asylum psychiatry in Bengal. *Indian Journal of History of Science, 39*(3), 247–277.

Facility Registry. (2023). *Ministry of health and family welfare, government of People's Republic of Bangladesh*. Retrieved April 04, 2023, from http://facilityregistry.dghs.gov.bd/index.php

Giasuddin, N. A., Levav, I., & Gal, G. (2015). Mental health stigma and attitudes to psychiatry among Bangladeshi medical students. *International Journal of Social Psychiatry., 61*(2), 137–147. https://doi.org/10.1177/0020764014537237

Government of The People's Republic of Bangladesh. (2022). National Mental Health Strategic Plan, 2020–2030.

Retrieved May 02, 2023, from https://dghs.gov.bd/sites/default/files/files/dghs.portal.gov.bd/notices/e27171cb_a80b_42d4_99ad_40095adef31b/2022-08-16-08-42-af8622e2c4936593dd45601b84f4920f.pdf

Haque, M. I., Chowdhury, A. B. M. A., Shahjahan, M., & Harun, M. G. D. (2018). Traditional healing practices in rural Bangladesh: A qualitative investigation. *BMC Complementary and Alternative Medicine, 18*(1), 62. https://doi.org/10.1186/s12906-018-2129-5

Islam, M. M., Ali, M., & Fenonia, P. (2001). Care seeking behavior of mentally ill: A qualitative and quantitative approach. *Bangladesh Journal of Psychiatry, 15*, 13–18.

Islam, R., & Howard, R. (1993). Psychiatry in Bangladesh. *Psychiatric Bulletin, 17*(8), 492–494. https://doi.org/10.1192/pb.17.8.492

Karim, M. R., Shaheed, F., & Paul, S. (2006). Psychiatry in Bangladesh. *Int Psychiatry: Bulletin of the Board of International Affairs of the Royal College of Psychiatrists, 3*(3), 16–18.

Kemp, C. G., Concepcion, T., Ahmed, H. U., Anwar, N., Baingana, F., Bennett, I. M., Bruni, A., Chisholm, D., Dawani, H., Erazo, M., Hossain, S. W., January, J., Ladyk-Bryzghalova, A., Momotaz, H., Munongo, E., Oliveira E Souza, R., Sala, G., Schafer, A., Sukhovii, O., Taboada, L., … Collins, P. Y. (2022). Baseline situational analysis in Bangladesh, Jordan, Paraguay, the Philippines, Ukraine, and Zimbabwe for the who special initiative for mental health: Universal health coverage for mental health. *PloS one, 17*(3), e0265570. https://doi.org/10.1371/journal.pone.0265570

Ministry of Health & Family Welfare, 2021. National Mental Health Survey 2019. Retrieved March 29, 2023, from http://nimh.gov.bd/wp-content/uploads/2021/11/Mental-Health-Survey-Report.pdf

Mullick, M. S. I. (2007). Teaching and training in psychiatry and the need for a new generation of psychiatrists in Bangladesh: Role of the royal college of psychiatrists. *Bulletin of the Board of International Affairs of the Royal College of Psychiatrists, 4*, 29–31.

Mullick, M. S. I., Khalifa, N., Nahar, J. S., & Walker, D.-M. (2013). Beliefs about Jinn, black magic and evil eye in Bangladesh: The effects of gender and level of education. *Mental Health, Religion and Culture, 16*(7), 719–729. https://doi.org/10.1080/13674676.2012.717918

Mental Health Act, 2018. Bangladesh. [Online]. Retrieved December 12, 2023, from http://bdlaws.minlaw.gov.bd/act-1273.html

National Institute of Advanced Nursing Education and Research (nd) Mental Health and Psychiatric Nursing. http://www.nianer.edu.bd/msn/advanced-specialties/mental-health-psychiatric/

Nuri, N. N., Sarker, M., Ahmed, H. U., Hossain, M. D., Beiersmann, C., & Jahn, A. (2018). Pathways to care of patients with mental health problems in Bangladesh. *International Journal of Mental Health Systems, 12*, 39. https://doi.org/10.1186/s13033-018-0218-y

Rabbani, G., Ahmed, H. U., Desai, G., & Bhugra, D. (2016). The Bangladesh perspective. In: D. Bhugra, S. Tse, R. Ng, & N. Takei (Eds.) *Routledge handbook of psychiatry in Asia* (pp. 39–48).

Sharma, S., & Varma, L. P. (1984). History of mental hospitals in Indian sub-continent. *Indian Journal of Psychiatry, 26*(4), 295–300.

Selim, N., & Satalkar, P. (2008). Perceptions of mental illness in a Bangladesh village. *BRAC University Journal, V*, 47–57.

World Health Organization. (2022a). Addressing mental health in Bangladesh. Retrieved May 03, 2023, from https://www.who.int/publications-detail-redirect/9789290210146

World Health Organization. (2022b). Mental Health Atlas 2020 Country Profile: Bangladesh. Retrieved on March 30, 2023, from https://www.who.int/publications/m/item/mental-health-atlas-bgd-2020-country-profile

World Health Organization. (2015). Bangladesh health system review. *Health Systems in Transition, 5*, 1–214.

World Health Organization. (2007). WHO-AIMS report on mental health system in Bangladesh. WHO Regional Office for South-East Asia. Retrieved May 05, 2023, from https://apps.who.int/iris/handle/10665/206149

World Population Review. (2023). *Muslim Majority Countries 2022*. Retrieved 18 May, 2023, from https://worldpopulationreview.com/country-rankings/muslim-majority-countries

# Chapter 4
# Biological Management of Psychiatric Disorders in Bangladesh

**S. M. Yasir Arafat and Noor Ahmed Giasuddin**

**Abstract** Biological or pharmacological management plays a vital role in mental health services in Bangladesh. To some extent, psychotropics are the core of management in the country. Psychotropics are becoming available in the country keeping with the pace of the global market. Although other methods of neuromodulation like deep brain stimulation are yet to get the momentum. Additionally, the use of electroconvulsive therapy has been decreasing day by day. This chapter elaborates on the historical aspects of psychotropics and available drugs including antipsychotics, antidepressants, psychostimulants, anxiolytics, sedatives, hypnotics, etc. other methods include electroconvulsive therapy in Bangladesh which is rarely used nowadays. We also discussed some potential barriers to biological treatment like stigma and poor mental health literacy along with possible ways out from this situation for better mental health services in Bangladesh.

**Keywords** Pharmacological treatment · Antidepressants · Antipsychotic · Mood stabilizer · Anxiolytic · Sedative-hypnotics · Electroconvulsive therapy · Anti-dementia · Stimulants · Bangladesh

## 4.1 Introduction

Psychiatric disorders are multifactorial. Therefore, the treatment of mental illness includes multiple modalities. The biopsychosocial model has been well-accepted while explaining mental disorders (Adler, 2009). Along with other modalities like psychotherapy and social interventions, biological measures have been proven as an important component of treatment. Before the 1930s, psychoanalysis played a vital role in the treatment of psychiatric disorders (Endler, 1988). In the next

S. M. Y. Arafat (✉)
Department of Psychiatry, Bangladesh Specialized Hospital Limited, Dhaka, Bangladesh
e-mail: arafatdmc62@gmail.com

N. A. Giasuddin
Department of Psychiatry, Magura Medical College, Magura, Bangladesh



S. M. Y. Arafat (ed.), *Mental Health in Bangladesh*,
https://doi.org/10.1007/978-981-97-0610-5_4

decade (1930s), there were several attempts to use somatointerventions like *insulin coma therapy*, *metrazol convulsive therapy*, psychosurgery, and electroconvulsive therapy (ECT) (Endler, 1988; Faedda et al., 2010). Since 1938, ECT has been used in multiple psychiatric disorders (Endler, 1988; Faedda et al., 2010) whilst the others have become obsolete. Chlorpromazine is the first antipsychotic invented in 1952 as a serendipity that stimulated a chemical revolution in the treatment of mental disorders (Majerus, 2019). After that newer molecules are emerging with better tolerability and acceptable side effect profile.

Mental health is a historically neglected component of health in Bangladesh. Although after the independence, the country made remarkable progress in economy and health, mental health is an under-prioritized entity in the country. There are huge out-of-pocket expenses, extremely low budgetary allocation, low mental health literacy, high stigma, and inadequate human resources affecting access to care (Arafat, 2024; Arafat et al., 2024). Mental health services were noted as asylum since 1815 in Dhaka and the first mental hospital was established in 1957 at Pabna (Arafat, 2024; Arafat et al., 2024). At that time, there were a few psychotropics and ECT were available at Pabna Mental Hospital for treating psychiatric patients. Over the years, the services have been expanded gradually. However, mental health services are still absent in primary and secondary care settings and are mainly available in tertiary-level hospitals in large cities (Arafat, 2024; Arafat et al., 2024). The treatment of mental illnesses is not a priority in any level of health care in the country as evidenced by previous studies. Moreover, there prevails nonscientific explanations of mental disorders like jinn, black magic, and availing religious leaders and traditional healers for care seeking (Mullick et al, 2013; Giasuddin et al., 2012). This chapter discusses the availability of psychotropics in the local market, the supply of medications at different levels of health care services, and uses of newer neuromodulation techniques in Bangladesh.

## 4.2 Mental Health Services and Access to Mental Health Care in Bangladesh

The epidemiology and burden of mental disorder has been discussed in Chap. 2 of this book (Mazumder, 2024). A brief depiction of mental health services is mentioned in Chap. 3 (Arafat, 2024). Another recently published chapter discusses mental health access in Bangladesh (Arafat et al., 2024). The latest mental health survey found that the prevalence of psychiatric disorders was 18.7% among adults with a 91% treatment gap in Bangladesh (Ministry of Health & Family Welfare, 2021). Access to mental health care is limited in the country because of the lack of adequate number of public mental health facilities, lack of sufficient skilled mental health professionals, poor financial sources for mental health care, lack of proper implementation of mental health policy, and social stigma (Arafat et al., 2024). About seventy percent of the population of Bangladesh lives in rural areas, but the majority of psychiatric beds are located in the capital Dhaka which measures to be five-fold than other parts of the country (Arafat et al., 2024; Bangladesh Bureau of Statistics, 2023; World Health Organization, 2007). Sixty-four percent of the health expenditure in the country comes from out-of-pocket payments and there is a lack of insurance coverage for mental disorders (World Health Organization, 2015). Psychotropic medications are not widely available in the country although the WHO has included several antipsychotics, anxiolytics, antidepressants, mood stabilizer drugs, and anti-epileptics in the list of essential drugs (World Health Organization, 2015). Less than 0.11% of the population of Bangladesh has access to essential psychotropic medication free of cost. The lowest cost of antipsychotics and antidepressants per day is USD 0.07 and USD 0.04 respectively (World Health Organization, 2015). The cost of psychotropic medication in Bangladesh is 2.5% of the minimum daily income which is near to the affordability of upper-middle-income countries (McBain et al., 2012). Psychiatrists are only posted at the tertiary care level in the country.

## 4.3 Available Pharmacotherapies

### *4.3.1 Psychotropics in Bangladesh Pharma Market*

We tried to collect the available information about the introduction of psychotropics in Bangladesh. We collected the information from personal communication with pharmaceutical companies. Then, we crosschecked with the IQVIA (merger with the Intercontinental Medical Statistics [IMS]) pharmaceutical products list which was collected through personal communication for the selected molecules (Table 4.1). We considered the first launching of molecule regardless of different strengths. We prioritize the molecule and launching year and request to deemphasize the brand and the company name. The list may exclude the recently launched as well as some older molecules that were imported previously. Additionally, the launching may be different from the IMS mentioned year. Some initial brands have been discontinued which may raise concerns. Data were cross-checked by two pharmaceutical managers. In some cases, several companies launched a molecule at the same time. Although we were meticulous in this edition, we will try to update the discrepancies (if any) in our next editions. Thioridazine was available in Bangladesh which was ceased later even though we could not find any specific year. Chlorpromazine and Zuclopenthixol were introduced in Bangladesh in 1986 and both generics are still available in the market and being used. Then gradual introduction happened as mentioned, Haloperidol in 1994 and Clozapine in 1999. Then, the entry of newer generation anti-psychotics happened gradually. We found that Clozapine is the first newer-generation antipsychotic launched in Bangladesh.

Currently, we have Fluphenazine, Zuclopenthixol, Flupenthixol, and Paliperidone preparations available as long-acting injections (LAIs). Previously, Risperidone LAI was being imported which was eventually ceased. Paliperidone monthly LAI is

**Table 4.1** Antipsychotics in Bangladesh market

| Generic | Brand | Company | Launching year |
|---|---|---|---|
| Oral preparations | | | |
| Amisulpride | Amipride | Beacon | 2020 |
| Aripiprazole | Aripra/Ariprazole | Incepta/General | 2005 |
| Brexpiprazole | Brexi | Eskayef | 2019 |
| Asenapine | Zukaria | Incepta | 2023 |
| Chlorpromazine | Opsonil | Opsonin | 1986 |
| Clozapine | Sizopin | Sun Pharma | 1999 |
| Flupentixol | Sentix | Eskayef | 2005 |
| Fluphenazine | Permival | Opsonin | 1993 |
| Haloperidol | Peridol | Square | 1994 |
| Iloperidone | Ilodon | Beacon | 2014 |
| Lurasidone | Luraprex | Square | 2015 |
| Olanzapine | Lopez/ Xytrex | General/ ACI | 2002 |
| Paliperidone | Palimax ER | ACI | 2017 |
| Pimavanserin | Serivan | Incepta | 2020 |
| Quetiapine | Quiet | Incepta | 2005 |
| Risperidone | Riscord/Rispolux | General/Sandoz | 2003 |
| Thioridazine | Melleril | Novartis | Year not known |
| Trifluoperazine | Telazin | SKF | 1995 |
| Ziprasidone | Zipradon | Drug Int | 2005 |
| Zuclopenthixol | Clopixol | Lundback | 1986 |
| Long acting anti-psychotics | | | |
| Flupentixol depot | Fluanxol | Lundback | 1981 |
| Fluphenazine depot | Fluphenazine | Rotex | 1996 |

expensive and may restrict its use. Among the anti-psychotics, Quetiapine has the highest sales volume (at least for the last 3 years) followed by Risperidone and Olanzapine. We checked the IMS sales data for the last quarters of 2020, 2021, and 2022. From these data, it was revealed that the sales of anti-psychotics were contracted in 2021 whereas there was noticeable growth in 2020 and 2022. This contraction can be explained by the COVID-19 pandemic and its restricting measures.

There are some popular combination medications in the market like Flupentixol and Melitracen, Amitriptyline and Chlordiazepoxide. These drugs have been frequently prescribed by general practitioners, and specialists from other disciplines.

Among the anti-depressants, Escitalopram has secured the highest sales volume followed by Mirtazapine, Duloxetine, and Sertraline (Table 4.2). Z-drugs (Zopiclone, Zolpidem, Zaleplon, Eszopiclone) are yet to gain popularity among prescribers and have been facing a continuous (at least for the last 3 years) contraction in sales (Table 4.3). A few brands of Z drug have been discontinued due to inadequate sales.

**Table 4.2** Antidepressants in Bangladesh market

| Generic | Brand | Company | Launching year |
|---|---|---|---|
| Agomelatine | Agotin | Beacon | 2012 |
| Amitriptyline | Amitril | Albert David | 1985 |
| Citalopram | Arpolax | Incepta | 2003 |
| Clomipramine | Anafranil | Sandoz | 1994 |
| Desvenlafaxine | Nevola | Ziska | 2015 |
| Duloxetine | Duloxen | Incepta | 2005 |
| Escitalopram | Nexcital | Unimed Unihealth | 2004 |
| Fluoxetine | Prolert | Square | 1995 |
| Fluvoxamine | Relafin | General | 2004 |
| Imipramine | Tofranil | Sandoz | 1990 |
| Levomilnacipran | Cipran | Renata | 2022 |
| Maprotiline | Ludiomil | Sandoz | 1985 |
| Milnacipran | Neocipran | Ibn Sina | 2012 |
| Mirtazapine | Mitrazin | General | 2003 |
| Nortriptyline | Nortin | Navana | 1999 |
| Paroxetine | Oxat | Square | 2004 |
| Sertraline | Setra | General | 2001 |
| Venlafaxine | Venlax/Venlaf | General/Orion | 2002 |
| Vilazodone | Vilazone | Renata | 2022 |
| Vortioxetine | Vortiox | Synovia | 2023 |

Tricyclic anti-depressants (TCA) were available in the market during the 1980s and 1990s whilst after 2000 there were a good number of other anti-depressants in the market. Fluoxetine was the first Selective serotonin reuptake inhibitor (SSRI) available in Bangladesh in 1995. Currently, there is a wide range of antidepressants available in the market (Table 4.2). It is important to consider that before introduction of molecules in Bangladesh pharma market, some of the drugs were being imported and used for treatment.

### *4.3.2 Electroconvulsive Therapy (ECT) in Bangladesh*

Since the early days of the establishment of psychiatric services in Bangladesh i.e. the starting of Pabna Mental Hospital in 1957, ECT has been used in Bangladesh. It was also available when the *National Institute of Mental Health* (NIMH) was founded. Over the decades, the practice and use of ECT has declined in the country. To the best of the authors' knowledge (based on personal communication) at the time of writing this chapter, there are four functioning ECT machines in Bangladesh in

**Table 4.3** Other psychotropics in Bangladesh market

| Generic | Brand | Company | Launching year |
|---|---|---|---|
| Mood Stabilizers | | | |
| Lamotrigine | Lamitrin | ACI Pharma | 2003 |
| Lithium | Lithosun | Sun Pharma | 2000 |
| Valproate | Valex | Incepta | 2000 |
| Benzodiazepines | | | |
| Alprazolam | Alzolam | Sun Pharma | 1999 |
| Bromazepam | Lexotanil/Bopam | Roche/Opsonin | 2002 |
| Clobazam | Frisium | Sanofi-Aventis | 1982 |
| Clonazepam | Rivotril | Roche | 1997 |
| Diazepam | Easium | Opsonin | 1985 |
| Flurazepam | Aluctin | Ambee Pharma | 1997 |
| Lorazepam | Lozicum | Incepta | 2002 |
| Midazolam | Dormicum | Roche | 1995 |
| Nitrazepam | Noctin | Ambee Pharma | 1998 |
| Oxazepam | Anoxa | Square | 2009 |
| Temazepam | Temixil | Renata | 2021 |
| Z Drugs | | | |
| Eszopiclone | S-Clon | Beximco | 2006 |
| Zaleplon | Eplon | Beximco | 2003 |
| Zolpidem | Nitrest | Sun Pharma | 2009 |
| Zopiclone | Imovane | Sanofi Aventis | 1995 |
| Sleep Enhancers | | | |
| Doxepin | Adnor | Apex Pharma | 2009 |
| Hydroxyzine | Atarax | ACI | 2001 |
| Ramelteon | Ramelta | Incepta | 2018 |
| Suvorexant | Somarant | Incepta | 2017 |
| Anti-dementics | | | |
| Rivastigmine | Exelon | Novartis | 2002 |
| Donepezil | Ameloss | Incepta | 2002 |
| Galantamine | Antial | ACI | 2011 |
| Memantine | Dementa | Ziska | 2010 |
| Anti-cholinergics | | | |
| Procyclidine | Perkinil | Square | 1990 |
| Trihexyphenidyl | Hexinor | Beacon | 2012 |
| Psychostimulants | | | |
| Armodafinil | Armoda | ACI | 2017 |
| Atomoxetine | Suev | Square | 2007 |
| Methylphenidate | Methyphen | General | 2020 |

public institutions (Menon et al., 2024). The institutions are NIMH, *Bangabandhu Sheikh Mujib Medical University* (BSMMU), *Sylhet MAG Osmani Medical College*, and Chattogram (Chittagong) Medical College. In the private clinic setting, ECT is available in Monojogot Center, Dhaka and at least one consultant uses ECT in a private clinic setting. Three ECT machines were purchased in *Rangpur Medical College* in 1999 and 2001 that were never been used and got burned later in an accidental fire. ECT was initially used in Barisal Medical College which has been ceased for more than a decade. There is an extreme dearth of research on ECT in Bangladesh. We did not find any study on any aspects of ECT in Bangladesh to date (Early September 2023) by an extensive search in PubMed, Embase, PsycINFO, Google Scholar, Google, and Bangladesh Journals Online (BanglaJOL). Personal communications were made to discuss the matter with Prof. Hidayetul Islam, on September 01, 2023. From personal communication, it was revealed that ECT was practiced in a private clinic (Dhaka Monorog Clinic) in the 1980s. It has been used in acute uncontrollable excitement, schizophrenia, mania, depression, catatonia, severe obsessive–compulsive disorder, postpartum psychosis, and conversion disorder. It had been used as out-patient basis also when necessary (Islam & Howard, 1993). The National Mental Health Strategic Plan, 2020–2030 mentioned a list of national essential medicines for common mental, neurological, and substance use disorders in Bangladesh (adapted from Government of The People's Republic of Bangladesh, 2022).

### *4.3.3 Other Insights: Neuromodulation*

Neuromodulation has been emerging as an option in several psychiatric disorders like depression, obsessive–compulsive disorder, and epilepsy. The first noted neuromodulation technique, Transcranial magnetic stimulation (TMS) was started in 2016 at *Ashiyan Medical College Hospital*, Dhaka (a private medical college) which was stopped later. Recently, another private mental hospital in Dhaka (*MindWell*) has started the TMS application. The *Institute of Neuro Development & Research* (INDR) uses Vagus Nerve Stimulation (VNS) and TMS for autism. VNS has been used for adult psychiatry at *Thikana Holistic Mental Health Care*. The modality is yet to be popularized in Bangladesh. And, currently, no other neuromodulation methods are available in Bangladesh.

## 4.4 Supply of Psychotropics in Bangladesh

**Box 4.1: Essential Psychotropics in Bangladesh (adapted from Government of The People's Republic of Bangladesh, 2021)**

1. Anti-depressants
    a. Fluoxetine

   b. Amitriptyline

2. Anti-psychotics
   a. Haloperidol
   b. Risperidone
   c. Chlorpromazine
   d. Fluphenazine
3. Anticholinergics
   a. Biperiden
   b. Trihexyphenidyl
4. Mood stabilizers
   a. Lithium
   b. Sodium valproate
   c. Carbamazepine
5. Anti-dementics
   a. Cholinesterase inhibitors-Donepezil, Galantamine
   b. Memantine
6. Epilepsy
   a. Carbamazepine
   b. Phenobarbital
   c. Phenytoin
7. Alcohol withdrawal- Diazepum
8. Opioid overdose- Naloxone
9. Opioid withdrawal
   a. Methadone
   b. Buprenorphine
   c. Morphine sulphate
   d. Clonidine
   e. Lofexidine
10. Prevent relapse in alcohol dependence
    a. Acamprosate
    b. Naltrexone
    c. Disulfiram

In 2022, Bangladesh launched its National Mental Health Strategic Plan (Government of The People's Republic of Bangladesh, 2022). It provides a list of psychotropics as essential in the country (Box 4.1). Among the recommended antidepressants, Amitriptyline is rarely used as anti-depressant, instead, it is used as an anxiolytic and hypnotic. Anti-epileptics (Box 4.1) are older with hidden side-effect profiles like hepatic enzyme induction, and Stevens-Johnson syndrome while newer generation drugs with acceptable side-effect profiles like levetiracetam are available. Among the four recommended anti-psychotics only Risperidone is a newer generation drug, recommended anticholinergic Biperiden is not available in Bangladesh. Also, Lofexidine and Disulfiram are not available in the country. Therefore, the provided psychotropics in the essential drug list are somewhat detached from the ground reality.

These psychotropic drugs are freely available based on prescriptions in Pabna Mental Hospital and the NIMH (Arafat et al., 2024). However, these are not freely available in general hospital settings and at the primary care level of the country (Arafat et al., 2024).

## 4.5 Current Challenges and Ways Forward

### *4.5.1 Current Challenges*

#### 4.5.1.1 High Stigma

There are proven pharmacological treatments for mental disorders, but availing the proven treatments become difficult because there exists negative social perception and stigmatization; these two factors proved to be the key obstacles to avail effective medications for individuals suffering from mental health problems (Shohel et al., 2022). Having a mental illness and seeking treatment for it has been stigmatized in the country (Hossain et al., 2014; Ministry of Health and Family Welfare, 2021). Persons with mental disorders (PMDs) find it difficult to discuss their issues with relatives and communities when they try to utilize available resources and medications. At the same time, social stigmas like labeling mental health problems as equal to madness impede the discussion of those issues with family members and communities (Shohel et al., 2022). Along with the community population, a higher level of stigma has been revealed among medical students (Giasuddin et al., 2015). There are negative attitudes of physicians toward psychiatrists as well as PMDs.

#### 4.5.1.2 Inadequate Mental Health Literacy

The concept of mental health literacy and its implication in treatment seeking behavior among PMDs has been poorly studied in Bangladesh. It is speculated that low mental health literacy is supposed to hinder the medication adherence for chronic disorders. This issue has been grossly neglected in the academic curriculum of schools. One study assessed the science books of primary and secondary schools and found the absence of contents related to mental health (Uddin, 2020). There are several studies on depression literacy in Bangladesh that Mental health literacy is a newer academic focus in Bangladesh (Arafat et al., 2017, 2018, 2019; Mali et al., 2018). Among the study participants, 65% of the nurses thought that anti-depressants are addictive (Mali et al., 2018). Other studies indicated that 71% of participants from various groups and about 80% of the university students thought that anti-depressants are addictive (Arafat et al., 2018, 2019). Due to the poor mental health literacy people visit traditional healers and other care providers like Ojha, Jhar-fuk, black magic removers which impose extra financial burden without benefit related to treatment.

#### 4.5.1.3 Polypharmacy

Prescribing multiple psychotropics is common in Bangladesh. Although there is lack of studies assessing the pattern at the national and/or regional level, as practicing psychiatrists in Bangladesh and based on our personal experience we observe that the majority of the psychiatrists in Bangladesh practice polypharmacy. It has been noted in academic settings as well as in the private chamber setting. It is possible that majority of the psychiatrists are not prescribing psychotropics judicially. One study assessed the prescription pattern in patients with schizophrenia and found that more than 45% of patients had been suggested by polypharmacy (Yang et al., 2018). There are notions (perhaps misbelief) that our psychotropics may contain the active ingredients in lower amounts than in the countries where the clinical trials were conducted and justify the overdoses (Arafat et al., 2024). There is a misconception among the general population in Bangladesh that psychiatrists use sedatives that make a person non-functioning. Perhaps this may happen by observing patients with multiple medications. This also reinforces stigma towards the biological treatment of psychiatric disorders in Bangladesh.

### *4.5.2 Ways Forward*

Stigma and discrimination contribute significantly to hindering the utilization of mental health services and available therapeutic interventions. It may be recommended to instill community-based awareness build-up to grow more positive perceptions about mental disorders. Mental Health Professionals (MHPs) have direct contact with PMDs and their families. Adequate psychoeducation to PMDs and their families, mass awareness build-up, as well as disregarding for non-scientific remedies such as Ojha, Jhar-fuk, and black magic will reduce the treatment gap to a great extent. A specific anti-stigma component is required to be put in the graduate curriculum as well as strategies to improve the existing attitude are required.

Media is the primary source of information for mental health (Hasan & Thornicroft, 2018; Qusar et al., 2022). So, both MHPs and media professions have roles in reducing social stigma and improving the utilization of available pharmacological interventions.

Additional research and interventions are warranted to improve the overall mental health literacy. Regular clinical audits could be a possible solution to reduce non-judicious prescriptions of multiple psychotropics (Arafat et al., 2024).

## 4.6 Conclusion

This chapter highlighted the biological management options for mental disorders in Bangladesh. We discussed the distribution and supply of psychotropics in Bangladesh which are moving with the global pharmaceutical inventions. Uses of ECT have been reduced in one end and in the other end, newer neuromodulation methods are yet to become popular. High stigma, low mental health literacy, and poly-pharmacy are the fundamental challenges in Bangladesh for continuing the biological management of psychiatric disorders. There is no alternative to formulate intervention measures like reducing stigma towards managing psychiatric disorders and raising mental health literacy at the community level for a better quality of life for PMDs in Bangladesh.

## References


Adler, R. H. (2009). Engel's biopsychosocial model is still relevant today. *Journal of Psychosomatic Research, 67*(6), 607–611. https://doi.org/10.1016/j.jpsychores.2009.08.008

Arafat, S. M. Y, Giasuddin, N. A., Mazumder, A. H. (2024). Access to mental health care in Bangladesh—Current status, potential challenges, and ways out. S. M. Y. Arafat, S. K. Kar, (Eds.) *Access to mental health care in South Asia—Current status, potential challenges, and ways out*. Springer Nature. https://doi.org/10.1007/978-981-99-9153-2_3

Arafat, S. M. Y. (2024). Mental health services in Bangladesh. S. M. Y Arafat, (Ed.) *Mental health in Bangladesh: From bench to community*. Springer Nature. https://doi.org/10.1007/978-981-97-0610-5_3

Arafat, S. M. Y., Shams, S. F., Chowdhury, M. H. R., Chowdhury, E. Z., Hoque, M. B., & Bari, M. A. (2017). Adaptation and validation of the Bangla version of the depression literacy questionnaire. *Journal of Psychiatry, 20*(4), 412. https://doi.org/10.4172/2378-5756.1000412

Arafat, S. M. Y., Ahmed, S., & Uddin, S. (2018). Depression literacy status in Bangladesh: A cross-sectional comparative observation. *Journal of Behavioral Health, 7*(2), 91–97. https://doi.org/10.5455/jbh.20171004090621

Arafat, S. Y., Al Mamun, M. A., & Uddin, M. S. (2019). Depression literacy among first-year university students: A cross-sectional study in Bangladesh. *Global Psychiatry, 2*(1), 31–36. https://doi.org/10.2478/gp-2019-0002

Bangladesh Bureau of Statistics. (2023). Post Enumeration Check (PEC) Adjusted Population. Population and Housing Census 2022. Retrieved October 23, 2023, from https://bbs.gov.bd/site/page/47856ad0-7e1c-4aab-bd78-892733bc06eb/Population-&-Housing

Endler, N. S. (1988). The origins of electroconvulsive therapy (ECT). *Convulsive Therapy, 4*(1), 5–23.

Faedda, G. L., Becker, I., Baroni, A., Tondo, L., Aspland, E., & Koukopoulos, A. (2010). The origins of electroconvulsive therapy: Prof. Bini's first report on ECT. *Journal of Affective Disorders, 120*(1–3), 12–15. https://doi.org/10.1016/j.jad.2009.01.023

Giasuddin, N. A., Chowdhury, N. F., Hashimoto, N., Fujisawa, D., & Waheed, S. (2012). Pathways to psychiatric care in Bangladesh. *Social Psychiatry and Psychiatric Epidemiology, 47*(1), 129–136. https://doi.org/10.1007/s00127-010-0315-y

Giasuddin, N. A., Levav, I., & Gal, G. (2015). Mental health stigma and attitudes to psychiatry among Bangladeshi medical students. *International Journal of Social Psychiatry., 61*(2), 137–147. https://doi.org/10.1177/0020764014537237

Government of The People's Republic of Bangladesh. (2022). National Mental Health Strategic Plan, 2020–2030.

Retrieved May 02, 2023, from https://dghs.gov.bd/sites/default/files/files/dghs.portal.gov.bd/notices/e27171cb_a80b_42d4_99ad_40095adef31b/2022-08-16-08-42-af8622e2c4936593dd45601b84f4920f.pdf

Hasan, M. T., & Thornicroft, G. (2018). Mass media campaigns to reduce mental health stigma in Bangladesh. *The Lancet. Psychiatry, 5*(8), 616. https://doi.org/10.1016/S2215-0366(18)30219-0

Hossain, M. D., Ahmed, H. U., Chowdhury, W. A., Niessen, L. W., & Alam, D. S. (2014). Mental disorders in Bangladesh: A systematic review. *BMC Psychiatry, 14*, 216. https://doi.org/10.1186/s12888-014-0216-9

Islam, R., & Howard, R. (1993). Psychiatry in Bangladesh. *Psychiatric Bulletin, 17*(8), 492–494. https://doi.org/10.1192/pb.17.8.492

Majerus, B. (2019). A chemical revolution as seen from below: The 'discovery'of neuroleptics in 1950s Paris. *Social History of Medicine, 32*(2), 395–413.

Mali, B., Akter, H., & Arafat, S. Y. (2018). Depression literacy among nurses: A cross-sectional observation in a tertiary care hospital of Bangladesh. *Malaysian Journal of Psychiatry, 27*(2), 14–19.

Mazumder, A. H. (2024). Epidemiology and Burden of Mental Disorders in Bangladesh. S. M. Y. Arafat (Ed.) *Mental health in Bangladesh: From bench to community*. Springer Nature. https://doi.org/10.1007/978-981-97-0610-5_2

McBain, R., Norton, D. J., Morris, J., Yasamy, M. T., & Betancourt, T. S. (2012). The role of health systems factors in facilitating access to psychotropic medicines: A cross-sectional analysis of the WHO-AIMS in 63 low- and middle-income countries. *PLoS Medicine, 9*(1), e1001166. https://doi.org/10.1371/journal.pmed.1001166

Menon, V., Kar, S. K., Gupta, S., Baminiwatta, A., Mustafa, A. B., Sharma, P., Abhijita, B., & Arafat, S. M. Y. (2024). Electroconvulsive therapy in South Asia: Past, present, and future. *Asian Journal of Psychiatry,* 92, 103875. https://doi.org/10.1016/j.ajp.2023.103875

Ministry of Health and Family Welfare. (2021). National Mental Health Survey 2019. Retrieved March 29, 2023, from http://nimh.gov.bd/wp-content/uploads/2021/11/Mental-Health-Survey-Report.pdf

Mullick, M. S. I., Khalifa, N., Nahar, J. S., & Walker, D.-M. (2013). Beliefs about Jinn, black magic and evil eye in Bangladesh: The effects of gender and level of education. *Mental Health, Religion and Culture, 16*(7), 719–729. https://doi.org/10.1080/13674676.2012.717918

Qusar, M. M. A. S., Hossain, R., Sohan, M., Nazir, S., Hossain, M. J., & Islam, M. R. (2022). Attitudes of mental healthcare professionals and media professionals towards each other in reducing social stigma due to mental illness in Bangladesh. *Journal of Community Psychology, 50*(7), 3181–3195. https://doi.org/10.1002/jcop.22823

Shohel, T. A., Nasrin, N., Farjana, F., Shovo, T. E., Asha, A. R., Heme, M. A., Islam, A., Paul, P., & Hossain, M. T. (2022). He was a brilliant student but became mad like his grandfather': An exploratory investigation on the social perception and stigma against individuals living with mental health problems in Bangladesh. *BMC Psychiatry, 22*(1), 702. https://doi.org/10.1186/s12888-022-04359-3

Yang, S. Y., Chen, L. Y., Najoan, E., Kallivayalil, R. A., Viboonma, K., Jamaluddin, R., Javed, A., Hoa, D. T. Q., Iida, H., Sim, K., Swe, T., He, Y. L., Park, Y., Ahmed, H. U., De Alwis, A., Chiu, H. F., Sartorius, N., Tan, C. H., Chong, M. Y., Shinfuku, N., … Lin, S. K. (2018). Polypharmacy and psychotropic drug loading in patients with schizophrenia in Asian countries:

Fourth survey of research on Asian prescription patterns on antipsychotics. *Psychiatry and Clinical Neurosciences*, *72*(8), 572–579. https://doi.org/10.1111/pcn.12676

Uddin, M. S. (2020). Mental health content in school science textbooks in Bangladesh. *The Lancet. Psychiatry*, *7*(3), e10. https://doi.org/10.1016/S2215-0366(20)30008-0

World Health Organization, 2007. WHO-AIMS report on mental health system in Bangladesh. WHO Regional Office for South-East Asia. Retrieved May 05, 2023, from https://apps.who.int/iris/handle/10665/206149

World Health Organization. (2015). Bangladesh health system review. *Health Systems in Transition*, *5*, 1–214.

# Chapter 5
# Psychosocial Management of Mental Disorders in Bangladesh

**Muhammad Kamruzzaman Mozumder**

**Abstract** The scope of professional support for mental health conditions is limited in Bangladesh. However, approaches to mental health service delivery as well as quality of service are steadily increasing. Although may not be considered a specialization in a strict sense, interest among the provider to work in a specific focused area has increased. Service delivery through digital platforms and increasing initiatives toward community mental health are generating hope towards increased access to services for people in need of mental health support. Despite opportunities, there are still challenges that need to be addressed for quality and ensuring access to psychological therapies in Bangladesh.

**Keywords** Bangladesh · Situation · History · Psychotherapy · Challenges · Transition

## 5.1 State of Mental Health Professionals in Bangladesh

The details of the prevalence of psychiatric disorders have been discussed in Chap. 2 of this book (Mazumder, 2024). According to the latest mental health survey, the prevalence of mental health problems is high among adults (18.7%) and children (12.6%). Lack of service providers, limited awareness, misconception, stigma and discrimination are also very common. These contribute to the extremely high (91%) treatment gap for mental illness in Bangladesh (Ministry of Health and Family Welfare, 2021; World Health Organization, 2020). Recent findings suggested an average 39.6 months (Nuri et al., 2018) delay in seeking psychiatric treatment All these data reflect serious concerns regarding access to mental health care for people with needs.

M. K. Mozumder (✉)
Department of Clinical Psychology, University of Dhaka, Dhaka, Bangladesh
e-mail: mozumder@du.ac.bd



S. M. Y. Arafat (ed.), *Mental Health in Bangladesh*,
https://doi.org/10.1007/978-981-97-0610-5_5

As of 2023, Bangladesh has 305 Psychiatrists,[1] 77 Clinical Psychologists,[2] 328 Assistant Clinical Psychologists,2 9 Counseling Psychologists,[3] 134 Assistant Counseling Psychologist3, 11 Educational Psychologists,3 135 Assistant Educational Psychologist3 and 170 professionals trained in mixed Clinical and Counseling Psychology[4] curriculum. Based on different sources the numbers vary as we see a bit of difference with the estimates mentioned in Chap. 3 (Arafat, 2024). These numbers further challenge the possibilities of reducing the treatment gap unless an innovative solution can be found. Additionally, these trained professionals are generally based in the bigger cities, creating a divide between rural and urban communities in terms of access to the service (Arafat et al., 2024).

The mhGAP training program, being implemented with support from WHO, is showing some hope. Para-professional-based community interventions being implemented and tested by BRAC, SAJIDA and other government and non-government organizations are also showing promise (BRAC, 2023).

## 5.2 Historical Development of Psychological Therapies in Bangladesh

The current state of psychological intervention is based on a foundation developed from a series of activities in the field of psychology and mental health. These milestone events acted as catalysts and triggered activities towards the next level in creating a supportive environment for the practice of psychological therapies to thrive. This section presents a detailed discussion of such milestone events. Figure 5.1 presents the key milestones.

**1940s.** ***Development of the Medistic Psychotherapy***. Developed by M. U. Ahmed, the Medistic psychotherapy was the first and only home-grown psychotherapy in Bangladesh (Ahmed, 1984). With a mix of psychodynamic and behavioural approaches, this therapy demonstrated usefulness, especially among patients with psychosomatic conditions (Ahmed, 1984).

**1962.** ***Psyche Mental Health Center. Dhaka.*** Psyche was the first dedicated psychotherapy clinic in Bangladesh. Although M. U. Ahmed has been practising his medistic psychotherapy for a long time, establishing Psyche as a psychological service center was a statement and surely a big milestone in establishing the practice of psychological therapies in Bangladesh.

**1956.** ***Department of Psychology, at Rajshahi University.*** Although psychology has been studied under the Department of Philosophy since the beginning of the

[1] Personal communication, Treasurer, Bangladesh Association of Psychiatrists.

[2] Personal communication, Chairman, Department of Clinical Psychology, University of Dhaka; and Chairman, Department of Clinical Psychology, Rajshahi University.

[3] Personal communication, Chairman, Dept. of Educational and Counselling Psychology, University of Dhaka.

[4] Course Teacher, Clinical and Counselling Psychology program, Jagannath University.

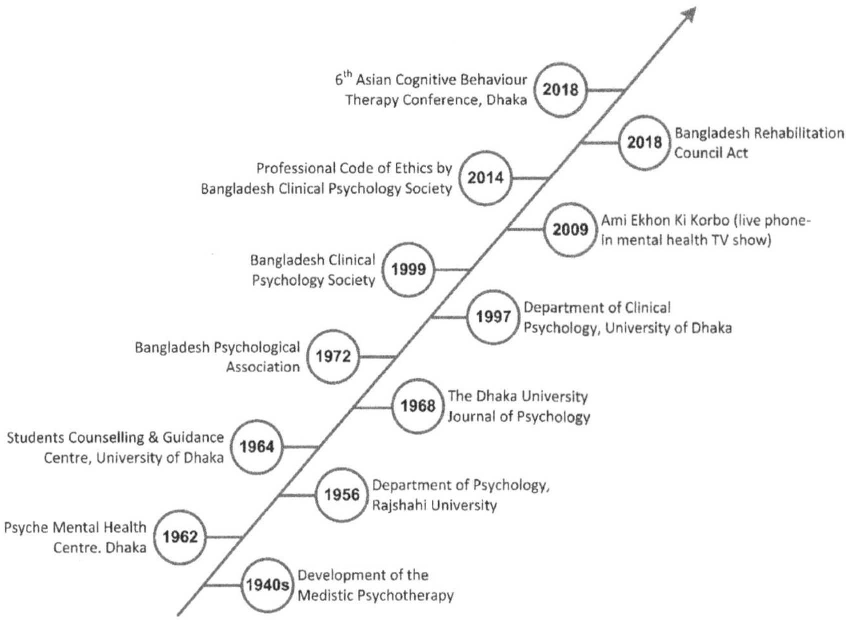


**Fig. 5.1** Timeline of the key milestones towards the growth of psychological therapies in Bangladesh

University of Dhaka in 2021; the first independent academic department to study psychology was established at Rajshahi University in 1956. This was followed by the establishment of the Department of Psychology at the University of Dhaka in 1965. These two departments led the graduate study program in psychology.

**1964.** ***Students Counseling and Guidance Center at the University of Dhaka.*** Initially started in 1964, the 'Guidance and Employment Bureau' provided counseling support to the students with the personal initiative of its director M. K. Ali. The centre was renamed as 'Student Counseling and Guidance Center' in 1969. The counseling service continued irregularly till 1998. Later in 1998, it became a regular service with support from the Department of Clinical Psychology. This was the first psychological support centre dedicated to the university student population in Bangladesh.

**1972.** ***Bangladesh Psychological Association.*** The Pakistan Psychological Association was formed in 1968 and later, after the independence of Bangladesh, it became the Bangladesh Psychological Association (BPA) in 1972. This was the first association of psychologists in Bangladesh.

**1968.** ***Dhaka University Journal of Psychology.*** Scientific journals are essential for developing the scientific credibility of any profession. The Dhaka University Journal of Psychology published in 1968 was the first academic journal of psychology in Bangladesh. This was soon followed by the Bangladesh Journal of Psychology, a flagship journal of BPA in 1972. However, both of them failed to maintain regularity as journals. The Bangladesh Psychological Studies, published first in 1991 with editorial leadership of Hamida Akhtar Begum, is continuing as a regular journal for psychological research in Bangladesh.

**1997.** ***Department of Clinical Psychology, at the University of Dhaka.*** The professional training program on applied psychology in Bangladesh was initiated by the establishment of the Department of Clinical Psychology at the University of Dhaka in 1997 under the leadership of M. Anisur Rahman. This initiated a transformation by bringing academic psychology knowledge into practical application in mental health service delivery. Based on the training model, syllabus and technical support from the University of London, UK, the required 3-year post-graduate training program was split into 1-year MS and 2-year MPhil study.

The department of educational and counseling psychology was established in the same university in 2011 offering MS and MPhil in educational psychology and counseling psychology. A combined 1-year Clinical and Counseling Psychology MS program was started in the Department of Psychology, Jagannath University in 2012 (Saha, 2022). A second graduate program in Clinical Psychology was started in 2015 at Rajshahi University (Saha, 2022).

**1999.** ***Bangladesh Clinical Psychology Society.*** Initially named the Bangladesh Clinical Psychology Association, this was the first professional organization for applied psychology in Bangladesh.

**2009.** ***Ami Ekhon Ki Korbo (the live phone-in mental health TV show*****).** Initiated by Mehtab Khanam, a professor at the University of Dhaka, this live phone-in mental health TV show created a sensation among the audience and soon many others started to follow this path. It is believed that these shows have significantly increased awareness about psychological treatment and have contributed to reducing the stigma around seeking treatment for mental health problems.

**2014. Professional Code of Ethics by** ***Bangladesh Clinical Psychology Society.*** Bangladesh Clinical Psychology Society drafted a professional code of ethics for its members. Later in 2016, a Bangla version of the code of ethics was also prepared. It marks the history of psychological service as these were the first documents ever produced by any psychological association in Bangladesh to protect the rights of the service recipients. A few other organizations also use these guidelines to ensure their ethical standard.

**2018.** ***6th Asian Cognitive Behavior Therapy Conference, Dhaka.*** The Bangladesh Clinical Psychology Society (BCPS) hosted the first-ever international conference specifically targeting only one model of therapeutic intervention. This Asian CBT conference was a huge success being attended by 667 delegates from 13 countries and demonstrated the strength of applied psychology in Bangladesh.

**2018.** ***Bangladesh Rehabilitation Council Act.*** Developed to protect the rights of people with disabilities, the Bangladesh Rehabilitation Council Act was an important milestone in introducing options for licencing for a range of professionals and service providers including applied psychology practitioners. This was the first government step toward regularization of the professional practices.

## 5.3 Approaches to Psychological Therapies in Bangladesh

Despite the growth of numerous therapeutic approaches across the world, choices are quite limited in Bangladesh. Over time, sporadic use of different therapeutic approaches has been observed, however, only a few received notable attention and focused practice by a larger group of practitioners. Some of these major psychological interventions practised in Bangladesh are discussed below.

### *5.3.1 Medistic Psychotherapy*

Medistic psychotherapy was probably the only indigenous psychotherapy ever developed in Bangladesh (Ahmed, 1984). For the first time in Bangladesh, it demonstrated the practical application of the theoretical knowledge of psychology and was heavily popularized by stage shows, the charismatic personality of its proponent M. U. Ahmed and his reader-friendly case studies published in weekly magazines. Although it promised excellent prospects in Bangladesh, Medistic psychotherapy has gradually lost its appeal and utility with the advent of modern psychotherapeutic approaches.

### *5.3.2 Psychodynamic Therapy*

Despite the huge popularity of Freudian concepts and theories in Bangladesh among mental health and allied professionals, psychodynamic therapy did not gain much attention as a therapeutic approach. It was only sporadically practised in Bangladesh by a few psychiatrists and psychology enthusiasts. Most notable among them was Dr. Nasirullah, a Bangladeshi-born British psychiatrist who after retirement, came to Bangladesh and started teaching and providing psychodynamic therapy through Bangabandhu Sheikh Mujib Medical University (BSMMU) in 1998. However, soon after his demise after a few years, it was seemingly lost again.

### *5.3.3 Client-Centered Therapy*

Client-centered approach is a common model of mental health service across Bangladesh. The most notable early practice of this approach was demonstrated by M. K. Ali, during his work as the director of the counseling and guidance centre at Dhaka University. The simplicity of the approach and lesser dependence on fancy techniques made this easy to train and practice. This model became heavily popularized through numerous trainings organized by the non-governmental organizations

(NGOs) as they started working on the well-being and rights of the people. With the strategic leadership of Khurshid Erfan Ahmed, co-founders of Ain o Salish Kendra (ASK), a local NGO, organized training on the Client-centered approach starting in 1996 by Philis Gilbert. At present, the basic principles of the Client-centered approach are embedded in the work of most practitioners. However, it is particularly popular among partially trained counselors who provide mental health services without rigorous academic training on mental health and service delivery.

### 5.3.4 Behavior Therapy

Although the techniques of behavior therapy have been widely used in Bangladesh, its use as a standalone therapy approach is rarely seen. In the present time, it is most commonly being used by professionals working with early childhood development (e.g. oppositional defiant disorder, conduct disorder, school phobia, nocturnal enuresis) and neurodevelopmental disability. Other groups such as addiction professionals, and professionals working with chronic mental health problems are also using behavioural techniques. Due to the rise of eclectic practice, almost all the mental health professionals working in Bangladesh make some use of behavioural techniques in their practice in phobia, obsessive–compulsive disorder (OCD).

### 5.3.5 Cognitive Behavior Therapy (CBT)

Bolstered by the integrated academic training in the clinical psychology program at the University of Dhaka since 1997, cognitive behavior therapy (CBT) became the first evidence-based intervention which we have rigorously trained and competent professionals in Bangladesh. With intensive training, practice and supervision of the professionals, CBT established its footing as a suitable therapeutic approach among Bangladeshi professionals. The structured approach of CBT is easy to train and has been well received by the service recipients. Its versatility in effectively treating different types of psychological disorders made CBT a popular choice, especially among evidence-based practitioners. Currently, CBT is probably the most or one of the most commonly used evidence-based therapeutic approaches in Bangladesh. The clinical psychology professionals in Bangladesh (approximately 350 professionals) are mostly reliant on CBT as their base model of intervention.

### 5.3.6 *Eye Movement Desensitization and Reprocessing (EMDR) Therapy*

First introduced by WHO at the end of 1999 through a series of training, EMDR was being practised by a handful of practitioners, however, it soon lost attention due to its perceived limited use for cases with trauma while other therapies were seemingly much easier to practice with a wider range of patients. A second impetuous of EMDR approach was seen in 2011, when HAP-Trauma Care in collaboration with the Department of Educational and Counseling Psychology organized a more intensive and well-designed training on EMDR. This training was designed for already trained and practising mental health professionals. The training was equipped with mandatory pre-EMDR preparatory training for the professionals on psycho-traumatology and post-training mandatory practice and supervision from the trainers.

### 5.3.7 *Transactional Analysis (TA)*

After CBT, TA probably had the second most rigorous training program in Bangladesh. Started with technical support from Ain o Salish Kendra in 2003, a group of professionals received a series of intensive training on TA through a decade of dedicated effort from P. K. Saru. TA had a structured design of training, practice, supervision and certification process. Currently, around 50 mental health professionals in Bangladesh are practising transactional analysis in their counseling work with a diploma in TA.

### 5.3.8 *Psychodrama*

First introduced in the country by an NGO named UTSA in 2003, psychodrama received considerable attention among mental health enthusiasts and professionals. Led by Herb Propper, a psychodrama trainer from the USA, its training and practice flourished in Bangladesh after 2005. Interest in Psychodrama shows a gradual decline after 2018. However, many practitioners trained in psychodrama utilize the specific components of its therapeutic techniques (such as empty chair, doubling and role reversal) in a blended form with other therapeutic approaches in their clinical work and training.

### 5.3.9 Narrative Therapy

Training on Narrative Therapy was first introduced in Bangladesh in 2005 by Ain o Salish Kendra. Trainers from the Dulwich Center, Australia provided two weeks of training for mental health service providers. Although many of the training recipients continued using this approach in therapeutic work, the interest was gradually lost. Narrative Therapy received a second impetus after 2015 when a group of clinical psychologists received training on the approach firstly as embedded with training on Systemic and Family Therapy and later as standalone training from UNK and Australia. Many practitioners are currently using techniques of narrative therapy in their clinical practice with cognitive behavior therapy and other models of interventions.

### 5.3.10 Dialectical Behavior Therapy (DBT)

Originally developed by Marsha Linehan as an effective therapy for borderline personality disorder (Linehan, 1987), DBT has been found useful with different other disorders and contexts of applications (Dimeff et al., 2007). DBT was officially introduced in Bangladesh in 2014 through a two-week orientation training offered by a Bangladeshi-born British Clinical Psychologist Farzeen Haque through the Nasirullah Psychotherapy Unit (NPU) of the Department of Clinical Psychology, at the University of Dhaka. Being manualized and instructive, DBT techniques have become very popular among mental health service providers who use these in clinical settings in a blended manner with their existing therapeutic models of intervention with borderline personality disorder, adjustment disorder, interpersonal relationship problems, trauma and suicidality in Bangladesh.

### 5.3.11 Systemic and Family Therapy

Mental health practitioners in Bangladesh have been practising some forms of family-informed therapy since the beginning of mental health service delivery where work with family was done to help individual clients. The true form of family therapy where the family as a whole is the focus of intervention started in 2015 with two British Systemic and Family therapists Glenda Freedman and Philip Messent. Subsequently, through intensive training and constant voluntary support from a pool of international experts, a group of mental health professionals became adept in Systemic and family therapy which has now been added as a major model of intervention in Bangladesh.

### *5.3.12 Interpersonal Therapy (IPT)*

Developed in the 1970s, IPT is a manualized time-limited intervention (see Weissman et al., 2017). IPT was introduced in Bangladesh through a collaborative effort of UNHCR and Columbia University to provide mental health support to the forcibly displaced Myanmar nationals, i.e., the Rohingya community, living in the camps. Introduced in 2020, IPT was added as an important alternative to the existing client-centered and cognitive behavioral approach of therapeutic work in the humanitarian crisis context.

### *5.3.13* Problem Management Plus (PM+)

Developed and endorsed by WHO, PM+ integrated problem-solving and behavioural treatment techniques to ensure easy learning and implantation by the psychological helpers (Dawson et al., 2015). Similar to IPT, PM+ was also specifically introduced in the humanitarian crisis context for the Rohingya community living in Bangladesh.

The therapeutic approaches discussed in this section are the most commonly used in Bangladesh. However, there are a few other approaches worth mentioning despite not being used by a large number of service providers. These include Play Therapy, Integrated Adapt Therapy (IAT), Art Therapy and Solution Focused Therapy.

## 5.4 Specialized Areas of Work

Over the decades of growth of psychological services in Bangladesh, there have been a few focused areas of work. Psychosocial service providers are working in these areas using a consistently better approach. The quality as well as reach of services are also enhancing constantly. A few of these areas are discussed below.

### *5.4.1 Addiction Counseling*

Addiction counseling is probably the specialized area of mental health service delivery where the highest number of psychological counselors work. Psychological counselling with people who use drugs started in the 'Bangladesh Rehabilitation and Assistance Center for Addicts (BARACA)' around 1989. Supportive counseling shadowing a client-centerd approach was used along with psychoeducation and skill-building support. Similar rehabilitation centres started to appear where the narcotic anonymous model became a popular approach. Mainstream psychological therapy using an evidence-based approach started to gain popularity in the addiction area in the year 2000 with its introduction through the collaborative study circles between CREA (a drug rehabilitation centre) and the Department of Clinical Psychology, University of Dhaka where concepts of addition and methods of intervention were discussed, debated and tested in clinical implementation.

With the rules published by the Government of Bangladesh in 2005, all the treatment and rehabilitation centres are mandated to have at least one mental health professional. This escalated the need for recruiting psychological counselors across the 300+ treatment centres. In recent times accredited training programs using the 'Universal Treatment Curriculum for Substance Use Disorders (UTC)' for addiction professionals have been initiated by the Department of Narcotics Control and the Dhaka Ahsania Mission (an NGO having a treatment facility for addiction). These trainings contributed a lot to improve the quality and comparability of service at the drug rehabilitation centres in Bangladesh.

### *5.4.2 Neurodevelopmental Disabilities*

Focused intervention on intellectual disability in Bangladesh started with the establishment of SWID Bangladesh, a collaborative initiative of parents, psychologists and philanthropists, in 1978. Later in 1984, the Bangladesh Protibondhi Foundation (BPF) was established to work with children with developmental disabilities. Child Development Center (CDC) was established in 1992 at Dhaka Shishu Hospital (DSH) which pioneered in evidence-based child development assessment and intervention practices. Currently, 35 CDCs are providing services at district-level tertiary hospitals. Although with variable and poorly defined training, a range of service providers work with children's neurodevelopmental disorders where assessment, psychological support and child development consultations are provided. The therapeutic approaches used by psychological support providers include supportive counseling, psychoeducation, applied behavior analysis, parent training and family counseling.

### *5.4.3 Sex Therapy*

Evidence-based psychological therapy for Psychosexual Dysfunction was first introduced in Bangladesh in 2001 by Mahmudur Rahman, a professor at the University of Dhaka, through the sex therapy clinic in the Marie Stopes Clinic. Since the beginning, the therapeutic work on psychosexual dysfunction mostly focused on the conjoint sex therapy approach developed by Master and Johnson (Masters & Johnson, 1966). However, after a decade, a group of mental health professionals started receiving training on more modern approaches to intervention through the European School of sexual medicine which has now been added to sex therapy practice. The practice of psychological therapy is being carried out by therapists in their personal clinical practice. Myths and myth-driven concerns around sexual aspects are a very common feature among patients seeking treatment for psychosexual dysfunctions (Miah et al., 2015; Mozumder & Rahman, 2004). Psychoeducation is therefore a major component in sex therapy with Bangladeshi clients where culture bound syndrome like Dhat syndrome is a common presentation (Maruf et al., 2024).

### 5.4.4 *Violence, Torture and Trauma*

Due to the developmental priorities, the government and NGOs are working closely to eliminate domestic and gender-based violence in Bangladesh. This has, therefore, developed as a core area of work for psychosocial service providers.

The Ministry of Women and Children Affairs (MOWCA) established the One-stop Crisis Centre (OCC) and National Trauma Counselling Centres (NTCC) to provide quality care to women and children affected by trauma and violence. The OCCs provide holistic care including medical, nursing, psychological, legal and vocational assistance to the victims of violence since 2001. Services from the National Trauma Counseling Center and its recent extension, the Regional Trauma Counselling Centres (RTCC) are focused on psychological support provision. NTCC and RTCC are well-equipped with trained mental health service providers. The practitioners working at OCC, NTCC and RTCC usually practice using cognitive behavior therapy, client-centered approach, dialectical behavior therapy and in some cases systemic and family therapy with the service recipients. MOWCA also operates a dedicated toll-free hotline for providing initial telecounseling support addressing violence and trauma.

NGOs in Bangladesh have good programs around psychological support for victims of gender-based violence. Research Dara suggests the effectiveness of psychosocial intervention in Bangladesh to reduce the impact of violence against women and children (Nath et al., 2018; Naved et al., 2018). Work around domestic violence in NGOs is generally fund-driven and hence often lacks sustainability. A decades-old study showed, that the claimed counseling services offered by them often lacked specificity and adequacy in terms of quality (see Deeba & Mozumder, 2006).

### 5.4.5 *Neuropsychology*

Clinical neuropsychology has been a recent addition to the mental health field of Bangladesh. A small group of professionals led by Shahnur Hossain at the Department of Clinical Psychology, University of Dhaka is working closely with supervision and support from UK-based experts, Graham Powell and David Quinn to develop this highly technical field of specialization. The team has acquired a number of assessment instruments and prepared adapted versions of many tools to be used in the assessment of the neuropsychological state of the person seeking service.

### 5.4.6 Refugee Mental Health

With the Rohingya influx in 2017, Bangladesh with its limited number of mental health professionals, was charged with the provision of psychosocial care to approximately one million forcibly displaced Myanmar nationals. With a concerted effort between the UN entities, international NGOs, local NGOs and government organizations, a range of psychosocial services coined together as mental health and psychosocial support services (MHPSS) started to emerge for the Rohingya community. The refugee mental health involved the provision of support through psychological first aid, individual and group counseling and specialized therapeutic intervention using already existing and new approaches to therapy. The new therapeutic approaches introduced through refugee care include Interpersonal Therapy (IPT: Weissman et al., 2017), Integrated Adapt Therapy (IAT; Tay et al., 2020) and Problem Management Plus (PM+ ; Dawson et al., 2015). The mental health services for the Rohingya community by different organizations are coordinated through the MHPSS working group with several smaller task groups. The situation and services around refugee mental health have been further discussed in Chap. 17 of this book (Hia & Mozumder, 2024).

### 5.4.7 Community Mental Health

With the centralization of mental health services in the big cities, increasing access to services can never be possible. Community mental health has been therefore being tried and tested across the country by the government as well as NGOs. The National Mental Health Policy 2022 emphasizes the promotion of community-based services for mental disorders (World Health Organization, 2020). BRAC has been trying different community-based interventions for over a decade. They started providing training to the volunteers on providing initial psychosocial support provision and referral, through their community empowerment project in 2013. BRAC is currently piloting an integrated approach to providing psychosocial support through para-professionals (para-counselors) at the community level. The initial analysis of the outcome indicated impressive results regarding the usefulness of the community-based service to the recipients (BRAC, 2023). SAJIDA Foundation has recently developed a 6-month intensive certificate course on community mental health care. They are also providing training to the project staff working at the community level on this module to ensure basic psychosocial support to the beneficiaries of their climate change project.

Most of the organizations engaged in community mental health service have a tiered approach to service delivery at the community level where community mobilizers or volunteers conduct the first screening and refer to the Para counselor who provides basic psychosocial care and may refer to mental health experts for intensive support if needed.

### 5.4.8 Psychological Therapy in Digital Platform

With advancement and innovation in the technological sphere, digital platforms have become a key contributor to mental health service delivery in Bangladesh. Digital aspects of mental health services have been discussed in Chap. 16 of this book (Muhammad & Arafat, 2024). Among the psychosocial service providers, Kan Pete Roi, Relaxy, Moner Bondhu, Moner Daktar and Mindly have gained popularity. Although some of these have been providing services for many years most of these have grabbed attention during the increasing demand for a non-contact-based approach to intervention during the COVID-19 pandemic (Chowdhury, 2021). Evidence demonstrates improvement in mental health from telemental health intervention (Arafat et al., 2024; Rahman et al., 2022).

Easy access and reduced waiting time have made services through digital platforms a desired option for many. However, service recipients as well as providers also reported challenges around disruption, privacy, technological difficulties, lack of control and limited non-verbal cues for communication associated with service delivered through digital platforms. Due to the lack of technological resources among many of the digital service providers, data breaches and other security concerns can be a major challenge for the growth and sustainability of service through digital platforms.

## 5.5 Challenges and Opportunities in Psychosocial Management

With 91% treatment gap in mental health (Ministry of Health and Family Welfare, 2021; World Health Organization, 2020), access to treatment for mental illness is a major concern in Bangladesh. Multiple factors play a role in this treatment gap. The challenges for access to mental health care have been discussed in Chap. 3 of this book (Arafat, 2024). Further, it has been discussed in a recently published another book chapter (Arafat et al., 2024). The challenges to practising psychological therapies in Bangladesh also add to these factors in reducing quality and access to treatment. The following section presents a range of challenges and opportunities generated through interviews with mental health professionals working in Bangladesh.

### 5.5.1 Beliefs About Supernatural Possession and Divine Punishment

For a large number of Bangladeshi communities, the mind–body relationship is vaguely constructed and people see them as separate. Many people interpret severe mental illness as possession of supernatural forces or as punishment from God for wrong deeds. Subequal, they chose to go to traditional healers including spiritual healers, religious leaders, or to shrines for recovery (Arafat et al., 2024). These practices delay access to modern treatment and increase further complexities of the problem and suffering for the patients and families.

### 5.5.2 *Dominance of Medical Model*

Although changing, the medical model still predominates in mental health care. Referrals for mental health problems are generally made for psychiatric medication. Even when the patients and the family members are referred to psychological therapy, they come with an expectation to get medicine. This creates a disconnect of the goal of intervention between psychological service providers and recipients.

### 5.5.3 *Stigma Around Mental Illness*

Stigma is a major barrier to accessing psychological services. Fear of being identified as insane or mad and of subsequent social humiliation and discrimination prevent people from accessing services and make them try hard to hide their conditions from others. However, in recent times an increased openness to accept and access psychological therapy has been observed especially among the younger generations.

### 5.5.4 *Poor Mental Health Literacy*

Except for the major conditions, mental health problems are often invisible from the outside. It takes a long time for the person and the family members to realize or identify that the person needs professional support. Even when they realize the need for support, they lack information about where to go for treatment. However, in recent times through awareness campaigns and media influence, people are increasingly becoming aware of the mental health needs and scope of services.

### 5.5.5 *Slow Impact of Psychological Therapies*

Psychological therapies take time to produce outcomes. While medication in most cases can demonstrate visible change in 2–6 weeks, psychological therapies usually take 2–4 months. This can be frustrating for the patients as well as family members. This often results in dropout from the psychosocial intervention creating a negative impression about the effectiveness of the psychological services.

### 5.5.6 Cost of Psychological Treatment

Psychosocial interventions are time-consuming and take a much longer per-patient time compared to the medical approach. In an attempt to make it professionally viable, the providers of psychosocial therapies charge a high amount as fees. This made the therapy an expensive option and a major barrier to access psychosocial support for most of the people in Bangladesh. This is also one of the reasons behind the lack of expansion of psychological services beyond the big cities of the country where people generally have comparatively lower financial capacity.

### 5.5.7 Lack of Regulation and Licensing

For maintaining standards in the quality of training and service delivery, regulation is a crucial component. This also ensures the protection of the rights of service recipients. It has been more than two decades since the formal introduction of psychological therapies in treating mental health conditions is introduced in Bangladesh. Despite several efforts by the Bangladesh Clinical Psychology Society, since 2010, the licensing system for clinical psychologists or other mental health service providers has not yet been established. However, the Bangladesh Rehabilitation Council Act 2018 has provisions of licensing for mental health professionals working in the area of rehabilitation.

The lack of regulations and licensing has resulted in poor quality unregulated training on psychological counseling throughout different institutions and organizations and more alarmingly, people having limited or no skills are providing psychological therapy across the country.

### 5.5.8 Lack of Skills Among Service Providers

Primarily due to the lack of regulations, anyone can claim him/herself as a mental health service provider. This has resulted in a wide range of service providers with a varied range of exposure and training to provide claimed psychosocial support. The service therefore also ranges from scientifically valid (i.e., evidence-based) to commonsense. Poorly trained or untrained providers also lack a proper understanding of the ethical concerns around service provision and thus pose a serious threat to the rights, safety and protection of the service recipients (see Islam & Mozumder, 2021).

### 5.5.9 Limited Availability of Supervisor

Clinical supervision is an important aspect and ethical imperative in maintaining the quality of mental health services. However, there is a lack of availability as well as interest among the service providers to get regular clinical supervision.

### 5.5.10 Limited Awareness and Scope of Continuing Professional Development

Considered a mandatory requirement among professional societies across the world, continuing professional development (CPD) is a major pathway for maintaining and enhancing professional competencies. Bangladesh is a low-resource country, and the opportunities for CPD are generally limited. At the same time, there is a lack of awareness among most service providers regarding the need and scope of CPD.

### 5.5.11 Lack of Integration and Coordination

Mental health care often requires a holistic approach. Psychological services alone are not enough to ensure the complete functioning and well-being of the patients. Due to limited inclusion in government services, providers of psychological therapies often work independently. A general lack of integration and coordination with allied services such as legal, educational, financial, shelter, protection and social care is, therefore, observed in Bangladesh.

### 5.5.12 Increasing Availability of Multiple Models of Intervention

In recent times alternative models of therapies have been introduced. These, as opportunities, enabled the service providers to choose and try the most suitable approach of intervention catering to the needs of the service recipients. This gave the recipients the freedom of choice and is likely to contribute to an improved therapeutic alliance between patients and providers.

### *5.5.13 Willing Contribution from Experts from Abroad*

Many international experts are willing to contribute and support in strengthening mental health service development and delivery in Bangladesh. Many others have already contributed or are continuing their support voluntarily. Their support in providing training, supervision and consultation has been extremely useful in reducing the gaps in mental health services.

### *5.5.14 Legislative Framework on Mental Health*

Focused initiatives in improving the mental health scenario in Bangladesh have resulted in the recent development of a series of policy documents including the Mental Health Act in 2018, the National Mental Health Policy 2022 and the National Mental Health Strategic Plan 2020–2030. Psychological approaches to intervention have been recognized in these documents. Though in a limited scope, the Bangladesh Rehabilitation Council Act 2018 is also a great initiative to introduce licensing.

### *5.5.15 Professional Identity as a Psychologist*

A few decades ago, psychology was generally considered a backward field of study with limited scope of utility. However, with the advent of applied branches of psychology, (e.g., clinical psychology, counseling psychology) it earned respect. Psychologists have now become a professional identity and in many cases a prestigious one.

## 5.6 Recent Transitions Around Psychosocial Management in Bangladesh

Transitions are usually challenging times that change the way things are done. Three major incidents in recent times have and are still playing roles in creating big shifts in the field of psychosocial management in Bangladesh. These are the Rohingya crisis, the COVID-19 pandemic and WHO's special initiative on mental health in Bangladesh.

### 5.6.1 Rohingya Crisis

The influx of Forcibly Displaced Myanmar Nationals (i.e., the Rohingya community) in 2017 resulted in a huge need for mental health professionals to address the psychosocial needs of their traumatized community seeking refuge in Bangladesh (see Islam & Mozumder, 2021). With the already limited number of available professionals in low-resource Bangladesh, the organization was bound to recruit individuals with no training or exposure in mental health to work with the Rohingya community. They were provided with limited training and sent to provide service. This was challenging; however, it demonstrated the possibility of providing service to individuals with limited skills and the value as well as a need for good quality training. The crisis also created a huge demand for qualified mental health professionals and increased interest among graduates towards pursuing psychosocial service delivery as a profession.

The need generated by the Rohingya crisis resulted in widespread training on Psychological First AID as a first-line service. A major contribution to the field of psychological therapy from the Rohingya Crisis is the introduction of a number of less resource-demanding therapeutic approaches namely Interpersonal Therapy (IPT: Weissman et al., 2017), Integrated Adapt Therapy (IAT; Tay et al., 2020) and Problem Management Plus (PM+; Dawson et al., 2015) in Bangladesh.

### 5.6.2 COVID-19 Pandemic

The COVID-19 pandemic has been a huge transitional factor across all aspects of life. While the stress associated with the novel situation increased the need for psychological support, the pandemic restrictions prevented people from accessing in-person services. The providers started to convert their in-person practices to online mode. It was a huge transition demonstrating the usefulness and suitability of digital platforms in providing psychological support. Individual therapists became confident in providing therapies through digital platforms. The organization working on mental health service delivery started exploring new or enhancing existing abilities in digital platforms. From the experience gained during the pandemic, the number of therapists and the frequency with which they use digital platforms has increased tremendously after the pandemic. This transition in mental health service delivery has enabled patients to form greater distances and disadvantaged conditions to reach psychological therapies at a much lower cost.

Additionally, the work of the mental health service providers during the pandemic situation enhanced a positive perception among general people towards psychological therapies and has demonstrated the importance and usefulness of psychological therapies in Bangladesh.

### *5.6.3 World Health Organization's Special Initiative for Mental Health, Bangladesh*

WHO's special initiative on mental health in Bangladesh is aimed at strengthening mental health systems across the country. The devised strategy includes innovations around the introduction of a separate Directorate for Mental Health, increasing demands for service, strengthening service delivery and ensuring the availability of mental health services in primary care facilities (World Health Organization, 2023). The special initiative is expected to bring mental health services at the community level. It has created an increased interest among the NGOs to introduce programs targeted at community-based mental health intervention.

Mental Health Gap Action Program (mhGAP) was introduced in Bangladesh in 2011 towards achieving universal health coverage by integrating mental health care into primary health care settings (Momotaz et al., 2019). With the WHO's special initiative on mental health in Bangladesh, the government is further enhancing the reach of the mhGAP training. Training of medical doctors on mhGAP has increased their knowledge and awareness about the mental health needs of the patients as well as the scope of referral and role of psychosocial therapies for patients with mental health conditions.

## 5.7 Conclusion

This chapter discussed the state and growth of psychological management of mental disorders in Bangladesh. Two of the transitional aspects namely the influx of Rohingya refugees and the pandemic have challenged mental health service delivery however, contributed to significant development in the area of service development and delivery. This reflects the core nature of psychology—growth through challenges. Several challenges and opportunities around psychological service delivery have also been presented and discussed. The question remains, are we equipped to provide psychosocial support for the mental well-being of the huge population of Bangladesh?

## References

Ahmed, M. U. (1984). *Learn to hypnotise and cure: Oriental method. Transition to medistic psychotherapy* (3rd ed.). Psyche Prokashani.

Arafat, S. M. Y., Giasuddin, N.A., Mazumder, A. H. (2024). Access to mental health care in bangladesh—Current status, potential challenges, and ways out. S. M. Y. Arafat, & S. K. Kar (Eds.), *Access to mental health care in South Asia—Current status, potential challenges, and ways out*. Springer Nature Singapore. https://doi.org/10.1007/978-981-99-9153-2_3

Arafat, S. M. Y. (2024). Mental Health Services in Bangladesh. S. M. Y. Arafat (Ed.) *Mental health in Bangladesh: From bench to community*. Springer Nature Singapore. https://doi.org/10.1007/978-981-97-0610-5_3

BRAC. (2023, Monday, 23 October 2023 00:00). *Mental health pilot intervention shows promising results at the community level*. https://www.brac.net/latest-news/item/1398-mental-health-pilot-intervention-shows-promising-results-at-the-community-level

Chowdhury, T. (2021). *As the epidemic of mental health gathers steam in Bangladesh, online and tele mental health services gain mainstream attention*. https://futurestartup.com/2021/04/28/online-and-tele-mental-health-services-gain-mainstream-attention/

Dawson, K. S., Bryant, R. A., Harper, M., Kuowei Tay, A., Rahman, A., Schafer, A., & van Ommeren, M. (2015). Problem management plus (PM+): a WHO transdiagnostic psychological intervention for common mental health problems. *World Psychiatry, 14*(3), 354–357. https://doi.org/10.1002/wps.20255

Deeba, F., & Mozumder, M. K. (2006). Psychological service analysis for victims of violence against women in Bangladesh: A nationwide survey. *Bangladesh Psychological Studies, 16*, 1–12.

Dimeff, L. A., Rizvi, S. L., & Koerner, K. (Eds.). (2007). *Dialectical behavior therapy in clinical practice: Applications across disorders and settings* (2nd ed.). Guilford Press.

Hia, M. S., & Mozumder, M. K. (2024). Mental health of vulnerable populations. S. M. Y. Arafat (Ed.) *Mental health in Bangladesh: From bench to community*. Springer Nature Singapore. https://doi.org/10.1007/978-981-97-0610-5_17

Islam, S., & Mozumder, M. K. (2021). Challenges to providing quality mental health services for forcibly displaced populations: The case of Rohingya refugees in Bangladesh. *Asian American Journal of Psychology, 12*(3), 234–240. https://doi.org/10.1037/aap0000195

Linehan, M. M. (1987). Dialectical behavior therapy for borderline personality disorder: Theory and method. *Bulletin of the Menninger Clinic, 51*(3), 261.

Masters, W. H., & Johnson, V. E. (1966). *Human sexual response*. Little, Brown.

Mazumder, A.H., (2024). Epidemiology and burden of mental disorders in Bangladesh. S. M. Y. Arafat (Ed.) *Mental health in Bangladesh: From bench to community*. Springer Nature Singapore. https://doi.org/10.1007/978-981-97-0610-5_2

Maruf, M. M., Saleem, T., & Arafat, S. M. Y. (2024). Dhat syndrome: A fact or myth. In S. K. Kar, S. M. Y. Arafat, V. Menon (Ed). *Dhat syndrome*. Springer. https://doi.org/10.1007/978-981-99-8870-9_15

Miah, M. A. A., Al-Mamun, M. A., Khan, S., & Mozumder, M. K. (2015). Sexual myths and behavior of male patients with psychosexual dysfunction in Bangladesh. *Dhaka University Journal of Psychology, 39*, 89–100.

Ministry of Health & Family Welfare, 2021. National Mental Health Survey 2019. Retrieved December 20, 2023, from http://nimh.gov.bd/wp-content/uploads/2021/11/Mental-Health-Survey-Report.pdf

Momotaz, H., Ahmed, H. U., Jalal Uddin, M. M., Karim, R., Khan, M. A., Al-Amin, R., … Kessaram, T. (2019). Implementing the mental health gap action programme in Cox's Bazar, Bangladesh. *Intervention Journal of Mental Health and Psychosocial Support in Conflict Affected Areas, 17*(2), 243–251. https://doi.org/10.4103/intv.Intv_14_19

Mozumder, M. K., & Rahman, M. M. (2004). A prevalence study of various male psycho-sexual dysfunctions and problems among individuals attending psychological services in a sex therapy clinic. *Bangladesh Psychological Studies, 14*, 71–88.

Muhammad, F., Arafat, S. M. Y. (2024). Technology-Based Interventions for Mental Health Support in Bangladesh. S. M. Y. Arafat (Ed.) *Mental health in Bangladesh: From bench to community*. Springer Nature Singapore. https://doi.org/10.1007/978-981-97-0610-5_16

Nath, S. R., Ali, R., Naomi, S. S., & Upoma, R. A. (2018). Impact of BRAC's coordinated approch in addressing violence against women and children.

Naved, R. T., Mamun, M. A., Mourin, S. A., & Parvin, K. (2018). A cluster randomized controlled trial to assess the impact of SAFE on spousal violence against women and girls in slums of Dhaka, Bangladesh. *Plos One, 13*(6), e0198926. https://doi.org/10.1371/journal.pone.0198926

Nuri, N. N., Sarker, M., Ahmed, H. U., Hossain, M. D., Beiersmann, C., & Jahn, A. (2018). Pathways to care of patients with mental health problems in Bangladesh. *International Journal of Mental Health Systems, 12*(1), 39. https://doi.org/10.1186/s13033-018-0218-y

Rahman, S., Amit, S., & Kafy, A. A. (2022). Impact of COVID-19 and telehealth on mental health in Bangladesh: A propensity score matching approach. *Spatial Information Research, 30*(3), 347–354. https://doi.org/10.1007/s41324-022-00434-9

Saha, A. K. (2022). Applied psychology in Bangladesh: Progress and prospect. *Mind and Society, 11*(02), 109–114. https://doi.org/10.56011/mind-mri-112-202212

Tay, A. K., Mung, H. K., Miah, M. A. A., Balasundaram, S., Ventevogel, P., Badrudduza, M., … Silove, D. (2020). An Integrative Adapt Therapy for common mental health symptoms and adaptive stress amongst Rohingya, Chin, and Kachin refugees living in Malaysia: A randomized controlled trial. *PLOS Medicine, 17*(3), e1003073. https://doi.org/10.1371/journal.pmed.1003073

Weissman, M. M., Markowitz, J. C., & Klerman, G. L. (2017). *The guide to interpersonal psychotherapy: Updated and expanded edition.* Oxford University Press. https://doi.org/10.1093/med-psych/9780190662592.001.0001

World Health Organization. (2020). *Bangladesh: WHO special initiative for mental health, Situational assessment.* W. H. Organization. https://www.who.int/docs/default-source/mental-health/special-initiative/who-special-initiative-country-report---bangladesh---2020.pdf?sfvrsn=c2122a0e_2

World Health Organization. (2023). *Bangladesh: WHO Special Initiative for Mental Health.* https://www.who.int/initiatives/who-special-initiative-for-mental-health/bangladesh

# Chapter 6
# Child and Adolescent Psychiatry in Bangladesh

**Rubaiya Khan and M. S. I. Mullick**

**Abstract** According to the latest mental health survey, the prevalence of mental illness among children and adolescents is 12.6% in Bangladesh. Though in recent times child and adolescent mental health services have undergone significant development in our country still it is not sufficient to meet the needs of the population. Child and adolescent mental health resources both in manpower and facilities are extremely scarce and maldistributed. Additionally, there is a lack of standard training and research in this field. Lack of awareness, high level of stigma and unfavorable beliefs, attitudes and behavior make the condition more complicated. Affordable, culturally suitable, local resources-based services can help to combat the condition. This chapter discusses the epidemiology of child psychiatric disorders, history, current status and challenges of child and adolescent mental health services in Bangladesh.

**Keywords** Child and adolescent psychiatry · Child mental health in Bangladesh · Child and adolescent psychiatric service · Epidemiology · Development

## 6.1 Introduction

Bangladesh is a low- and middle-income country with a total population of 169.8 million people, of whom 38.6% have age below 18 years (Bangladesh Bureau of Statistics, 2022). Just like other developed countries, this group is very susceptible to developing psychiatric disorders too. According to recent global epidemiological estimates, up to one in fifth children and adolescents experience a disabling psychiatric disorder (World Health Organization, 2000). About 50% of all adult mental disorders start by the age of 14 years and 75% by 25 years (Kessler et al.,

R. Khan (✉)
Department of Psychiatry, Khwaja Yunus Ali Medical College and Hospital, Sirajganj, Bangladesh
e-mail: rubaiya1201@gmail.com

M. S. I. Mullick
Independent Researcher, Dhaka, Bangladesh

 
S. M. Y. Arafat (ed.), *Mental Health in Bangladesh*,
https://doi.org/10.1007/978-981-97-0610-5_6

2005, 2007). Throughout the world, the third most common cause of death among adolescents is suicide (World Health Organization, 2001).

It has been seen mental health problems affect all domains of life of a child. Children and adolescents who suffer from mental health problems frequently struggle with their academics. They have lower school attendance and poor academic results. The dropout rate is much higher among them (Dalsgaard et al., 2020). As a result, they usually have lower occupational achievement. It has a serious negative impact on their physical health and well-being and they experience a lower quality of life (Dey et al., 2012). Moreover, childhood psychiatric disorders have long-term impacts as well. In one study it was found that high externalizing and internalizing behavioral problems in childhood are related to increased risk of mortality even in adulthood (Jokela et al., 2009). Childhood mental disorders have a huge adverse impact on families also. It increases the risk of developing mental disorders of other family members too. One study showed siblings of affected children have an increased rate of both internalizing and externalizing problems (Krzeczkowski et al., 2022). Child psychiatric disorders have a significant economic burden. It has an adverse effect on the country's productivity, economic stability and progress (Smith & Smith, 2010). Early interventions for child and adolescent mental health (CAMH) problems significantly prevent developmental impairment and adulthood continuity and decrease disease burden.

## 6.2 Epidemiology and Cultural Perspective of Child Psychiatric Disorder in Bangladesh

### *6.2.1 Epidemiology*

The first epidemiological study of child mental health was done in 2005 and it revealed that 10.9–20.8% of children aged 5–10 had psychiatric disorders. It indicates over 5 million individuals had psychiatric disorders causing them significant distress and impairment. The prevalence varied among rural, urban and slum areas which were 15.4%, 10% and 19.5% respectively. Among total diagnoses behavioral disorders (8.9%) and anxiety disorders (8.1%) were the most common psychiatric disorders in all three areas (Mullick & Goodman, 2005).

Another study done by Rabbani et al. in 2009 revealed the prevalence of mental disorders, mental retardation (MR), epilepsy and substance related disorder (SRD) were 18.4%, 3.8%, 2.0% and 0.8% respectively. Enuresis (3.0%) was the most prevalent psychiatric disorder followed by somatoform pain disorder (1.9%), communication disorder (1.6%), obsessive–compulsive disorder (1.3%), generalized anxiety disorder (1.3%), oppositional defiant disorder (1.0%), conduct disorder (1.0%), attention deficit hyperactivity disorder (1.0%), bipolar mood disorder(1.0%), depressive disorder (1.0%), autistic disorder (0.9%), conversion disorder (0.8%), phobic disorder(0.7%), dissociative disorder(0.4%), schizophrenia (0.1%). The prevalence of psychiatric disorders varied according to age. Among the children of 5–11 years prevalence of epilepsy (2.6%) and mental retardation (4.6%) were more whereas adolescents aged 12 and more had more mental disorders (21.2%) and substance abuse (2.1%) (Rabbani et al., 2009).

In the year 2018–2019 National Mental Health Survey was carried out which showed the prevalence of psychiatric disorders in children between the age of 7–17 years was 12.6%. NDDs (5.1%) were the most frequent diagnosis, followed by anxiety related disorders (4.7%), disruptive, impulse control and conduct disorders (1.7%), depressive disorders (0.4%), sleep wake disorders (0.4%), and schizophrenia spectrum disorders (0.2%), bipolar disorder (0.1%), and obsessive–compulsive and related disorders (0.1%). Among individual psychiatric disorders Intellectual disability disorder was the most prevalent one followed by Enuresis (1.6%) Attention-Deficit / Hyperactivity Disorder (ADHD) (1.1%), Conduct Disorder (0.9%), Social Phobia (0.7%), Specific Phobia (0.6%), Oppositional defiant disorder (ODD (0.6%), Generalized Anxiety Disorder (0.4%), Conversion Disorder (0.4%) and Language Disorder (0.4%) (Ministry of Health and Family Welfare, 2021).

A study done from July 2012–February 2013 in three prime tertiary hospitals of Dhaka showed that 18% of children aged 5–16 years old attending pediatric outpatient departments have a mental illness. Behavioral problems, emotional problems and developmental disorders were identified in 9.0%, 15.0% and 0.4% respectively. The most prevalent psychiatric disorder was hyperkinetic disorder, which occurred in 5.0% of cases (Jesmin et al., 2016).

There is limited information about psychiatric disorders in preschool children of Bangladesh. A study conducted in Bangladesh indicated that 11.9% of 3–4-year-olds in an urban sample had psychiatric problems. Among them, 4.4% had emotional disorder, 5.6% had conduct disorder and 1.9% had hyperactivity. Emotional disorder was more common among girls and behavioral disorder was more common among boys. In most of the cases, there were multiple psychiatric disorders (Mullick & Islam, 2020). The epidemiological aspects have also been discussed in Chap. 2 of this book (Mazumder, 2024).

### 6.2.2 *Cultural Perspective in the Presentation of Disorders*

Somatoform disorder is frequently seen in children and adolescents of Bangladesh. The commonest somatic symptom among children is discomfort, burning sensation or pain in the abdomen whereas in adolescents headache is the most common somatic symptom. Other common somatic symptoms include body weakness, tiredness, fatigue, burning of hands, feet or all over the body, feverish feeling, feeling of hotness in the head or ear etc. The tendency of increased somatization can be due to stigma and negative attitudes of parents and caregivers towards mental health. Young people with depressive disorder and anxiety disorder also frequently present with somatic symptoms in this country (Mullick, 2002).

One study indicated Autism was less prevalent but it is gradually increasing in Bangladesh (Rahman, 2010). According to a systematic review, Bangladesh's autism spectrum disorder prevalence is predicted to be between 0.2 and 0.8% (Hossain et al., 2017). A study done in 2018 on 13–17 years old adolescents showed, 36.6% of adolescents attending urban and semi-urban schools reported having depression symptoms (Anjum et al., 2022). Whereas in another study it was found that depression is less common in 5–10 years old children. Obsessive–compulsive disorder (OCD) is relatively higher among children of this age group in Bangladesh than in developed countries (Mullick & Goodman, 2005). Regarding the pattern of OCD, contamination obsession followed by miscellaneous obsessions (pathological doubt and religious obsession) is the main content of obsession whereas washing/cleaning followed by checking are the most common types of compulsion (Chowdhury et al., 2016; Mullick et al., 2017).

Conversion disorder is proportionately high in this culture. A study done among 52 outpatients between four to sixteen years of age showed fainting attacks, motor symptoms and sensory symptoms are the most common presenting symptoms of conversion disorder followed by mute and other somatic symptoms (Khanam et al., 2002).

In the past few years, there have been few incidents of mass psychogenic illness among school children. The most common symptoms are abdominal pain, headache, body aches, nausea, generalized weakness and fatigue, chest pain, burning sensation of the body, dizziness and dry mouth (Tarafder et al., 2016).

Recently there have been changes in the trend of psychiatric disorder with a high rate of suicide, self-harm and substance use among the adolescents of Bangladesh. A population-based nationwide survey conducted by National Institue of Mental Health (NIMH, World Health Organization (WHO, Bangladesh), and Non-communicable Diseases Control, Ministry of Health, Bangladesh among adolescents aged 10–24 years showed 4.7% of the participants had suicidal ideation and 1.5% had suicidal plans and history of suicide attempt at least once (NIMH, 2021). Another study found that the rate of suicidal behavior, suicidal plan, suicidal attempt and suicidal behavior among adolescents of Bangladesh over previous 12 months were 4.2%, 5.4%, 4.2% and 8.95% respectively (Marthoenis & Arafat, 2022). Substance use among adolescents is also significantly prevalent nowadays. A recent study showed the prevalence of substance use among 7 years and above children and adolescents is 2.9% (Alam et al., 2018). A Few new problems like the internet and other behavioral addictions, cyber bullying have also emerged in the past few years among the young population of the country (Hassan et al., 2020; Mallik and Radwan, 2020).

## 6.3 History of Service Development of Child and Adolescent Psychiatry in Bangladesh

The historical aspects of Child and Adolescent Psychiatry (CAP) in Bangladesh have been reported by Arafat and his colleagues in 2020. The initiation of mental health services for children and adolescents in Bangladesh started in 1975 with the opening of a child guidance clinic at *Dhaka Medical College Hospital* (DMCH). In December 1977, a group of professionals, social workers and parents of children with intellectual disabilities founded the *Society for Welfare of the Intellectually Disabled* (SWID), an organization that works to raise social awareness towards disabled people, by supporting their socialization and education, as well as by protecting their legal rights, social security, entertainment, employment, rehabilitation and dignity. The *Bangladesh Protibondhi Foundation* (BPF), a non-profit, non-government humanitarian organization, was founded in 1984 to empower children with developmental disabilities to become self-reliant, independent and valuable members of the communities. Then in 1991, *Dhaka Shishu (Child) Hospital* started its child development center. In the following year *Institute of Child and Mother Health (ICMH)* was established. In *Chattagram Maa-O-Shishu (mother & child) Hospital*, a child development center was opened in 1998. In the same year, a child mental health clinic in *Bangabandhu Sheikh Mujib Medical University* (BSMMU) was also established. Another milestone was achieved in the following year when child and adolescent psychiatry was started as a separate wing in BSMMU. In the same year, *Child Development Center* was started at the *International Center for Diarrhoeal Disease Research, Bangladesh* (ICDDR, B). Another significant event in the history of child and adolescent psychiatry of Bangladesh was the initiation of the Department of Child, Adolescent and Family Psychiatry at NIMH Dhaka in 2001. *Bangladesh Association for Child and Adolescent Mental Health (BACAMH)*, a national organization for professionals working in the field of child and adolescent mental health, was established in 2008. The purpose of the organization is to promote mental health among children, adolescents and families through training, services, research, advocacy, peer support and national and international collaboration. In order to enable persons with neurodevelopmental disabilities to live with dignity as a part of society *Neuro-Developmental Disability Protection Trust* was established in 2013. The main aims of the trust are to provide physical, emotional and financial support as far as possible to disabled persons, to provide them with appropriate education and technical knowledge and to empower them socially. The *Shuchona Foundation*, a non-profit organization dedicated to advocacy, research, and capacity building was founded in 2014 with a focus on mental health and neurodevelopmental disorders (NDDs) (Arafat et al., 2020).

## 6.4 Current Status of Child and Adolescent Psychiatry in Bangladesh

### *6.4.1 Child and Adolescent Psychiatric Service*

Child psychiatric services are given at different levels throughout the country. However, the existing service is insufficient in comparison to the vast amount of need.

- At sub-specialist level:
  - BSMMU: There is a separate wing of child and adolescent psychiatry in the department of psychiatry. Out of 40, 10 beds are specially allocated for child and adolescent patients. There is a specialized child and adolescent mental health clinic (CAMHC) where patients under the age of 18 years with mental health problems are assessed, diagnosed and treated. The clinic works on outpatient department (OPD) basis only on Wednesday of every week for two hours. The department also runs ADHD clinic every Sunday 11 am to 1 pm with the aim to provide specialized care to the patients with ADHD. Besides these specialized clinics, there is psychiatric OPD where along with adult patients, child and adolescent patients with mental health problems are consulted every day of the week except Fridays and government holidays.
  - NIMH: There is a separate child adolescent and family department where 20 beds are reserved for children and adolescents. There is a special outpatient department for below 18 years of old patient too. The OPD runs every day except Fridays and government holidays.
  - *Institute for Pediatric Neurodisorder and Autism (IPNA)* provides outpatient and inpatient services to children with autism and other neurodevelopmental disabilities. In addition, they have a school to provide intensive education for children with autism.
  - There are *Child Development Centers* (CDCs) in some government and private hospitals where along with general assessments, assessments by psychometric tools are conducted to diagnose Autism, Intellectual Disability and other neurodevelopmental disorders.
- Specialist level:
  - In government and private medical colleges in Bangladesh, there are psychiatric OPDs where children and adolescents with mental disorders are consulted by Psychiatrists. Some of them have an inpatient psychiatry department and specialized child and adolescent mental health clinic too.
  - Besides this, Pediatricians, Neurologists and Pediatric neurologists of different hospitals are providing treatment for neurodevelopmental and psychiatric disorders too.
  - A very limited number of schools have psychologists who are providing psychotherapy to these young people.

- Non-Specialist Level:

  In different community clinics, upazila health complex general practitioners are providing some services.

### 6.4.2 *Training and Courses on Child and Adolescent Psychiatry*

- Postgraduate courses and training:
  - Currently, in Bangladesh, 5 years Doctor of Medicine (MD) course on child and adolescent psychiatry is offered by BSMMU. It started from the year of 2016. Initially, there were 3 seats only in BSMMU. In the following year, seats were increased to 7 and from the year 2023 residency training in Child and Adolescent Psychiatry has started at NIMH, Dhaka.
  - Bangladesh College of Physicians and Surgeons has also started a 5-year fellowship program on Child and Adolescent from 2022.
- Undergraduate course and training:
  - Undergraduate medical students are placed in the Psychiatry department where they get a practical understanding of young people with psychiatric disorders but the duration and extent of the training is inadequate.
- Courses and training for allied professions
  - MPhil and MS are available in clinical, educational and counseling psychology at Dhaka University.
  - Diploma and Bachelor courses and training are available in Occupational Therapy, Speech and Language therapy at the Center for the Rehabilitation of the Paralyzed (CRP).
- Other trainings:
  - Through World Health Organization's Mental Health Gap Action Program (mhGAP) evidence-based principles for treating mental, neurological and substance use disorders are provided to non-specialist health workers. One of the modules of mhGAP is Child and Adolescent Mental and Behavioral Disorders which covers presentations, assessments and all aspects of care, from general principles of care to specific pharmacological, psychological and social interventions for developmental, emotional and behavioral disorders of children and adolescents.
  - IPNA has been running a 6 months long certificate course on Autism and other neurodevelopmental disabilities since 2019 with the aim to provide training to physicians, psychologists, special educators, teachers of mainstream and special schools, developmental therapists, occupational therapists and parents

to acquire the specialized knowledge and skills they need to work with patients with autism and NDDs.

- Some psychiatrists, child and adolescent psychiatrists and psychologists are organizing seminars, conducting workshops in different schools for the students, teachers and parents in order to create awareness and provide training on child mental health.

### 6.4.3 Human Resources

Regarding the human resources available for service provision currently, there are only 12 Child and Adolescent Psychiatrists and about 350 psychiatrists in Bangladesh (Arafat, 2024). Among the Psychiatrists, only a few have specialized training in child mental health from different countries. The total number of mental health workers in CAMH services is 384 which is 0.64 per 100,000 population (World Health Organization, 2022). A significant number of these professionals work in Dhaka creating an extreme disproportion in the distribution of human resources between urban and rural areas (Arafat et al., 2024).

### 6.4.4 Research in Child and Adolescent Psychiatry

There have been advancements in the field of Child psychiatry in recent years. Some of the widely used psychometric tools related to child mental health like- *Strengths and Difficulties Questionnaire (SDQ)* (Mullick & Goodman, 2001), *Development and Wellbeing Assessment (DAWBA)* (Mullick & Goodman, 2005), *Parenting Style and Dimensions Questionnaire (PSDQ)* (Arafat, 2018) are validated in Bangla. A few new scales like *Dhaka Stress Scale* (Mullick et al., 2019) have been developed. Some epidemiological surveys on child and adolescent psychiatric disorders have been carried out in the last few years. Using different validated scales a good number of researches on child psychiatric disorders are being carried out.

### 6.4.5 Child Mental Health Legislation and Policy

In recent times neurodevelopmental disorders have been given high priority by the Bangladesh government. In order to ensure the rights and interests of people with neurodevelopmental disorders, the government of Bangladesh has accepted *Neuro-Development Disability Protection Trust Act* 2013 and *Neuro-Development Disability Protection Trust Rules* 2015.

## 6.5 Current Challenges and Ways Forward

The treatment gap of child psychiatric disorders has been estimated as 94.3% by the recent national mental health survey (Ministry of Health and Family Welfare, 2021). A WHO conference on Caring for Children with Mental Disorders in 2003 identified a number of barriers to care, including a lack of resources, stigma, inadequate transportation, inefficient communication, a lack of health literacy and public awareness of mental disorders among adolescents.

Despite some limitations, low-income countries have some benefits too. Its distinctive strength is its relatively stable traditional society, high level of family cohesion, strong support from the family and neighborhood, warm relationships between teachers and students, and potential manpower including parents, teachers, child health workers, primary care physicians, social workers, counselors, traditional healer, religious leader and volunteers (Mullick & Giasuddin, 2010).

### *6.5.1 Lack of Resources*

Bangladesh has a very limited number of psychiatrists and there is a severe shortage of child and adolescent psychiatrists. Moreover, the available manpower in mental healthcare is inequitably distributed across the country with a high proportion in Dhaka city. The scarcity and disproportionate distribution of mental health professionals are obstacles to providing mental health care (Arafat et al., 2024).

To deal with the situation, a standard model for delivering a child and adolescent mental health service (CAMHS) should be adapted. Mullick and Giasuddin proposed a model of Child and Adolescent Mental Health Services (CAMHS) for low-income countries like Bangladesh in 2010 with the level of care mentioned in Table 6.1.

The authors (Mullick & Giasuddin, 2010) also mentioned some possible strategic actions. They are

- Integration of CAMHS with existing health, mental health and child health services.
- Best utilization of existing CAMHS.
- Establishing child psychiatry and pediatric liaison
- Developing school-based service.
- Creating multidisciplinary team
- Providing training to the allied professionals and potential manpower
- Enhancing governmental initiative and support
- Increasing participation of Non-governmental organizations (NGOs)
- Involvement of the community
- Offering coordinated services through health, education and social agencies

**Table 6.1** Proposed model for delivering a child and adolescent mental health service in Bangladesh (adapted from Mullick & Giasuddin, 2010)

| Level of care | Infrastructure | Service delivered by/Human resources |
|---|---|---|
| Primary level—non-specialist level | Outdoor and outreach facilities of Primary health centers and community clinic | General practitioners (GPs), primary health workers, health counselors, trained child mental health workers, trained teachers and parents |
| Secondary level—non-specialist/ Specialist level | Outdoor, indoor facilities of general hospitals and specialist clinics | Specially trained GPs, pediatricians, neurologists, general psychiatrists, psychologists, behavioral scientists, social welfare workers etc. |
| Tertiary level—sub-specialist level | Outdoor, indoor facilities of specialist hospitals and specialist clinics | Child and adolescent psychiatrists, child and adolescent clinical psychologists, child and adolescent psychiatric social workers and psychiatric nurses with specialization in child and adolescent psychiatry |

### 6.5.2 *Lack of Adequate Standard Training*

At the undergraduate level, students have very inadequate exposure to psychiatry and psychiatry is evaluated very flexibly as part of medicine which causes general physicians (GPs) low capability to meet the community need for psychiatric care. Postgraduate psychiatry and child and adolescent psychiatry programs are standard but the number of production of professionals every year is very limited. To overcome this undergraduate medical students should be adequately trained and compulsorily evaluated in psychiatry including child & adolescent psychiatry. The psychiatry part of MBBS course curriculum should be more enriched. More doctors should be enrolled in postgraduate psychiatry and child and adolescent psychiatry courses and training centers for child and adolescent psychiatry should be increased. Child and adolescent training should be strengthened in general psychiatry training. Adequate space for child and adolescent psychiatry should be created in general pediatrics and pediatric neurology postgraduate courses. Existing courses and training need to be reviewed for better utilization. Courses in psychiatric nursing and child psychotherapy can be started. Need-based short training on child mental problems can be offered to GPs, school personnel, social workers and volunteers. More training of the trainers can be arranged to offer training and supervision to the manpower. Apart from providing clinical care, child psychiatrists need to take part in leadership and training other manpower for the development of community-based child mental health care (WHO, 2003).

### 6.5.3 Lack of Research

Research on mental health is very limited in Bangladesh. Considering the severity of the issue in the nation, the amount of research done on mental disorders is inadequate (Arafat et al., 2024). More research needs to be done to understand the disease burden, psychopathology of disorders, to provide evidence-based treatment and to plan more appropriate services. By making investments in these areas, mental disorders in children and adolescents can be prevented, diagnosed earlier and with greater accuracy, and treated more effectively and affordably (Skokauskas et al., 2019).

### 6.5.4 Distant Services

Distant Services is another important obstacle to getting mental health care (WHO, 2003). This is also supported by the National Mental Health Survey as it revealed that the time taken on the way to reach mental health facilities was 8.1 h. Transportation for community outreach clinics, home visits and telepsychiatry can solve the problem to some extent (Mullick & Giasuddin, 2010).

### 6.5.5 Stigma Related to Mental Health

According to the National Mental Health Survey, 14.1 days are taken to take the first psychiatric consultation for child mental disorder. Stigma, negative attitude toward mental health and lack of knowledge about mental health have negative impacts toward help-seeking behavior. This can be overcome by promoting Mental Health Literacy Programs and inclusion of mental health in school curriculums (Ministry of Health and Family Welfare, 2021). Mass media can play an important role in increasing mental health awareness and reducing stigma too (Arafat et al., 2024).

Bangladesh is a country where 90% of the population is Muslim (World Population Review, 2022). In one study done among Muslims of Dhaka city it was found that 44% of participants believed jinn could cause mental health difficulties and a significant number among them sought help from religious personnel. So it is recommended to educate religious figures about mental disorders to establish appropriate referrals (Khalifa et al., 2012; Mullick et al., 2013).

## 6.6 Conclusion

Child and adolescent psychiatry in Bangladesh is in its early stages of development. Though in the last few years, it has made significant advancements yet most of the children and young people are out of mental health coverage. In comparison to the needs of the population, services are inadequate. To reduce the gap between service need and service delivery it is necessary to develop feasible, affordable and need-based services as early as possible. It is important to identify the strengths, resources, challenges and opportunities of the country while planning a service system. Potential collaboration and networking among concerned national and international communities is recommended to achieve the goal.

## References

Alam, M. F., Sarkar, M., Alam, M. T., Ahmed, H. U., Bhowmik, A. D., & Roy, S. (2018). Prevalence of substance use in Bangladesh. *Bangladesh Journal of Psychiatry, 32*(1), 1–8. https://bapbd.org/docs/journal/46.pdf

Anjum, A., Hossain, S., Sikder, T., Uddin, M. E., & Rahim, D. A. (2022). Investigating the prevalence of and factors associated with depressive symptoms among urban and semi-urban school adolescents in Bangladesh: A pilot study. *International Health, 14*(4), 354–362. https://doi.org/10.1093/inthealth/ihz092

Arafat, S. M. Y., Giasuddin, N. A., & Mazumder, A. H. (2024). Access to mental health care in Bangladesh—Current status, potential challenges, and ways out. In S. M. Y. Arafat, & S. K. Kar (Eds.) *Access to mental health care in South Asia—Current status, potential challenges, and ways out*. Springer Nature. https://doi.org/10.1007/978-981-99-9153-2_3

Arafat, S. M. Y. (2024). Mental Health Services in Bangladesh. S. M. Y. Arafat (Ed.) Mental health in Bangladesh: From bench to community. Springer Nature. https://doi.org/10.1007/978-981-97-0610-5_3

Arafat, S. Y. (2018). Validation of Bangla parenting style and dimension questionnaire. *Global Psychiatry, 1*(2), 95–108. https://doi.org/10.2478/gp-2018-0011

Arafat, S. Y., Mullick, M. S., & Islam, H. (2020). Development of psychiatric services in Bangladesh. *Asian Journal of Psychiatry, 47*. https://doi.org/10.1016/j.ajp.2019.101870

Bangladesh Bureau of Statistics. Population and Housing Census. 2022. Retrieved October 30, 2023, from https://bbs.portal.gov.bd

Chowdhury, M. H. R., Mullick, M. S., & Arafat, S. M. (2016). Clinical profile and comorbidity of obsessive-compulsive disorder among children and adolescents: A cross-sectional observation in Bangladesh. *Psychiatry Journal*. https://doi.org/10.1155/2016/9029630

Dalsgaard, S., McGrath, J., Østergaard, S. D., Wray, N. R., Pedersen, C. B., Mortensen, P. B., & Petersen, L. (2020). Association of mental disorder in childhood and adolescence with subsequent educational achievement. *JAMA Psychiatry, 77*(8), 797–805. https://doi.org/10.1001/2Fjamapsychiatry.2020.0217

Dey, M., Landolt, M. A., & Mohler-Kuo, M. (2012). Health-related quality of life among children with mental disorders: A systematic review. *Quality of Life Research, 21*, 1797–1814. https://doi.org/10.1007/s11136-012-0109-7

Hassan, T., Alam, M. M., Wahab, A., & Hawlader, M. D. (2020). Prevalence and associated factors of internet addiction among young adults in Bangladesh. *Journal of the Egyptian Public Health Association, 95*, 1–8. https://doi.org/10.1186/s42506-019-0032-7

Hossain, M. D., Ahmed, H. U., Jalal Uddin, M. M., Chowdhury, W. A., Iqbal, M. S., Kabir, R. I., Chowdhury, I. A., Aftab, A., Datta, P. G., Rabbani, G., & Hossain, S. W. (2017). Autism Spectrum disorders (ASD) in South Asia: A systematic review. *BMC Psychiatry, 17*, 1–7. https://doi.org/10.1186/s12888-017-1440-x

Jesmin, A., Mullick, M. S. I., Rahman, K. M. Z., & Muntasir, M. M. (2016). Psychiatric disorders in children and adolescents attending pediatric outpatient departments of tertiary hospitals. *Oman Medical Journal, 31*(4), 258. https://doi.org/10.5001/omj.2016.51

Jokela, M., Ferrie, J., & Kivimäki, M. (2009). Childhood problem behaviors and death by midlife: The British national child development study. *Journal of the American Academy of Child and Adolescent Psychiatry, 48*(1), 19–24. https://doi.org/10.1097/CHI.0b013e31818b1c76

Kessler, R. C., Amminger, G. P., Aguilar-Gaxiola, S., Alonso, J., Lee, S., & Üstün, T. B. (2007). Age of onset of mental disorders: A review of recent literature. *Current Opinion in Psychiatry, 20*(4), 359–364. https://doi.org/10.1097/YCO.0b013e32816ebc8c

Kessler, R. C., Berglund, P., Demler, O., Jin, R., Merikangas, K. R., & Walters, E. E. (2005). Lifetime prevalence and age-of-onset distributions of DSM-IV disorders in the national comorbidity survey replication. *Archives of General Psychiatry, 62*(6), 593–602. https://doi.org/10.1001/archpsyc.62.6.593

Khalifa, N., Hardie, T., & Mullick, M. S. (2012). *Jinn and psychiatry: Comparison of beliefs among Muslims in Dhaka and Leicester*. Publications Archive.

Khanam, M., Mullick, M. S. I., Nahar, J. S., & Salam, M. A. (2002). Conversion disorder in children and adolescents—A clinical study. *Bangladesh Journal of Psychiatry, 16*(2), 26–31.

Krzeczkowski, J. E., Wade, T. J., Andrade, B. F., Browne, D., Yalcinoz-Ucan, B., Riazi, N. A., Yates, E., Tagalakis, A., & Patte, K. A. (2022). Examining the mental health of siblings of children with a mental disorder: A scoping review protocol. *PLoS ONE, 17*(9), e0274135. https://doi.org/10.1371/journal.pone.0274135

Mallik, C. I., & Radwan, R. B. (2020). Adolescent victims of cyberbullying in Bangladesh-prevalence and relationship with psychiatric disorders. *Asian Journal of Psychiatry, 48*, 101893. https://doi.org/10.1016/j.ajp.2019.101893

Marthoenis, M., & Yasir Arafat, S. M. (2022). Rate and associated factors of suicidal behavior among adolescents in Bangladesh and Indonesia: Global school-based student health survey data analysis. *Scientifica*. https://doi.org/10.1155/2022/8625345

Mazumder, A. H. (2024). Epidemiology and burden of mental disorders in Bangladesh. In S. M. Y. Arafat (Ed.) Mental health in Bangladesh: From bench to community. Springer Nature Singapore. https://doi.org/10.1007/978-981-97-0610-5_2

Ministry of Health and Family Welfare. (2021). National Mental Health Survey. Retrieved October 30, 2023, from https://nimh.gov.bd/wp-content/uploads/2021/11/Mental-Health-Survey-Report.pdf

Mullick, M. S. I., Khalifa, N., Nahar, J. S., & Walker, D.-M. (2013). Beliefs about Jinn, black magic and evil eye in Bangladesh: The effects of gender and level of education. *Mental Health, Religion and Culture, 16*(7), 719–729. https://doi.org/10.1080/13674676.2012.717918

Mullick, M. S., Chowdhury, M. H. R., & Arafat, S. Y. (2017). Phenomenology of obsessive-compulsive disorder in children and adolescents: A cross-sectional observation in Bangladesh. *Jentashapir Journal of Health Research, 8*(4), e63414. https://doi.org/10.5812/jjhr.63414

Mullick, M. S., & Giasuddin, N. A. (2010). A strategic proposition for child and adolescent mental health services in low income Countries. *Bangladesh Journal of Psychiatry, 24*(1).

Mullick, M. S. I., & Goodman, R. (2001). Questionnaire screening for mental health problems in Bangladeshi children: A preliminary study. *Social Psychiatry and Psychiatric Epidemiology, 36*, 94–99. https://doi.org/10.1007/s001270050295

Mullick, M. S. I., & Goodman, R. (2005). The prevalence of psychiatric disorders among 5–10 year olds in rural, urban and slum areas in Bangladesh: An exploratory study. *Social Psychiatry and Psychiatric Epidemiology, 40*, 663–671. https://doi.org/10.1007/s00127-005-0939-5

Mullick, M. S., & Islam, M. (2020). The prevalence of psychiatric disorders among 3–4 year olds in an urban sample in Bangladesh. *Asian Journal of Psychiatry, 54*, 102368. https://doi.org/10.1016/j.ajp.2020.102368

Mullick, M. S., Algin, S., Islam, M., Phillipson, A., Nahar, J. S., Morshed, N. M., Chowdhury, H. R., & Shahid, S. F. B. (2019). Dhaka stress scale-adult: A scale for assessing psychosocial stressors among adults. *Bangabandhu Sheikh Mujib Med Univ J, 12*, 119–127. https://doi.org/10.3329/bsmmuj.v12i3.43328

Mullick, M. S. I. (2002). Somatoform disorders in children and adolescents. *Bangladesh Medical Research Council Bulletin, 28*(3), 112–122. PMID: 14509383.

National Institute of Mental Health. (2021). Epidemiology of suicide and suicidal behavior among youth and adolescents in Bangladesh (Project Report). https://doi.org/10.13140/RG.2.2.27542.52801

Rabbani, M. G., Alam, M. F., Ahmed, H. U., Sarker, M., Chowdhury, W. A., Zaman, M. M., et al. (2009). Prevalence of mental disorders, mental retardation, epilepsy and substance abuse in children. *Bangladesh Journal of Psychiatry, 23*, 12–54.

Rahman, M. M. (2010). Autism spectrum disorders. *Journal of Bangladesh College of Physicians and Surgeons, 28*(3), 143.

Skokauskas, N., Fung, D., Flaherty, L.T., Von Klitzing, K., Pūras, D., Servili, C., Dua, T., Falissard, B., Vostanis, P., Moyano, M.B., & Feldman, I. (2019). Shaping the future of child and adolescent psychiatry. *Child and Adolescent Psychiatry and Mental Health, 13*(1), 1–7. https://doi.org/10.1186/s13034-019-0279-y

Smith, J. P., & Smith, G. C. (2010). Long-term economic costs of psychological problems during childhood. *Social Science and Medicine, 71*(1), 110–115. https://doi.org/10.1016/j.socscimed.2010.02.046

Tarafder, B. K., Khan, M. A. I., Islam, M. T., Mahmud, S. A. A., Sarker, M. H. K., Faruq, I., Miah, M. T., & Arafat, S. M. (2016). Mass psychogenic illness: Demography and symptom profile of an episode. *Psychiatry Journal*. https://doi.org/10.1155/2016/2810143

World Health Organization. (2000). *The world health report 2000: health systems: Improving performance*. World Health Organization. https://books.google.com.bd/books?hl=en&lr=&id=luqgKK2euxoC&oi=fnd&pg=PR7&dq=world+health+report+2000&ots=sOh35bbJP9&sig=AuYoWgFeDG3teLvUZ1tPYWZYfjc&redir_esc=y#v=onepage&q=world%20health%20report%202000&f=false

World Health Organization. (2001). The World Health Report 2001: Mental health: new understanding, new hope. https://books.google.com/books?hl=en&lr=&id=GQEdA-VFSIgC&oi=fnd&pg=PR9&dq=world+health+report+2001&ots=d3PzXJfhrE&sig=gVDYTToBbRRbzrTqmDCXlObiFuA

World Health Organization (2003). Caring for children and adolescents with mental disorders: Setting WHO directions. https://iris.who.int/bitstream/handle/10665/42679/9241590637.pdf

World Health Organization. (2022). Mental Health Atlas 2020 country profile: Bangladesh. Retrieved October 12, 2023, from https://www.who.int/publications/m/item/mental-health-atlas-bgd2020-country-profile

World Population Review. (2022). Muslim Majority Countries 2022. Retrieved October 27, 2022, from https://worldpopulationreview.com/countryrankings/muslim-majority-countries

# Chapter 7
# Substance Use and Mental Health Conditions: Co-existence of Dual Problems in Bangladesh

**Mohammad Muntasir Maruf, Antara Chowdhury, and Md. Rahanul Islam**

**Abstract** Substance use is currently an important public health as well as social issue in Bangladesh. At the same time, psychiatric disorders are also of growing concern in the country. However, there is a dearth of research regarding the dual diagnosis of substance use and psychiatric disorders in Bangladesh. Available research indicates that psychiatric disorders or mental health conditions are frequent both as a risk factor and a comorbidity of substance use. There are some tertiary care centers in government level and many legal and illegally established drug addiction treatment centers which deal with persons with substance abuse with or without mental health conditions. The assessment and management process including available services for the dual problems are neither satisfactory nor coordinated. Recently the *Mental Health Act* and the *Narcotics Control Act* have been enacted to aid in the process of management of the problem. Still, there are many barriers in providing effective services for the co-occurring disorders. To deal with the dual problems successfully, further research, skilled manpower, raising awareness, adequate and integrated services and intersectoral collaboration are needed. This chapter discusses the current scenario, challenges and future directions for better services regarding the issue.

**Keywords** Substance use · Drug addiction · Dual diagnosis · Psychiatric comorbidity · Mental health conditions · Co-occurring disorder · Bangladesh

---

M. M. Maruf (✉) · A. Chowdhury
Department of Addiction Psychiatry, National Institute of Mental Health, Dhaka, Bangladesh
e-mail: marufdmc@gmail.com

Md. R. Islam
Central Drug Addiction Treatment Centre, Tejgaon, Dhaka, Bangladesh



S. M. Y. Arafat (ed.), *Mental Health in Bangladesh*,
https://doi.org/10.1007/978-981-97-0610-5_7

## 7.1 Introduction

The terms ‘dual diagnosis’, ‘comorbidity’, ‘co-occurring disorder’ are used commonly and sometimes interchangeably to refer to the coexistence of a substance use disorder and one or more psychiatric disorders in the same individual. This condition is common across psychiatric and substance dependent populations and could be considered more as an expectation than an exception when assessing persons with both the disorders. Recent systematic reviews and meta-analysis showed that comorbidity between substance use disorders (SUDs) and other psychiatric disorders specially schizophrenia, bipolar disorder and depressive disorders are highly prevalent in both hospital and community-based samples and rates are more or less same over time (Hunt et al., 2016a, 2016b, 2018, 2020).

There are several proposed general explanations for the high rates of dual diagnosis of substance use disorders and other psychiatric disorders. One assumption is that substance abuse causes psychiatric disorders. In some cases, substance use may be an attempt to ameliorate the symptoms of the psychiatric disorders as self-medication. Some psychiatric disorders and SUDs share same etiological factors including genetic vulnerability. However, in comparison to either disorder, various researches reported more negative consequences of dual diagnosis, including poor motivation to change, poor treatment compliance, slower improvement in response to treatment, high drop out from long term programs, frequent relapses, increased suicide risk or aggression, social exclusion, poor self-care, homelessness, possible incarceration, unemployment, injury, higher rates of physical comorbidities including HIV, hepatitis, cardiovascular, hepatic, and gastrointestinal disease. All of these contribute to a greater health burden, which diminishes the capacity of the health care system to manage the patients appropriately. Therefore, assessment and cohesive management plans that can address both the substance use disorders and psychiatric disorders are recommended in case of dual diagnosis, to provide appropriate treatment, and other cares to accommodate the individual’s social and vocational needs. For this, the current situation analysis regarding dual diagnosis in the country is necessary to develop appropriate strategy to combat the conditions.

Substance use is currently an important public health and social issue in Bangladesh. Due to its geographic location in the central point of the world’s largest growing narcotics zone: the ‘golden crescent’ and the ‘golden triangle’, and the production of illicit substances by neighboring countries, Bangladesh is in high risk of easy availability of substances which contributes to its increasing substance use related problems (Kamal et al., 2018). On the other hand, psychiatric disorders are also of growing concern in the country. The latest national mental health survey reported that 18.7% of the population has been suffering from psychiatric disorders (Ministry of Health and Family Welfare, 2021a, 2021b). However, little has been identified about substance abuse and mental disorders in the country. In this chapter, we begin with the prevalence of substance use in Bangladesh. Then, mental health conditions are explored as a risk factor and as a comorbidity of substance use. Mental health conditions include psychiatric disorders and other psychiatric symptoms which could not be labeled as a disorder according to any diagnostic instrument. We also discuss about the available services, assessment and management steps, legal aspects and organizations working for the dual diagnosis. Future direction for establishing effective and feasible services are proposed.

## 7.2 Epidemiology of Substance Abuse in Bangladesh

According to the Department of Narcotics Control (DNC), an increasing trend of substance use has been observed in Bangladesh over the past two decades. In the last twelve years, there was more than five-fold rise in the number of patients having treatment in government drug addiction centers including Central Drug Addiction Treatment Center (CTC) city (DNC, 2023).

Though there is no precise estimation, on the basis of different statistics, it is stipulated that more than 6 million people are abusing or dependent on substance in Bangladesh (DNC, 2023). According to the nationwide community-based survey conducted by the *National Institute of Mental Health* (NIMH), the prevalence of substance use disorders was 3.3% among the adult population. Among the population aged 12–17 years and 7–11 years, the prevalence was found 1.5% and 0.2% respectively (Ministry of Health and Family Welfare, 2021a, 2021b). Despite various estimations and findings, there are concerns about under-reporting that hides the real gravity of the problem.

There are wide variations in the findings regarding the most frequently used substances and epidemiology of substance users or persons with substance use disorders published in various reports by different government institutions, non-government organizations (NGOs) and empirical studies due to the differences in study design, settings, population and sampling. Studies found cannabinoids, methamphetamine and opioids as commonly used substances among the abusers taking treatment in CTC, various drug rehabilitation centers and in community, cannabis being the most common in community and CTC and methamphetamine (yaba) or opioids being the most common in drug rehabilitation centers (DNC, 2022; Ministry of Health & Family Welfare, 2021a, 2021b; Hawlader et al., 2020; DNC, 2018b; Kamal et al., 2018; DNC, 2017, Maruf et al., 2016).

## 7.3 Relationship of Substance Use and Mental Health Conditions in Bangladesh

### *7.3.1 Mental Health Conditions or Psychological Issues as Risk Factors for Substance Use*

The relation of substance use and mental health conditions are bidirectional. Mental health conditions can be a consequence of substance use or substance use increases the risk of various psychiatric disorders. On the other hand, psychiatric disorders or some mental health issues can make an individual vulnerable for using substances or develop dependency on substances. Study results show that secondary substance use disorders may be lessened significantly through the prevention of primary psychiatric disorders (Swendsen et al., 2010).

In most of the studies, most influencing risk factors for substance use in Bangladesh include peer pressure, availability of drugs, curiosity, pleasure seeking etc. Some also mentioned of unemployment, failure in love, and family conflict (DNC, 2022; DNC, 2018b; Kamal et al., 2018; Zaman et al., 2015). Few studies investigated or found mental health conditions as contributing factors for substance use in Bangladesh. A study conducted in Chattogram and Noakhali regions of the country reported that one-fourth of the respondents became addicted to substance due to psychological causes while about two-third (65.5%) due to various social and cultural causes (Patoari, 2021). Among the psychiatric symptoms or psychological issues, depression, frustration, sorrow, worrying about a personal problem, loneliness, to feel relaxed, to enhance sexual performance, to get amusement have been mentioned as the reasons of substance use by the respondents (DNC, 2022; Patoari, 2021; DNC 2018b; Kamal et al., 2018; Zaman et al., 2014; Maruf et al., 2012). Depression was significantly associated with the number and duration of abusing substances, the age of first use and the first substance used (Zaman et al., 2014). Excessive smartphone use and late-night sleeping were significantly associated with substance use in high school-going adolescents (Moonajilin et al., 2021). In a case-control study, the association of substance use with personality traits was investigated which reported that psychoticism was the most common trait among the substance users and it was found significantly higher among the substance users who had history of trouble with legal authorities (Roy et al., 2010).

### *7.3.2 Psychiatric Comorbidities in Persons with Substance Use*

To the best of our knowledge, no nationwide community-based study has been conducted to assess the burden of other psychiatric disorders among the persons with substance use disorders in the country. In a hospital-based study, among the patients with substance use disorders ($n = 9143$), 11% had comorbid mental disorders, among which depressive disorder was the most common. Interestingly, frequency of personality disorders was found very low (antisocial personality disorder—0.7%, borderline personality disorder—1.3%) compared to other psychiatric disorders among the persons with substance use disorders (Table 7.1). Moreover, dementia was found in 1.3% of the respondents. Considering various substances separately, prevalence of mental disorders was found highest among cocaine users (36.6%). Prevalence of overall mental disorders among alcohol, cannabis, amphetamine, opioids, sleeping pills and tobacco users were found at 12.2%, 12.1%, 10.7%, 6.3%, 15%, and 11% respectively. Among the users of alcohol, cannabis and amphetamine separately, depressive disorders were the most common psychiatric disorders for all the groups (among alcohol users—21.4%, cannabis users—32.5%, amphetamine users—58.3%), followed by schizophrenia spectrum and other psychotic disorders (19%) for alcohol, and anxiety disorders for both cannabis (17.5%) and amphetamine (16.7%) users. Among sleeping pill users, anxiety disorders (33.3%) were the most common, followed by bipolar and related disorders (22.2%) (Ahmed et al., 2020).

Comorbid psychiatric disorders were found among about one-third of the hospitalized methamphetamine abusers and more than one-fourth of opioid users (Maruf et al., 2013, 2021). Few studies were conducted among the adolescent substance users. In both a hospital-based and a juvenile correction center-based study, more than three-fourth of the male adolescents were suffering from psychiatric disorders (Khan et al., 2021a, 2021b; Maruf et al., 2015a, 2015b).

Some studies reported psychiatric symptoms, not disorder, among the substance users where among the other symptoms, anxiety, depression and insomnia were commonly found (Table 7.1) (Zaman et al., 2014; DNC, 2018b; Sarker et al., 2023; Islam & Hossain, 2017).

Comorbid substance use is prevalent commonly in patients with psychiatric disorders. Very few studies in Bangladesh determined the rate of substance use among the persons with psychiatric disorders. One study reported that about one-third of the depressed adult male patients had lifetime history of substance use except tobacco and caffeine. Commonly used substances were benzodiazepines (72.9%), alcohol (25.0%), cannabis (22.9%) and opioids (20.8%). When tobacco was considered, about half of the respondents were current smokers. Suicidal attempts were significantly higher among depressed substance users (Maruf et al., 2012). History of lifetime substance use was reported in 14.7% of the persons with obsessive compulsive disorder, where alcohol (68.2%) was the most common substance, followed by cannabis (63.6%), sedatives (22.7%) and amphetamine (18.2%) (Khanom, 2023). Lifetime substance use was found in 10% of female juvenile offenders with psychiatric disorders (Maruf et al., 2015a, 2015b).

**Table 7.1** Psychiatric disorders or symptoms among the persons with substance use

| Year | Author | Study population | Comorbid psychiatric disorders or symptoms |
|---|---|---|---|
| 2023 | Sarker et al. | Community people (12–35 years) abusing substances in Pabna, a northern district | Anxiety—32%<br>Depression—32%<br>Aggressiveness—26%<br>Sleep problems—26% |
| 2022 | Maruf et al. | Hospitalized methamphetamine abusers | Overall psychiatric disorders—29.6%<br>Personality disorders—17.4%<br>Anxiety disorders—7.8%<br>Depressive disorders—6.1%<br>Bipolar and related disorders—4.3%<br>Obsessive compulsive and related disorders—4.3%<br>Schizophrenia spectrum and other psychotic disorders—3.5% |
| 2021 | Khan et al. | Adolescent (11–17 years) male substance users in two drug addiction treatment center | Overall psychiatric disorders—77.1%<br>Among psychiatric disorders:<br>Conduct disorder—31.4%<br>ADHD—21.4%<br>ODD—18.5%<br>Depressive disorders—17.1% |
| 2020 | Ahmed et al. | Substance abusers seeking treatment in 13 government hospitals where psychiatric consultations are available | Overall psychiatric disorders—11.0%<br>Among psychiatric disorders:<br>Depressive disorders—32.0%<br>Somatic symptoms disorders—16.0%<br>Anxiety disorders—15.7%<br>Schizophrenia spectrum and other psychotic disorders—6.0%<br>Bipolar and related disorders—5.1% |
| 2019 | DNC | Substance users in government treatment center | Cranky mood—64.7%<br>Sleeping problems—52.6%<br>Fatigue—50.5%<br>Depression—41.8%<br>Decreased working capacity—37.3%<br>Worries/fear—33.8% |

(continued)

**Table 7.1** (continued)

| Year | Author | Study population | Comorbid psychiatric disorders or symptoms |
|---|---|---|---|
| 2017 | Islam and Hossain | Substance users (recent graduates, civil servants, and civil society members) | Insomnia—20.0%<br>Hallucination—20.0%<br>Sexual problem—15.0%<br>Abnormal behavior—10.0% |
| 2015 | Maruf et al. | Male juvenile offender with substance use | Psychiatric disorders—77.4% |
| 2014 | Zaman et al. | Substance users undergoing detoxification as outpatients in the government treatment center | Depression—92%<br>(moderate depression—55%<br>severe depression—4%<br>extreme depression—3%)<br>Insomnia—91%<br>Reduced appetite—69%<br>Violence—62% |

## 7.4 Treatment-Seeking Behavior of the Substance Users with Mental Health Conditions

There are few studies which reported the behavior and pattern of treatment-seeking of substance users and individuals with psychiatric disorders separately. Despite the high prevalence of substance related problems, most people do not seek professional help. A country-wide study reported that one-third of the substance users got admitted to any rehabilitation center for the management of their problem; and among those treatment-seekers, less than one-third (29.8%) were hospitalized voluntarily (DNC, ). In a study conducted in Pabna, a northern district of Bangladesh, 89% of the substance users did not receive any treatment for their addiction, might be due to poor knowledge and unavailability of treatment facilities. Among the respondents who got treatment, majority received short term treatment and relapsed (Sarker et al., 2023). Even among the graduates, civil servants and civil society members, more than three-fourth (79%) of the substance users did not take any treatment (Islam & Hossain, 2017). Two hospital-based studies conducted among the individuals with opioid use disorders and amphetamine use disorders found that more than two-thirds (69.9% and 69.6% respectively) of the participants were hospitalized against their will (Maruf et al., 2013; Maruf et al., 2021). Another study found that more than 90% of the substance users were brought to the hospital involuntarily (Soron et al., 2017).

The latest National Mental Health Survey found that persons with addictive disorder had the lowest interest in treatment-seeking compared to the other psychiatric disorders. Only 4.8% of the persons with addictive disorder sought healthcare services. Family history of psychiatric illness increased the probability of treatment-seeking by around 6%. Patients with more severe symptoms mostly sought treatment (Huque et al., 2023).

The barriers for treatment-seeking specifically for substance abuse in Bangladesh have not been systematically explored so far. Regarding mental health care overall, scarcity of public mental healthcare facilities and skilled mental health professionals, limited financial resource allocation, high social stigma are generally the barriers to treatment-seeking (Hasan et al., 2021).

Besides, concerns about the service providers' inappropriate professional practices including hurried communication, judgmental attitude, unscientific approaches, and breach of confidentiality can also be regarded as the constraints for the poor treatment-seeking behavior (Shultana, 2022). Same factors can be considered as barriers in help-seeking in substance abuse in addition to the high treatment costs, poor coordination among various concerned departments of the health sectors, and inadequate advocacy about seeking services. Therefore, unless extreme disruption in personal, social or professional life happens due to substance use and/or psychiatric disorders, persons remain reluctant to seek treatment. Meanwhile, they adopt various types of alternative coping including help-seeking from traditional healers, and some transient relief from these approaches in turn hinders appropriate treatment-seeking. In other cases, some traditional practices cause physical and psychological problems, further complicating the prognosis (Hossain et al., 2014). Lack of motivation to control or cut down substance use may be a contributing factor to the refusal or avoidance of treatment for many persons with dual diagnosis.

## 7.5 Available Services for Managing Patients with Dual Diagnosis

Various qualified and semi-qualified professionals provide health care services in Bangladesh with backgrounds in allopathy and alternative care. They provide their services in the government, as well as private sectors. Besides, there are many unqualified, traditional and informal healthcare providers in the country (Ministry of Health & Family Welfare, 2021a, 2021b). For the management of dual diagnoses of substance use disorder and any mental health condition, persons seek help from any of these providers.

### *7.5.1 Government Services*

**Primary and Secondary Healthcare**

In the primary and secondary health care settings at government services, there is no provision of specialized mental health care, let alone services for substance abuse. However, with the initiatives of the World Health Organization, Directorate General of Health Services of Bangladesh and NIMH, many physicians and nurses of primary and secondary care have been trained on mental health issues including substance abuse. Patients with dual diagnoses can have outpatient services from trained physicians. At Upazilla Health Complex part of primary health care and Zilla Sadar Hospital part of secondary health care manage cases of intoxication as a component of emergency service. However, there is no position for psychiatrist or any other mental health professional at primary and secondary level and after emergency management referral for psychiatric assessment is rare.

**Tertiary Healthcare**

**CTC, Dhaka**—The CTC is the official nodal tertiary care for substance use disorder treatment at the government level which started its journey under the Directorate of Health under the control of the Ministry of Health in August 1988. In July 1990, the center was transferred to the President's Secretariat from being under the control of the Ministry of Health. In October 1991, the Center was transferred from the President's Secretariat to the Directorate of Narcotics Control under the Ministry of Home Affairs. In the inpatient department of CTC, there are 90 beds for adult males, 24 beds for adult females and 10 beds for children and adolescents. Besides, there are 3 Divisional Drug Addiction Treatment Centers in Chattogram, Rajshahi and Khulna having 25 inpatient beds in each center (DNC, 2023).

**Mental Hospital, Pabna**—Mental Hospital Pabna, about 210 km distant from the capital Dhaka was established in 1957. In that hospital, there is a 30-bed addiction unit established in 1988.

**National Institute of Mental Health, Dhaka**—In NIMH, there is a department of Addiction psychiatry dedicated to the management of persons with substance use disorders with or without mental health conditions. The department has 15 inpatient beds for males. It runs a specialized clinic for substance abuse and other behavioral addictions weekly (NIMH, 2023).

**Department of Psychiatry in BSMMU and medical colleges:** In the department of Psychiatry in BSMMU and medical colleges, there is no dedicated inpatient bed only for substance abuse. However, patients with psychiatric disorders with comorbid substance use disorders can get inpatient treatment, if indicated, in BSMMU and medical colleges having psychiatric inpatient beds.

### *7.5.2 Private Services*

Psychiatrists and psychologists provide outpatient services for mental health conditions including substance abuse in their private chambers. Currently, there are 365 DNC-approved non-government drug addiction treatment and rehabilitation centers having 4996 inpatient beds for substance abusers in Bangladesh (DNC, 2023). Besides, there are many illegal and unlicensed treatment centers, known as rehab centers for the management of substance abuse, run mainly by informal care providers. Non-government psychiatric hospitals, licensed from DGHS, also manage inpatient substance abusers with comorbid mental health conditions.

### 7.5.3 Procedure of Hospitalization

According to the Mental Health Act, 2018, there are three types of admission for the patients with mental disorders including drug addiction—voluntary, non-protesting and involuntary admission. According to the act, adult patients can be hospitalized voluntarily, if indicated by psychiatrists or physicians, for their desired treatment. Consent of guardian or relative is needed in case of minor (age <18 years). A guardian or relative may apply for admission for a non-protesting patient who is incapable of giving an opinion about their admission or treatment and the patient may be admitted by a responsible medical practitioner after proper assessment. The involuntary admission is permitted, with or without an application by a guardian or legal authority, if a psychiatrist judges it necessary considering the severity of the person's condition and relevant matters (Karim & Shaikh, 2021). Experience from the government and non-government drug addiction treatment centers, majority of the patients with substance abuse are hospitalized involuntarily as it happens during crisis mostly like intoxication, suicidal attempts, violence, encounter with law enforcing officials or they deny their problems. Even in the cases of voluntary admission, the consent of a legal guardian is sought by most of the treatment centers.

According to the act, Mental Health Review and Monitoring Committee at district-level is the authority to review the rationality of hospitalization of the patient and to decide about the long duration of inpatient stay (more than 3 months) (Karim & Shaikh, 2021). However, the committee in each district is yet to be formed. Therefore, practically, the decision depends on the psychiatrist, where available, and the legal guardians.

### 7.5.4 Assessment and Management of Patients with Dual Problems in Bangladesh

To formulate an effective treatment plan, systematic assessment is the core and is the first step to proceed further. For systemic assessment and referral, there are several steps as screening, assessment of recovery capital, investigations, advanced assessment and referral. But this systematic procedure is not followed in the country. In most cases, parents or legal guardians suspect or come to know about the patient's substance abuse and take him/ her to the physician/ psychiatrist or other health care providers for assessment or hospitalization. In CTC and some other non-government centers, Bangla translation of '*Alcohol, Smoking and Substance Involvement Screening Test* (ASSIST)' is used as a screening tool, of Addiction Severity Index to assess severity of substance abuse and validated Bangla 'Brief Assessment of Recovery Capital-10' to assess recovery capital. But in most other centers and private chambers, assessment is done through history taking and mental state examination. Then, on the basis of availability and feasibility, routine investigations and drug screening or dope tests are done. In NIMH, CTC, Pabna mental hospital, BSMMU and in some medical colleges and few private diagnostic centers, quantitative laboratory analyzes of urine samples are not available to detect recent use of a particular substance rather than using strips for qualitative tests in urine only. Few private diagnostic centers perform using semi-quantitative tests by enzyme immunoassay to determine opioids, cannabinoids, benzodiazepine, and methamphetamine except alcohol and new psycho-active substances. Regarding management, detoxifications are dealt with general physicians or psychiatrists, on the basis of their local availability. In the government centers, long duration of hospital stay is discouraged. Therefore, mostly detoxification remains the aim for hospitalization besides psychoeducation. Psychosocial management is provided as outpatients in government centers. CTC provide family psycho-education on every Wednesday (DNC, 2023). The sessions are conducted according to a semi-structured outline, delivered as a 4 week program where anyone who missed a session could catch up if s/he just joined the missed session which will be repeated next month. Each session is conducted by chief consultant, resident psychiatrist, rehabilitation officer, occupational therapist, and matron (junior) with support from social welfare department.

Most of the private centers follow a modified version of therapeutic community model incorporating 12-steps approach of Narcotics Anonymous and network therapy for the inpatient substance abusers, where recruiting process of the patients is not structured or systematic. In some NGO-run centers, residential and abstinence-oriented treatment programs are provided which include detoxification initially, usually for 2 weeks. During the program, regular health check-ups, clinical care and counseling (with or without family members) are conducted including basic education on sexual health, STI prevention and substance related harms. Life skills and vocational training are provided towards the end of the program (Maehira et al., 2013). Informal care providers, known as peer counselors or support staffs, provide psychosocial management in most centers. In the government tertiary centers and some private centers, psychologists are available, though very few in number, to deal with these issues. There is no licensed motivational interviewing practitioner in Bangladesh except one psychiatrist who has completed an online training.

There are some established self-help support groups in Bangladesh to aid in the management of substance abusers. There are 18 Narcotics Anonymous (NA) groups in Dhaka, 2 in Chittagong and one in Sylhet. There is only one Alcoholics Anonymous (AA) group currently running in Dhaka. There is no mutual self-help group for caregivers of substance abusers in Bangladesh.

Mental health conditions of the substance abusers are assessed and managed by psychiatrists in the government tertiary care centers and some of the private centers in divisional levels. But these issues are generally ignored or maltreated in most of the private centers.

### 7.5.5 Opioid Substitution Therapy in Bangladesh

The 1st OST program in Bangladesh started in 2010 approved as a pilot project. Currently, ICDDR,B, Save the Children, CARE and Ashokta Punarbashan Sangstha are running opioid substitution therapy (OST) in the form of *Methadone Maintenance Treatment* (MMT). They have 2600 injectable substance abusers in the MMT program under direct supervision of DNC. The program is running in 17 centers, 9 of which are situated in Dhaka. Besides, there are MMT centers in Cumilla, Gazipur, Narayanganj and Rajshahi.

### 7.5.6 Diagnostic Norms and Jargons Used in Substance Abuse Field

During primary assessment, recording diagnosis is not the common practice in Bangladesh not only in the field of psychiatry but also other medical specialties. Drug addiction, abuse and SRD are interchangeable terms most frequently used by different allied professionals including psychiatrists of Bangladesh to describe substance use disorder. Being a member of commonwealth nation though Bangladesh is officially supposed to use the *International Classification of Diseases* (ICD 10/11) in practice nearly all clinicians follow the *Diagnostic and Statistical Manual of Mental Disorders* (DSM 5) to generate diagnosis. But in case of legal communication with court and law authority following the ICD 10 is the norm as per Directorate General of Health of Bangladesh.

After publishing DSM 5 in 2013 diagnostic norms and terms have been changed. The term previously used in DSM IV like substance dependence, substance abuse till now visible in available treatment or discharge paper by some clinicians to describe or record the current term substance use disorder.

In addition to medical doctor there are numerous service providers working in substance use disorder field from diverse educational background. Some of them work with different title like peer counsellor, programmer (who runs 12 step based semi-structured program in inpatient), educator etc. Among them there are some jargons frequently used like B.C (bad company), pull up, rescue/caught (involuntary admission) etc.

## 7.6 Laws Related to Substance Abuse and Mental Health Conditions

According to the constitution of Bangladesh, the state is committed to provide medical care in case of sickness or disability. Clause 18 (Public health and ethics) of the constitution mentions that the state shall take effective measures to prohibit the use of alcohol and other narcotic drinks and herbs injurious to health, except for medical needs or other needs specified by law. Despite the presence and correlation of different laws of Bangladesh, law and policy related to the treatment of substance abuse and mental health conditions are predominantly guided by the Narcotics Control Act and the Mental Health Act, both enacted in 2018.

Box 7.1: Some important laws and rules related to substance abuse in Bangladesh

- Alcohol Control Rules, 2022
- Rules for establishment and maintenance of Drug addiction treatment centers, drug addiction rehabilitation centers and drug addiction counseling centers in non-government sector, 2021
- Narcotics Control Act (2018) (amended in 2020)
- Mental Health Act (2018)
- Bangladesh Rehabilitation Council Act, 2018
- Road Transport Act, 2018
- Rights and Protection of Persons with Disabilities Act, 2013
- Children Act, 2013
- Bangladesh Medical and Dental Council Act, 2010
- Smoking and Use of Tobacco Products (Control) Act, 2005

### *7.6.1 Narcotics Control Act (2018)*

It is an act to make provisions for the control, reduction of supply and demand, prevention of abuse and smuggling of narcotic drugs, and the treatment and rehabilitation of drug addicts. This act has been passed by the parliament of Bangladesh by repealing the Narcotics Control Act, 1990. The new act contains 70 clauses divided into 7 chapters. Definitions and clauses related to treatment have been described in the first and seventh chapters. According to the act, DNC is responsible for conducting any research or survey for the collection of any information relating to narcotics, taking measures related to the production, supply, use and control of narcotic drugs, taking necessary measures regarding the treatment and rehabilitation of drug addicts, the establishment and monitoring of drug addiction treatment and rehabilitation centers (DNC, 2018a, 2018b). The act made provision of dope tests for admission in institutions for higher education and sports and appointment if government services (DNC, 2023). According to the act, the courts dealing with drugs offence have the choice to offer rehabilitation to a person with drug addiction issues if he/ she has not been involved with any other drug-related criminal offence; however, in reality, this discretion has not been implemented properly (Rahman, 2019). Moreover, criminalization of person who are suffering from substance use disorder may attribute in increasing stigma in society and be a barrier to access health care.

### *7.6.2 Mental Health Act (2018)*

In the MHA 2018, which was passed replacing the 105-year-old Lunacy Act 1912, a distinction between mental disorder and mental illness has been made. 'Mental disorder' includes intellectual disability, drug addiction and other clinically recognized psychiatric conditions, that hamper normal living, whereas 'mental illness' is the kind of mental disorder excluding intellectual disability and drug addiction. The act allows the government to operate related rehabilitation centers by private agencies alongside establishing separate psychiatric units in the government medical college hospitals and district-level hospitals (Karim & Shaikh, 2021).

## 7.7 Non-government Organizations Working in the Field of Substance Use and Mental Health

There is no NGO working specifically or only with the individuals with dual diagnosis of substance use disorders and psychiatric disorders. There are some organizations working in the field of mental health primarily, which by default deal with the persons with comorbid substance use. On the other hand, the organizations, primarily dealing with substance use disorders, also address some aspects of mental health conditions. However, to our current knowledge, there is no organization emphasizing both issues with same vigor. There are 79 NGOs working on various aspects of substance abuse in Bangladesh. Among the organizations, *Bangladesh Rehabilitation and Assistance Center for Addicts (BARACA), Ashokti Punorbashon Nibash (APON), Dhaka Ahsania Mission* (DAM), etc. are mentionable names, which are involved in awareness building and research activities in these fields apart from providing direct service to the persons with the disorders.

### *7.7.1 Bangladesh Rehabilitation and Assistance Center for Addicts (BARACA)*

*BARACA is a NGO which started its journey in 1988 as the* central project of Caritas Bangladesh. It established the first drug treatment and rehabilitation center in Bangladesh, later added 4 drop-in centers and two night shelters. *Moreover, it organizes awareness programs, voluntary counseling and testing for the persons with substance use (BARACA).*

### 7.7.2 *Ashokti Punorbashon Nibash or Addiction Rehabilitation Residence (APON)*

Brother Ronald Drahozal, an American citizen and a Holy Cross Brother of St. Joseph Province, Bangladesh founded APON on the 1st of October, 1994. At first, this center was started on a temporary basis in Dhaka, later on in July 2007, APON Center has been shifted and started running its own permanent premises around 27 km away from Dhaka and named as "Apongaon". APON provides long term treatment and rehabilitation services for the male, female and children (minor) substance abusers. However, APON is the only Addiction Rehabilitation Residence which runs a school in their premises dedicated for the children they are treating and most of them are street children. They offer a six and half months rehabilitation program adapting the principles of the 12 steps of Narcotics Anonymous and therapeutic community and other related activities, especially group sessions.

### 7.7.3 *Dhaka Ahsania Mission (DAM)*

DAM launched a program on drug prevention and control in 1990 which was reorganized in 2004 to be known as 'Addiction Management and Integrated Care' (AMIC). Besides establishing drug addiction treatment and rehabilitation centers for men in Gazipur and Jashore and for women in Dhaka, it arranges awareness programs on substance use issues. The Global Center for Credentialing and Certification (GCCC) of Colombo Plan has recognized DAM as an Education Provider for enhancing the capacity of professionals in the treatment of substance use disorders which also addresses co-occurring disorders (Dhaka Ahsania Mission, 2023).

### 7.7.4 *Other Organizations*

Among other organizations, Sajida Foundation in Dhaka and Ashokta Punorbashon Songstha (APOSH) in Rajshahi are also renowned. There are many registered and unregistered local drug rehab centers in various districts of Bangladesh, which provide treatment to the persons with substance use disorder with or without mental health conditions as well as organize awareness programs on a small-scale. Local psychiatric clinics also do the same alongside providing treatment to psychiatric patients with or without substance use disorders.

## 7.8 Current Status of Research on Substance Use with Psychiatric Disorders

Though there are separate national level surveys regarding psychiatric disorders and substance use besides some local or single health- care facility-based studies, there is a paucity of research regarding the dual diagnoses of substance use disorders and psychiatric disorders (Table 7.2). The small-scale, hospital or rehab center-based studies have several short-comings including small sample size, convenient or purposive sampling methods, and lack of use of proper diagnostic tool which restricts the generalizability of their findings. The issues in two specific nationwide studies claiming to investigate both substance use and psychiatric disorders in a relatively large-scale will be described a bit more here.

The nationwide community-based survey conducted by NIMH, Dhaka to determine the prevalence and risk factors of substance use, in Bangladesh claimed to use ASSIST (Ministry of Health & Family Welfare, 2021a, 2021b). ASSIST obtains information from clients about lifetime use of substances, and use of substances and associated problems over the last 3 months. In the NIMH study, one-fourth (25.2%) of the respondents were claimed to be 'screen positive cases' in the study, but it was not clear whether it was applicable for lifetime use or use over last 3 months. No risk score or risk category, which ASSIST determines, was mentioned. Moreover, though the methods of the study claimed that diagnosis of substance use disorders was confirmed following DSM 5 criteria by research psychiatrists, the prevalence of substance use, not 'disorders', was found 3.3% among the adult population—according to the summary, objectives and results. The prevalence of substance use was found 2.9% among respondents irrespective of age group despite 25.2% screen positive cases. This study also explored the prevalence of mental disorders among adults (13.7%) and among children (17.3%.), thoughthe prevalence or association of mental disorders with substance use was not reported. Five focus group discussions were conducted as a part of qualitative assessment in this study, but the total number of participants, process of data analysis and presentation of the findings for this part was not clear as frequency and percentage of some 'factors as causes of substance use' were presented (Ministry of Health & Family Welfare, 2021a, 2021b).

Another cross sectional study conducted in the inpatient and outpatient departments of psychiatric settings of 13 selected hospitals in Bangladesh explored the prevalence and pattern of comorbid mental illnesses in substance use disorders (Ahmed et al., 2020). Inclusion criteria was not clear in the study. In the method it was claimed that inclusion criteria was—'lifetime history of any substance use' and also in the result section and tables, mostly 'lifetime substance use' was mentioned. But in the methods, it was mentioned that during the study period, all the patients (19663) who visited the 13 settings, were interviewed and 9143 of them were included as they were seeking treatment for their addiction problems at that time which indicates that the participants were current substance abusers. MINI International Neuropsychiatric Interview (MINI) was used for screening purpose in the study, though MINI is a structured diagnostic psychiatric interview. Again, the number of screen positive

**Table 7.2** Recent (2014–2023) published articles in which both substance use disorders and psychiatric disorders or symptoms were addressed

| Author and year | Study type | Study place | Study population | Sampling technique | Sample size | Investigated issue related to dual diagnosis |
|---|---|---|---|---|---|---|
| Sarker et al. (2023) | Cross sectional | Pabna | Community people (12–35 years age) | Random | 600 | Psychiatric symptoms among substance users |
| Maruf et al. (2022) | Hospital records analysis | A private deaddiction clinic in Dhaka | Hospitalized methamphetamine abusers | Consecutive | 115 | Frequency and types of psychiatric disorders |
| Moonajilin et al. (2021) | Cross sectional | Savar, Dhaka | High school-going adolescents | 3 stage cluster sampling | 424 | Risk factors of substance use |
| Patoari (2021) | Cross sectional + qualitative | Chattogram and Noakhali | Male substance abusers | Convenient | 136 | Psychological aspects of substance abuse |
| Khan et al. (2021a, 2021b) | Cross sectional | Two drug addiction treatment centers, Dhaka | Adolescent male with substance use | Convenient | 70 | Psychiatric comorbidity |
| Ahmed et al. (2020) | Cross sectional | Government psychiatric hospitals, medical colleges and CTC | Treatment-seeking patients with substance use disorders | Consecutive | 9143 | Psychiatric morbidity |
| Islam and Hossain (2017) | Cross sectional | Bangladesh | Substance users (100) and non-users (100) | Purposive | 200 | Mental health issues as risk factor and consequences |
| Islam and Biswas (2015) | Cross sectional | Drug addiction treatment center in Mymensingh | Substance users | Purposive | 38 | Psychological factors as a reason |
| Maruf et al. (2015a, 2015b) | Cross sectional | Juvenile development Center, Gazipur | Male juvenile offenders | Consecutive | 138 | Psychiatric disorder in substance use |
| Maruf et al. (2015a, 2015b) | Cross sectional | Juvenile development Center, Gazipur | Female juvenile offenders | Consecutive | 43 | Substance use in psychiatric disorders |
| Zaman et al. (2014) | Cross sectional | CTC, Dhaka | Male substance users in detoxification | Convenient | 300 | Psychosocial illness |

samples was not mentioned. According to data collection technique, at first, research psychiatrists confirmed the diagnose of mental disorders according to DSM 5 criteria before taking detailed socioeconomic and related clinical and substance use related information from the respondents. Besides the 'others' category, 20 types of psychiatric disorders (either single disorder or group of disorders) were found comorbid, though standard MINI diagnose 17 common psychiatric disorders. Again, though the frequency of 'schizophrenia spectrum and other psychotic disorders' was estimated as a whole, the frequency of 'delusional disorder' (which is a disorder in the category of 'schizophrenia spectrum and other psychotic disorders') was separately mentioned in the calculation of total frequency. Same was done for 'panic disorder' and 'specific/social phobia' whereas the frequency of 'anxiety disorders' as a whole was estimated.

## 7.9 Challenges of Management of Substance Abuse with Mental Health Conditions in Bangladesh

Persons with dual diagnoses encounter unique challenges compared to the persons having either mental health conditions or substance use disorders. Their risk of homelessness, confinement and relapse are particularly high. Moreover, one condition, specially if untreated, can worsen the other. Therefore, management strategies should comprehensively address and deal with all the conditions (Substance Abuse & Mental Health Services Administration, 2020). Developing and disseminating such services for co-occurring disorders in Bangladesh, like in many other low-or-middle-income countries (LMIC), can be challenging due to a variety of social, cultural, economic, and healthcare system factors. The significant challenges are as follows:

### *7.9.1 Poor Awareness Along with High Stigma*

High social stigma attached to both mental health conditions and substance use disorders and poor literacy regarding mental health issues can be important determinants that hamper the treatment of co-occurring disorders in the country. Various studies reported the high prevalence of mental health stigma and misconceptions in Bangladesh which act as barriers to accessing mental health care (Faruk et al., 2023; Ministry of Health & Family Welfare, 2021a, 2021b; Nuri et al., 2018). According to a study conducted on the relapsed patients taking treatment in drug addiction centers, almost two-thirds of the substance abusers perceived social stigma, more than half experienced bullying, and half of the participants felt isolated from society and lack of additional support (Hawlader et al., 2020).

### 7.9.2 *Inadequate and Separate Services for Mental Health and Substance Abuse*

Available mental health services and services for substance abuse are significantly inadequate compared to the needs of the distressed. Services for both the conditions are negligible in primary and secondary health care. In tertiary health care settings, there are few service providing institutions, which have been discussed in the relevant part of the chapter, but drug addiction and mental health services remain largely separated. CTC and the other government drug addiction treatment centers are under the direct control of DNC, a part of the Ministry of Home. Private drug addiction treatment/rehabilitation centers are also licensed and monitored by DNC. The requirements for running the centers are different from the criteria of a psychiatric clinic/hospital mentioned by Directorate General of Health Services (DGHS) under Ministry of Health and Family Welfare. Therefore, if any clinic/hospital wants to provide inpatient services for both substance abuse and mental health conditions, it needs to take legal clearance from both DNC and DGHS, which is a cumbersome and lengthy process. There is lack of coordination between the two ministries.

### 7.9.3 *Lack of Skilled Manpower*

Available personnel in mental healthcare and services for drug addiction in Bangladesh is limited and skewed in distribution. Very few healthcare professionals in Bangladesh are trained in providing psychiatric services (0.49%) let alone substance abuse. There are only 270 psychiatrists and 565 psychologists in the country, the majority being working in the urban areas (World Health Organization, 2020). There is scarcity also in other related manpower including psychiatric social worker, psychiatric nurses, case manager, recovery coach, ward boy etc. to run a service for dual problems. To fill up the gap and to create personnel with at least basic level training on management of substance abuse incorporating co-occurring disorders, CTC has been conducting training based on 'Universal Treatment Curriculum' of International Center for Credentialing and Education of Addiction Professionals since 2013 for persons from different background including psychiatrist, doctor, clinical psychologist, psychologist, nurse, recovering addict, clinic owner, etc. However, though more than 2300 persons got basic level training, only 54 of them cleared the basic level examination for becoming *International Certified Addiction Professional* (ICAP) and only 1 person completed the next level among the 4 levels of ICAP examination.

### 7.9.4 Negligible Budget

The fund availability for the management of co-occurring disorders, research on substance abuse and mental health services are undeniably insufficient. Less than 0.5% of total government health budget is devoted to mental health in Bangladesh, 67% of which are allocated for mental hospitals (Islam & Biswas, 2015). In non-government settings, large groups or companies show less interest on investing in mental health and drug addiction services. A major share of the budget of DNC is devoted to the legal aspects of drug addiction. Therefore, co-occurring disorders suffer a deficiency of funding overall.

### 7.9.5 Complicated System of Care

Service-providers and the persons suffering from co-occurring disorders alike may find it challenging to navigate the complex treatment procedures for the dual problems. The treatment consists of outpatient and inpatient treatment, medication, individual, group and family counseling, follow-up with psychiatrist and psychologist, as well as additional services, mutual support and other programs. Navigating through this multi-sectoral process can lead to delays and drop outs in treatment, especially in a LMIC like Bangladesh where there is a lack of facilities and skilled professionals.

### 7.9.6 Poor Research and Data Quality

Countrywide epidemiological study to identify the actual burden of dual diagnoses, even the frequency of substance related disorders, has not been conducted in Bangladesh. A community-based study estimated the frequency of lifetime substance users, and a multiple center-based study reported the frequency of comorbid psychiatric disorders in substance abusers, but the quality of data in those studies is questionable, which has been discussed in the relevant part of this chapter. The number of yearly service users from CTC and other government drug addiction treatment centers under DNC are found, but those do not contain the information regarding co-occurring disorders. DNC publishes the information regarding the amount of seized drugs and the number of cases and arrests for drug dealing and other drug-related legal actions, but those are not of significant help from the clinical ground.

### *7.9.7 Lack of Clarity and Discrepancy in Existing Laws*

Bangladesh has limited policies and regulations in place to govern treatment programs for co-occurring disorders and the quality of care provided. Substance abuse is criminalized from a legal perspective. Moreover, there are discrepancies in the definitions of some related terms including mental disorder, mental illness, drug addiction, mental hospital, drug addiction treatment center/ rehabilitation center, mental health professionals, psychologist etc. among the various laws related to mental health and substance abuse. Issues of co-occurring disorders are not addressed properly in the existing laws. There is also a lack of clarity and discrepancies in the laws regarding the establishment and maintenance of healthcare centers for the dual problems (Mental Health Act, 2018; Narcotics Control Act, 2018).

## 7.10 Future Direction for Services Development in Bangladesh

### *7.10.1 Integration of Services for Substance Abuse and Mental Health Conditions*

In the Integrated Treatment approach, one or more specialists contribute in each multidisciplinary treatment team in the healthcare center. They cross-train other team members to circulate information and skills about managing patients with dual problems. Working in multidisciplinary teams also ensures that management strategy addresses the individual's goals related to both substance abuse and mental health conditions. Integrated treatment for substance abuse and mental health conditions is associated with decreased substance use, improvement in psychiatric problems and functioning, reduced hospitalization, more stable housing, fewer incarcerations, and better quality of life (SAMSA, 2020). Besides tertiary care settings, primary health care centers in government level are also appropriate places of integration. This could increase access to and retention in treatment and better health outcomes. Early diagnosis and brief behavioral change counseling in primary care can be effective in managing substance abuse before it turns to dependency. The strength of primary care is in its providers' skills to deal with the range of healthcare issues associated with substance abuse (Kaswa, 2021).

### 7.10.2 Developing Skilled Manpower

Measures need to be taken to develop skilled manpower working in the field of co-occurring disorders. Every year, around 30 psychiatrists are entering in professional field completing any kind of post-graduation course, which does not allow to meet the country's need of psychiatrists. Physicians should be encouraged more to take psychiatry as a career choice and proper incentives should be there. More MD (Psychiatry) courses should be arranged in old and reputed government medical colleges. Related graduation and post-graduation courses should be made available and expanded for the other professionals working in the field. Opportunities of job for psychologists, occupational therapists, social workers and related others should be made in healthcare centers dealing with co-occurring disorders. Basic training for all concerned professionals including peer counselors and case managers in private drug addiction centers, based on 'Universal Treatment Curriculum' of International Center for Credentialing and Education of Addiction Professionals may be conducted by NIMH and Mental Hospital, Pabna in addition to CTC and DAM. Besides, more emphasis should be given on mental health and substance abuse in undergraduate medical curriculum to have general physicians capable of dealing with co-occurring disorders in primary care.

### 7.10.3 Intersectoral Collaboration

Intersectoral collaboration is necessary since the risk factors for substance abuse and mental health conditions are linked with many areas. A whole-of-society method works including government sectors or departments, non-government and community groups and facilitates exchange of knowledge and experience and sharing of substance and mental health-related data and research among them. Collaboration among the professionals such as psychiatrists, other clinicians, psychologists, nurses, social workers, researchers, media professionals, and social scientists is important. Collaboration specially among the Ministry of Health and Family Welfare, Ministry of Home Affairs, Ministry of Social Welfare, Ministry of Education, Ministry of Youth and Sports among others are imperative for the effective management including prevention of substance abuse issues comorbid with mental health conditions. There should be synchronization in the initiatives of government, non-government and voluntary organizations working in the field of substance abuse and mental health. Support from international organizations should be incorporated effectively in this regard.

### 7.10.4 Information and Communication Technology (ICT)-Based Management

Considering the substantial gap between the number of individuals seeking treatment for co-occurring disorders and the capacity to offer adequate and timely health support in terms of available professionals, ICT-based solutions or e-health appear to offer cost effective and efficient opportunities for clinicians, health administrators and decision-makers to expand service availability and reduce treatment gap. Interventions can be offered via different approaches, including telephone counseling and web-based video conferencing tools, self-directed desktop therapeutic tools, web-based text communication (email, chat, forums), as well as e-Health. Though there are limitations related to digital literacy, safety and confidentiality and other issues, ICT-based interventions for mental health issues and some addictive behaviors have proved to be effective in various countries (Fonseca & Osma, 2021; Guo et al., 2023).

### 7.10.5 Quality Data and Research

There should be a national guideline for the management of co-occurring disorders formulating feasible pharmacological and psychosocial approaches considering the country's economic socio-cultural and legal context. This guideline should be evidence-based and prepared following a standard process. Quality research following sound methodology and ethical principles are important to generate reliable data that can be the basis of the standards of care. For quality research, adequate funding to the legitimate and trustworthy research projects is essential.

### 7.10.6 Raising Awareness

To decrease stigma and increase awareness regarding substance abuse and mental health conditions, community level efforts are necessary targeting the local political and religious leaders, teachers of schools and colleges, journalists and youth. Awareness campaigns should target a public audience and be conducted through an organized process of communication to draw people's attention to the fact that substance abuse with comorbid mental health conditions is a serious public health issue which is controllable and preventable. Advocacy targeting the policy makers and authority personnel aims to bring about changes such as decriminalization of substance related disorders and multi-sectoral collaboration. It may also help to decrease stigma and negative attitudes among people with co-occurring disorders.

### *7.10.7 Reform of the Existing Laws and Regulations*

Substance related disorders are mental health issues rather than legal problems only. Decriminalization of the persons with substance related disorders must be prioritized so that these populations can have their access to treatment instead of punishment. Legal process of establishment and maintenance of healthcare facilities should be hassle-free and consumer-friendly. Reform and revise of various laws and regulations related to co-occurring disorders including Mental Health Act (2018) and Narcotics Control Act (2018) in accordance with international standards, and the constitution of Bangladesh is the pivotal area to focus on to overcome current and future challenges as strategy directs actions.

## 7.11 Conclusion

In Bangladesh, mental health is a neglected entity. Substance use is also stigmatized and seen more from a legal ground than medical. Though comorbidities of substance use and mental health conditions are commonly prevalent in Bangladesh, the services for the management of the conditions are inadequate. There is a lack of skilled manpower, health care facilities and financial resources to deal with the dual problem. Poor awareness, high stigma, separate and poorly coordinated services for mental health and substance abuse, complicated system of care, lack of clarity and discrepancies in local laws and regulations etc. are other significant barriers in proper management of the dual issues. Moreover, a dearth of research may be failing to reveal the gravity of the real situation to the policymakers. Good quality research with trustworthy data, proper training for human resources, intersectoral collaboration for integrated services addressing both the issues, ICT-based management, awareness building in the community and revision of concerned laws and regulations should be the priorities for effective service delivery for the individuals with co-occurring disorders in Bangladesh.

## References

Ahmed, H. U., Alam, M. T., Sarkar, M., Alam, M. F., Hossain, M. D., Bhowmik, A. D., Khan, N. M., Uddin, M. M. J., Royle, R. K. S., Khan, M. Z. R., Sarkar, A. A., Hossain, R., Islam, M. R., Podder, B. R. R., Kalam, M., Acharjee, P., & Hossain, M. J. (2020). Psychiatric comorbidity among the patients with substance use disorders in Bangladesh. *Archives of NIMH, 3*(1), 7–12.

*Bangladesh Rehabilitation and Assistance Center for Addicts.*Retrieved October 16, 2023, from https://www.baracabd.org

Department of Narcotics Control. (2017). *Baseline study on drug addiction in Bangladesh.* (Project report). Dhaka: Ministry of Home, Bangladesh. Retrieved October 10, 2023, from https://dnc.gov.bd/site/files/f20344f2-c63b-4761-9535-ff4f49b97cf8

Department of Narcotics Control. (2018). *Annual drug report Bangladesh 2018*. Dhaka: Ministry of Home, Bangladesh. Retrieved November 9, 2023, from https://dnc.gov.bd/site/view/annual_reports/

Department of Narcotics Control. (2018). Cause and victim of drug addiction and way forward for establishment of adequate treatment and rehabilitation facilities at private sector in Bangladesh. (Project report). Dhaka: Ministry of Home, Bangladesh. Retrieved October 10, 2023, from https://dnc.gov.bd/site/files/f20344f2-c63b-4761-9535-ff4f49b97cf8

Department of Narcotics Control. (2022). Annual drug report Bangladesh 2022. Ministry of Home, Bangladesh. Retrieved October 19, 2023, from https://dnc.gov.bd/site/view/annual_reports/

Department of Narcotics Control. (2023). Annual report 2022–23. Dhaka: Ministry of Home, Bangladesh. Retrieved November 9, 2023, from https://dnc.gov.bd/site/view/annual_reports/

Dhaka Ahsania Mission. Retrieved October 16, 2023, from https://www.amic.org.bd

Faruk, M. O., Khan, A. H., Chowdhury, K. U. A., Jahan, S., Sarker, D. C., Colucci, E., & Hasan, M. T. (2023). Mental illness stigma in Bangladesh: Findings from a cross-sectional survey. *Global Mental Health (cambridge, England), 10*, e59. https://doi.org/10.1017/gmh.2023.56

Fonseca, A., & Osma, J. (2021). Using information and communication technologies (ICT) for mental health prevention and treatment. *International Journal of Environmental Research and Public Health, 18*(2), 461. https://doi.org/10.3390/ijerph18020461

Guo, H., Yang, H., Yuan, G., Zhu, Z., Zhang, K., Zhang, X., Lu, X., Zhang, J., Du, J., Shi, H., Jin, G., Hao, J., Sun, Y., Su, P., & Zhang, Z. (2023). Effectiveness of information and communication technology (ICT) for addictive behaviors: An umbrella review of systematic reviews and meta-analysis of randomized controlled trials. *Computers in Human Behavior, 147*, 107843. https://doi.org/10.1016/j.chb.2023.107843

Hasan, M. T., Anwar, T., Christopher, E., Hossain, S., Hossain, M. M., Koly, K. N., Saif-Ur-Rahman, K. M., Ahmed, H. U., Arman, N., & Hossain, S. W. (2021). The current state of mental healthcare in Bangladesh: Part 1—An updated country profile. *Bjpsych International, 18*(4), 78–82. https://doi.org/10.1192/bji.2021.41

Hawlader, M. D. H., Nabi, M. H., Hussain, A., Al Amin, S. U., Zaman, S., & Masud, I. (2020). Legal and social consequences of substance use: Results from a nationwide study in Bangladesh. *Journal of Ethnicity in Substance Abuse*, 1–11. Advance online publication. https://doi.org/10.1080/15332640.2020.1846008

Hossain, M. D., Ahmed, H. U., Chowdhury, W. A., Niessen, L. W., & Alam, D. S. (2014). Mental disorders in Bangladesh: A systematic review. *BMC Psychiatry, 14*, 216. https://doi.org/10.1186/s12888-014-0216-9

Hunt, G. E., Large, M. M., Cleary, M., Lai, H. M. X., & Saunders, J. B. (2018). Prevalence of comorbid substance use in schizophrenia spectrum disorders in community and clinical settings, 1990–2017: Systematic review and meta-analysis. *Drug and Alcohol Dependence, 191*, 234–258. https://doi.org/10.1016/j.drugalcdep.2018.07.011

Hunt, G. E., Malhi, G. S., Cleary, M., Lai, H. M., & Sitharthan, T. (2016a). Comorbidity of bipolar and substance use disorders in national surveys of general populations, 1990–2015: Systematic review and meta-analysis. *Journal of Affective Disorders, 206*, 321–330. https://doi.org/10.1016/j.jad.2016.06.051

Hunt, G. E., Malhi, G. S., Cleary, M., Lai, H. M., & Sitharthan, T. (2016b). Prevalence of comorbid bipolar and substance use disorders in clinical settings, 1990–2015: Systematic review and meta-analysis. *Journal of Affective Disorders, 206*, 331–349. https://doi.org/10.1016/j.jad.2016.07.011

Hunt, G. E., Malhi, G. S., Lai, H. M. X., & Cleary, M. (2020). Prevalence of comorbid substance use in major depressive disorder in community and clinical settings, 1990–2019: Systematic review and meta-analysis. *Journal of Affective Disorders, 266*, 288–304. https://doi.org/10.1016/j.jad.2020.01.141

Huque, R., Azad, A. K., Ahmed, H. U., & Amin, M. R. (2023). Mental health care seeking behavior in Bangladesh: Evidence from the National Mental Health Survey 2019. (preprint). https://doi.org/10.21203/rs.3.rs-2736863/v1

Islam, A. & Biswas, T. (2015). Mental health and the health system in Bangladesh: Situation analysis of a neglected domain. *American Journal of Psychiatry and Neuroscience, 3*(4), 57–62. https://doi.org/10.11648/j.ajpn.20150304.11

Islam, A., & Hossain, M. F. (2017). Drug abuse and its impact on Bangladesh. *International Journal of Sociology and Anthropology, 9*(11), 143–156. https://doi.org/10.5897/IJSA2016.0736

Kamal, M., Huq, N., Mali, B., Akter, H., & Arafat, S. M. Y. (2018). Epidemiology of substance abuse in Bangladesh: A narrative review. *Journal of Mental Disorders and Treatment, 4*, 165. https://doi.org/10.4172/2471-271X.1000165

Karim, M. E., & Shaikh, S. (2021). Newly enacted mental health law in Bangladesh. *Bjpsych International, 18*(4), 85–87. https://doi.org/10.1192/bji.2021.1

Kaswa, R. (2021). Primary healthcare approach to substance abuse management. *South African Family Practice: Official Journal of the South African Academy of Family Practice/primary Care, 63*(1), e1–e4. https://doi.org/10.4102/safp.v63i1.5307

Khan, N. M, Mullick, M. S. I., & Hussain, S. (2021). Psychiatric comorbidity among adolescents with substance use disorder. *American journal of psychiatry and neuroscience, 9*(3), 98–106. https://doi.org/10.11648/j.ajpn.20210903.14

Khan, S. I., Khan, M. N. M., Irfan, S. D., Rumayan Hasan, A. M., Ross, A. G., Horng, L. M., Lachowsky, N., Knudson, G., & Azim, T. (2021b). The effects of methamphetamine use on the sexual lives of gender and sexually diverse people in Dhaka, Bangladesh: A qualitative study. *Archives of Sexual Behavior, 50*(2), 479–493. https://doi.org/10.1007/s10508-020-01674-2

Khanom, S. (2023). Substance use disorder among patients with obsessive compulsive disorder. FCPS dissertation (unpublished).

Maehira, Y., Chowdhury, E. I., Reza, M., Drahozal, R., Gayen, T. K., Masud, I., Afrin, S., Takamura, N., & Azim, T. (2013). Factors associated with relapse into drug use among male and female attendees of a three-month drug detoxification-rehabilitation programme in Dhaka, Bangladesh: A prospective cohort study. *Harm Reduction Journal, 10*, 14. https://doi.org/10.1186/1477-7517-10-14

Maruf, M. M., Alam, M. T., Khan, N. M., Khan, M. Z. R., Begum, K., Mamun, A. A., & Chowdhury, M. W. A. (2012). Substance abuse among male patients with major depressive disorder. *Bangladesh Journal of Psychiatry, 26*(1), 54–63.

Maruf, M. M., Jahan, N., Bhowmik, A. D., Syed, S. E., Alam, M. T., Rahman, F., Sarker, M., & Khan, M. Z. R. (2013). Opioid use: Sociodemography and some related factors. *Bangladesh Journal of Psychiatry, 27*(1), 20–27.

Maruf, M. M., Jahan, N., Khan, M. Z. R., Haq, A. I., Akhter, J., Rishad, M. M., & Kamal, M. (2021). Co-morbidities and family history among methamphetamine users. *Bangladesh Medical Journal, 50*(2), 15–20. https://doi.org/10.3329/bmj.v50i2.61173

Maruf, M. M., Khan, M. Z. R., & Jahan, N. (2016). Pattern of substance use: Study in a de-addiction clinic. *Oman Medical Journal, 31*(5), 327–331. https://doi.org/10.5001/omj.2016.66

Maruf, M. M., Rahman, F., Khan, M. Z. R., & Jahan, N. (2015). Psychiatric morbidity and substance abuse among male juvenile offenders in Bangladesh. *Life: International journal of health and life-sciences, 1*(1), 161–171. https://doi.org/10.20319/lijshls.2015.s11.161171

Maruf, M. M., Rahman, F., Khan, M. Z. R., & Jahan, N. (2015). Socio-demography, substance abuse and offence among inmates with psychiatric disorders in female juvenile centre, Bangladesh. *People: International Journal of Social Sciences, 1*(1), 500–508. https://doi.org/10.20319/pijss.2015.s21.500508

Mental Health Act. (2018). Bangladesh. [Online]. Retrieved October 12, 2023, from https://legislativediv.gov.bd/site/page/3c13bbde-76b4-41fc-89cab738dd04a0bb

Ministry of Health and Family Welfare. (2021). National Mental Health Survey 2019. (project report). Dhaka: Ministry of Health and Family Welfare, Bangladesh. Retrieved October 29, 2023, from http://nimh.gov.bd/wp-content/uploads/2021/11/Mental-Health-Survey-Report.pdf

Ministry of Health and Family Welfare. (2021). Prevalence and associated factors of substance use in Bangladesh. (Project report). Dhaka: Ministry of Health and Family Welfare, Bangladesh.

Retrieved October 29, 2023, from https://nimh.gov.bd/english/wp-content/uploads/2021/11/Substance-Use-Full.pdf
Moonajilin, M. S., Kamal, M. K. I., Mamun, F. A., Safiq, M. B., Hosen, I., Manzar, M. D., & Mamun, M. A. (2021). Substance use behavior and its lifestyle-related risk factors in Bangladeshi high school-going adolescents: An exploratory study. *PLoS ONE, 16*(7), e0254926. https://doi.org/10.1371/journal.pone.0254926
Narcotics Control Act. (2018). Bangladesh. [Online]. Retrieved October 12, 2023, from https://legislativediv.gov.bd/site/page/3c13bbde-76b4-41fc-89cab738dd04a0bb
National Institute of Mental Health. (2023). Retrieved October 29, 2023, from https://nimh.gov.bd/english/
Nuri, N. N., Sarker, M., Ahmed, H. U., Hossain, M. D., Beiersmann, C., & Jahn, A. (2018). Pathways to care of patients with mental health problems in Bangladesh. *International Journal of Mental Health Systems, 12*(1), 39. https://doi.org/10.1186/s13033-018-0218-y
Patoari, M. M. H. (2021). Socio-cultural, psychological and family aspects of drug addiction of adolescents and its impact: An analysis from Bangladesh perspective. *Journal of Advanced Research in Social Sciences and Humanities, 6*(1), 1–14. https://doi.org/10.26500/JARSSH-06-2021-0101
Rahman, K. F. (2019). Is punitive action enough to prevent abuse of drug?. The daily star. Retrieved November 10, 2023, from https://www.thedailystar.net/law-our-rights/law-analysis/news/punitive-action-enough-prevent-abuse-drug-1697473
Roy, J., Morshed, N. M., Qusar, M. M. A. S., Nahar, J. S., Miah, M. A. S., Shah, M. A., Shams, S. F., Shahid, S. F. B., Ikbal, M. M., & Khanom, M. M. (2010). Personality traits of substance users in Bangladesh. *BSMMU Journal, 3*(2), 76–81. https://doi.org/10.3329/bsmmuj.v3i2.7056
SAMSA. (2020). Substance use disorder treatment for people With co-occurring disorders.
Sarker, A. K., Raju, F. R., Sultana, M. P., Milon, M. M. M., & Akter, S. (2023). Exploration of drug addiction prevalence among young generation of Pabna district, Bangladesh. *Journal of Drug Delivery and Therapeutics, 13*(3), 78–84. https://doi.org/10.22270/jddt.v13i3.5764
Shultana. F. (2022). Exploring barriers in seeking mental health services. M.phil thesis.
Soron, T. R., Siddike, P. M. A., Ahmed, H. U., & Chowdhury, C. A. (2017). Social and family determinants of substance abuse among the patients of two hospitals in Bangladesh. *Journal of Addiction Research and Therapy, 8*, 340. https://doi.org/10.4172/2155-6105.1000340
Substance Abuse and Mental Health Services Administration. (2020). Substance use disorder treatment for people with co-occurring disorders: Treatment Improvement Protocol (TIP 42). Department of Health and Human Services, US. https://store.samhsa.gov/sites/default/files/SAMHSA_Digital_Download/PEP20-02-01-004_Final_508.pdf
Swendsen, J., Conway, K. P., Degenhardt, L., Glantz, M., Jin, R., Merikangas, K. R., Sampson, N., & Kessler, R. C. (2010). Mental disorders as risk factors for substance use, abuse and dependence: Results from the 10-year follow-up of the National Comorbidity Survey. *Addiction (ablngdon, England), 105*(6), 1117–1128. https://doi.org/10.1111/j.1360-0443.2010.02902.x
World Health Organization. (2020). Bangladesh WHO special initiative for mental health situational assessment. https://www.who.int/docs/default-source/mental-health/special-initiative/who-special-initiative-country-report---bangladesh---2020.pdf?sfvrsn=c2122a0e_2
Zaman, B., Ahmed, S. M., Hossain, M. M., & Kamal, M. M. (2015). Psychosocial illness among the drug abusers undergoing detoxification in Dhaka, Bangladesh. *South East Asia Journal of Public Health, 4*(2), 36–41. https://doi.org/10.3329/seajph.v4i2.23693

# Chapter 8
# Community Psychiatry in Bangladesh: Development and Current Status

**Md. Enayet Karim, Rahanul Islam, Atiqul Haq Mazumder, and S. M. Yasir Arafat**

**Abstract** Community psychiatry is the practice of providing mental health services in the community rather than in long-term institutions. It aims to improve the quality of life and human rights of people with mental disorders or disabilities. Bangladesh faces many challenges in implementing effective and accessible community psychiatric services. These include a lack of resources, a high treatment gap, a low awareness, and a strong stigma. The country has recently adopted new policies and laws to promote community psychiatry, such as the *Mental Health Act* 2018 and the *Mental Health Policy* 2019. These policies emphasize a psychosocial approach, decentralization, and community participation. The country also plans to establish 18,000 community clinics to provide primary care services, including mental health screening, identification, and counseling. Moreover, some innovative initiatives have been launched, such as the "First Day-centers Meaningful Social Access for Persons with Mental Health Needs" project and telepsychiatry. These initiatives aim to provide comprehensive and holistic care to people with mental health needs in the community. However, more efforts are needed to overcome the existing barriers and gaps in community psychiatric services in Bangladesh.

**Keywords** Bangladesh · Community psychiatry · Bangladesh psychiatry · Mental health · Psychiatric services · Human resource

Md. E. Karim
Department of Psychiatry, MH Samorita Hospital & Medical College, Dhaka, Bangladesh

R. Islam
Central Drug Addiction Treatment, Resident Psychiatrist, Dhaka, Bangladesh

A. H. Mazumder
Department of Adult Psychiatry, National Institute of Mental Health, Dhaka, Bangladesh

S. M. Y. Arafat (✉)
Department of Psychiatry, Bangladesh Specialized Hospital Limited, Dhaka, Bangladesh
e-mail: arafatdmc62@gmail.com



S. M. Y. Arafat (ed.), *Mental Health in Bangladesh*,
https://doi.org/10.1007/978-981-97-0610-5_8

## 8.1 Introduction

The concept of community psychiatry may be recognized when we consider the historical aspect of modern mental health services delivery in Europe and the USA (Farooq & Minhas, 2001). Deinstitutionalization is the practice of transitioning individuals diagnosed with mental disorders or developmental disabilities from long-term psychiatric institutions to more integrated community mental health services (Eisenberg & Guttmacher, 2010). It started in the late twentieth century, when psychiatric drugs made it easier to treat psychotic symptoms and social-political movements advocated for patient rights. It also helped governments save money by closing many psychiatric hospitals (Fakhoury & Priebe, 2007). It resulted in the cessation of many mental hospitals, with persons with mental illness increasingly receiving care at home settings, in clinics and hospitals, or sometimes not receiving care at all. Some patients did not receive adequate care in the community or became homeless or criminals (Lamb & Bachrach, 2001).

The historical roots of 'community psychiatry' can be traced back to countries like England, France, Italy, and the USA, where it evolved based on specific principles and the existing pattern of mental health services in these Western nations. In 1963, the *Community Mental Health Act* (CMHA) was passed by Congress and signed by President Kennedy. The aim of the CMHA was to reduce the number of institutionalized patients by fostering autonomous and community psychiatry centers (Erickson, 2021). This led to a significant push towards community psychiatry in the high income countries, resulting in the emergence of various programs. However, the growth and implementation of community psychiatry as a service in national strategies differ between low and middle income and high income countries.

The effective engagement of individuals grappling with chronic mental health issues is crucial for any intervention or service to be successful in the society. Communities possess distinct knowledge about their circumstances and needs, which, when combined with scientific expertise, is essential for the delivery of effective and accessible services (Bouras, 2017). The creation and quality evaluation of services for screening, prevention, testing, and treatment by groups of drug users and other relevant populations can aid in ensuring the effectiveness of services designed to address the needs of individuals marginalized due to various chronic psychiatric conditions.

## 8.2 History of Community Psychiatry in Bangladesh

Prior to 1947, under British governance, the development of psychiatric services adhered to the asylum model, and at that time, the concept of community psychiatry was not yet established. Although the movement towards community psychiatry began in India in the early 1950s (Chadda, 2012), the path in Bangladesh (previously known as East Pakistan) followed a different trajectory.

The psychiatry movement in Bangladesh began after the establishment of the first mental hospital in the Pabna district in 1957 (Arafat et al., 2024, 2024a, b). Interestingly, this mental hospital largely embodied the asylum philosophy, given its remote location, isolation, focused treatment for psychosis patients, and absence of other medical specialties. It had several cottages where the patient's caregivers could stay with them within the hospital grounds, often for extended periods of time.

Post the liberation war in 1971, Bangladesh has experienced various stages of progress. This began with family care for mentally ill individuals within the premises of a single mental hospital, leading to the establishment of satellite clinics and a national mental health program. Other initiatives have included medical camps, efforts by non-government organizations and the media, mental health services for populations affected by disasters, and weekly private practice sessions by psychiatrists and psychologists in various remote districts.

## 8.3 Legal Frameworks and Policy for Community Psychiatry in Bangladesh

In a bid to safeguard the dignity of individuals with psychiatric disorders, providing mental health services, ensure their property rights, and support their rehabilitation, Bangladesh replaced the 105-year-old Lunacy Act of 1912 with the Mental Health Act (2018). This Act, which consists of 31 sections, will ensure the supervision and coordination of matters related to mental health and the responsibilities assigned to the government (Mental Health Act, 2018). While this law discourages prolonged hospital stays, it doesn't contain a specific clause addressing community psychiatry.

The new *Mental Health Policy*, endorsed by the Ministry of Health in 2019, signifies a transition from a biomedical to a biopsychosocial treatment approach. This policy emphasizes the development of decentralized and community-based mental health care, as well as support for individuals living with mental illness (World Health Organization, 2021).

## 8.4 Generic Mental Health Services in Bangladesh

The mental health services delivery has been mentioned in Chap. 3 of this book (Arafat, 2024a). It has been further elaborately discussed in another book chapter by Arafat and his colleagues (Arafat et al., 2024, 2024a, b). The health system reaches the community individuals by existing public, private, and non-governmental organization (NGO)-supported health services, hospitals, health centers and clinics through all administrative levels from capital to unions and wards. The national budget for mental health services is less than 0.05% of total health expenditure and 60% of the budget is directed to mental hospitals (World Health Organization, 2021).

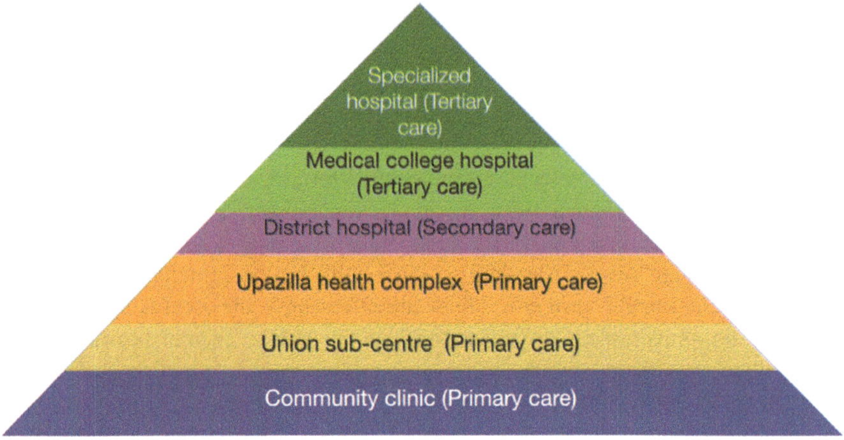


**Fig. 8.1** Health service delivery levels in Bangladesh (adapted from Arafat et al., 2024, Arafat, S. M. Y.,2024a, b; Facility Registry, 2023; Government of the People's Republic of Bangladesh, 2022)

Since the independence, Bangladesh has developed a well-structure health services care delivery system between the community and the specialist level (Fig. 8.1). It included community clinic, Upazila Health Complex (UHC), District (Sadar) Hospital, Medical Colleges and specialized institutions, and medical universities. It has been planned to develop 18,000 community clinics (one for every six thousand people), so that community level health care services can be available within a distance of half-an hour walk. However, currently, 13,707 community clinics are providing health care services to the community people in the country. Along with this established structure, health services delivery persons deliver different domiciliary health services. The clinics are managed by the *Community Clinic Management Committee*. There are staffs for three different services i.e., health and disease, population service, and community health care. The clinics are managed at union level and there are 4700 unions in Bangladesh (Fig. 8.1).

The next level of service delivery has been provided by UHC at Thana level followed by Sadar hospitals at district level. At the Government level health services, usually, psychiatric patients are referred to secondary and tertiary care level services. Unfortunately, there is no allocated post for mental health specialist (Psychiatrist) at secondary level care in Bangladesh (Arafat et al., 2024, 2024a, b; Government of the People's Republic of Bangladesh, 2022). Treatment of psychiatric emergencies with inpatient care is available at tertiary care level and specialized institutions such as public and private medical college hospitals, *National Institute of Mental Health and Hospital* (NIMH), and the Mental Hospital at Pabna.

## 8.5 Community Psychiatric Services

Community-based mental health services refer to services provided outside of a hospital setting within the community, regardless of whether it's an urban or rural area. These services utilize resources available in the community and are aided, supported, and supervised by mental health professionals. They are integrated with both primary health care and general health services. The reflection of the community psychiatric services includes the available number of community-based outpatient services outlets like community psychiatric centers, additional outpatient facilities like day care services, and psychiatric community residential services for adults.

A psychiatric community residential service is a non-clinical, community-focused establishment that provides accommodation for individuals with psychiatric illness. Typically, the services cater to individuals with comparatively manageable state of psychiatric illness that do not require intensive and active psychiatric management. They encompass supervised residential facility, unstaffed group homes, group homes managed by few residential or visiting staff, hostels with daytime staffs, hostels with whole day staff, residential facility with whole day nursing services, halfway houses, and therapeutic communities. The services may include facilities for specific populations like children and adolescents or elderly. Probably, *Organization of Training in Mental Health* (OTMH) started by Prof. Dr. Hidayetul Islam in 1978 was the first community psychiatry initiative in Bangladesh (Chowdhury et al., 2024). OTMH gained popularity specially for its training activity for the general physicians. Subsequently, he established *Dhaka Monorog Clinic* and *Institute of Community Mental Health* (ICMH) in 1983 which was registered in 1984 (Arafat et al., 2020). ICMH arranged 60 days of training for social welfare students. It also had other training activities (Islam, 2019).

### *8.5.1 Day-Centers*

The "First Day-centers Meaningful Social Access for Persons with Mental Health Needs" project is a three-year initiative that commenced in 2018. It is operated by the Center for the Rehabilitation of the Paralyzed (CRP) and funded by the Kadoorie Charitable Foundation (KCF). The project, located at CRP-Ganakbari and CRP-Mirpur, which are 40 km and 13 km away from Dhaka respectively, works primarily in two areas: individual support and community awareness building. It offers mental health care support and comprehensive psychosocial rehabilitation to individuals with mental health needs through two day-centers. These centers deliver services using a multi-disciplinary team approach. After clients complete their rehabilitation at the day-center, the staff follows up with them via phone calls, video calls, and occasional home visits (CRP, 2023).

A psychiatric day care service is an establishment that generally provides care to psychiatric patients during the daytime. These facilities typically: (1) service groups of users simultaneously rather than one-on-one, (2) expect users to remain at the facility beyond their face-to-face interactions with staff (meaning the service isn't merely based on users attending appointments and leaving immediately afterwards), and (3) require attendances that last half a day or whole day. Such facilities include day-centers, day care centers, sheltered workshops, clubhouses, drop-in centers, employment/rehabilitation workshops, and social firms. Special day treatment facilities for children and adolescents, as well as those for other specific groups like the elderly, are also included (CRP, 2023).

### 8.5.2 *Telepsychiatry*

Telepsychiatry is a pioneering approach in the realm of psychiatry, and its significance and popularity are on the rise in Bangladesh. Considering the recent national mental health survey, approximately 16.8% of the country's population is grappling with mental disorders. However, the number of mental health care providers is insufficient. Therefore, telepsychiatry serves as an effective tool to readily reach out to the community (Ministry of Health & Family Welfare, 2021).

Telepsychiatry in Bangladesh is still in its early stages and is largely considered a branch of telemedicine rather than a standalone service. However, its significance and popularity have started to emerge (Islam, 2020). Since June 2016, Thikana Psychiatric and Drug Addiction Clinic's lead psychiatrist, Dr. Atiqul Haq Mazumder, has been providing telepsychiatry services through *FaceTime* (Mazumder, 2022). The COVID-19 pandemic has accelerated the adoption and importance of telepsychiatry among the general populace. By mid-2020, telemedicine in Bangladesh became a trusted mode of communication between patients and doctors, not only in psychiatry but across all medical fields. A functioning setup at NIMH allows doctors from the UHC to consult with psychiatrists (Arafat et al., 2024, 2024a, 2024b).

## 8.6 Research on Community Psychiatry in Bangladesh

The Dasherkandi project studies were perhaps the earliest studies in Bangladesh involving the community population of a village near Dhaka (Chowdhury et al., 1981; Alam et al., 1982). In 2011, a pilot project aimed at strengthening the primary health care (PHC) system for the treatment of mental and neurological disorders was initiated in Sonargaon Upazila, Bangladesh. The project's goal was to identify children experiencing Generalized tonic–clonic seizures (GTCS) in the community and manage them with phenobarbitone, or carbamazepine as a secondary drug for cases unresponsive to phenobarbitone. All children aged 5–14 (11,669 in total) in two unions of Sonargaon Upazila were evaluated (World Health Organization, 2013). Initially, the treatment gap was 87%. At present, almost all children needing medication are receiving treatment, reducing the treatment gap to 5%. However, the latest prevalence study indicates a persistent 91% treatment gap for mental disorders in Bangladesh (Ministry of Health & Family Welfare, 2021).

## 8.7 Gaps in Community Psychiatric Services and Ways Forward

We mentioned earlier in this book and chapter, there is no post of psychiatrist in primary and secondary care level services in Bangladesh (Fig. 8.1) (Government of The People's Republic of Bangladesh, 2022). Psychiatry has been neglected in the undergraduate curriculum of medical education in the country (Arafat, 2024b). There is a significant deficiency in both services and manpower in the field of mental health. As of 1992, more than 90% of the population was not covered by services, and no significant changes were observed by 2019. In Bangladesh, there is a 91% treatment gap for mental disorders (Ministry of Health & Family Welfare, 2021). The mental health gap in Bangladesh is further exacerbated by the lack of awareness and the prevalent stigma surrounding mental health.

There are no available services at the community level for issues related to children and adolescents, sub-normality, and drug abuse. Also, the services for other types of mental disorders are extremely insufficient and poor. There is a noticeable shortage of psychiatrists, social workers, occupational therapists, and psychologists. Many patients are compelled to turn to traditional healers like spiritualists, hekim, kabiraj, and quitek, who are not equipped to treat severe mental health patients properly. At the district level, there are no designated positions for psychiatrists in the government structure. Additionally, the availability of psychotropic drugs at the community level is still not widespread, and certain drugs are not only hard to find but also costly (Arafat et al., 2024, 2024a, b). Community-based mental health services can be hindered by the stigma and social distancing towards individuals with mental health conditions.

Strong attention from the policy makers is warranted for the establishment of community psychiatry in Bangladesh. Integration of mental health services with primary health care structure could be a potential area recognized by the World Health Organization (Arafat et al., 2018). Augmented funding and research should be focused in the country. Changes in undergraduate medical curriculum could be prioritized. It's worth noting that psychiatric care in resource-limited settings like Bangladesh could be enhanced by training primary healthcare workers to provide mental health education to their communities (Abayomi et al., 2012). To achieve the Sustainable Development Goals and reduce the vast treatment gap, various initiatives are needed, both strategically and practically. This includes creating culturally appropriate service demand baseline data and developing different manuals for psychosocial interventions.

## 8.8 Conclusion

Community psychiatry is in the rudimentary state in Bangladesh with substantial challenges. These include insufficient funding, a deficit of skilled manpower, and a significant 91% treatment gap for mental disorders. Existing services, provided by government, private, and NGO-sponsored providers, are supported by only 0.05% of the overall health budget. Despite initiatives like the "First Day-centers Meaningful Social Access for Persons with Mental Health Needs" project and the adoption of telepsychiatry, issues persist. Problems are exacerbated by a lack of awareness, widespread stigma, and unavailability of community services for specific demographics and disorders. To enhance psychiatric care, strategies involving training primary healthcare workers in mental health education, developing culturally appropriate service demand data, and creating psychosocial intervention manuals are vital. In addition, the expansion of community clinics and specialized hospitals, as well as the effective implementation of policies emphasizing community-based services, will play a crucial role in addressing these challenges.

## References


Abayomi, O., Adelufosi, A. O., & Olajide, A. (2012). *Changing Attitude to Mental Illness among Community Mental Health Volunteers in South-Western Nigeria, 59*(6), 609–612. https://doi.org/10.1177/0020764012448781.

Alam, M. N., Kabir, M. Z., Ali, S. M., & Chowdhury, A. K. (1982). Dasherkandi project studies–health of the under fifteen. *Bangladesh Medical Research Council Bulletin, 8*(2), 39–46.

Arafat, S. Y., Roy, S., & Huq, N. (2018). Integrating mental health into primary health care in Bangladesh: Problems and prospects. *Mental Health and Addiction Research, 3*(2), 1–2.

Arafat, S. M. Y., Mullick, M. S. I., & Islam, H. (2020). Development of psychiatric services in Bangladesh. *Asian Journal of Psychiatry, 47*, 101870. https://doi.org/10.1016/j.ajp.2019.101870.

Arafat, S. M. Y., Giasuddin, N. A., Mazumder, A. H. (2024). Access to mental health care in Bangladesh–current status, potential challenges, and ways out. In S. M. Y. Arafat, S. K. Kar (Eds.), *Access to mental health care in South Asia-current status, potential challenges, and ways out*. Springer Nature Singapore. https://doi.org/10.1007/978-981-99-9153-2_3

Arafat, S. M. Y. (2024a). Mental health services in Bangladesh. In S. M. Y. Arafat (Ed.), *Mental Health in Bangladesh: From Bench to Community*. Springer Nature Singapore. https://doi.org/10.1007/978-981-97-0610-5_3

Arafat, S. M. Y. (2024b). Psychiatric education and research system in Bangladesh. In S. M. Y. Arafat (Ed.), *Mental health in Bangladesh: From bench to Community*. Springer Nature Singapore. https://doi.org/10.1007/978-981-97-0610-5_12

Bouras N. (2017). Social challenges of contemporary psychiatry. *Psychiatrike = Psychiatriki*, 28(3), 119–202. https://doi.org/10.22365/jpsych.2017.283.199.

Chadda, R. K. (2012). Six decades of community psychiatry in India. *International Psychiatry, 9*(2), 45–47. https://doi.org/10.1192/s1749367600003106.

Chowdhury, A. K., Alam, M. N., & Ali, S. M. (1981). Dasherkandi project studies. Demography, morbidity and mortality in a rural community of Bangladesh. *Bangladesh Medical Research Council bulletin, 7*(1), 22–39.

Chowdhury, N. F., Fariduzzaman, A. M., Arafat, S. M. Y. (2024). Prominent figures in psychiatry in Bangladesh. In S. M. Y. Arafat (Ed.), *Mental health in Bangladesh: From bench to community*. Springer Nature Singapore. https://doi.org/10.1007/978-981-97-0610-5_1

CRP. (2023). Meaningful Social access for persons with mental health needs project. https://www.crp-bangladesh.org/crp-project/meaningful-social-access-persons-mental-health-needs-project. Retrieved November 16, 2023.

Eisenberg, L., & Guttmacher, L. B. (2010). Were we all asleep at the switch? A personal reminiscence of psychiatry from 1940 to 2010. *Acta Psychiatrica Scandinavica, 122*(2), 89–102. https://doi.org/10.1111/j.1600-0447.2010.01544.x.

Erickson, B. (2021). Deinstitutionalization through optimism: The community mental health act of 1963. *American Journal of Psychiatry Residents' Journal, 16*(4), 6–7. https://doi.org/10.1176/appi.ajp-rj.2021.160404.

Fakhoury, W., & Priebe, S. (2007). Deinstitutionalization and reinstitutionalization: Major changes in the provision of mental healthcare. *Psychiatry, 6*(8), 313–316. https://doi.org/10.1016/j.mppsy.2007.05.008.

Farooq, S., & Minhas, F. (2001). Community psychiatry in developing countries–a misnomer? *Psychiatric Bulletin, 25*(6), 226–227. https://doi.org/10.1192/pb.25.6.226.

Government of The People's Republic of Bangladesh. (2022). National Mental Health Strategic Plan, 2020–2030. https://dghs.gov.bd/sites/default/files/files/dghs.portal.gov.bd/notices/e27171cb_a80b_42d4_99ad_40095adef31b/2022-08-16-08-42-af8622e2c4936593dd45601b84f4920f.pdf. Retrieved May 02, 2023.

Islam, M. H. (2019). *Jibone colar pothe*. Academic Press and Publishers Library.

Islam, M. A. (2020). Telepsychiatry. *Archives of NIMH, 3*(2), 01–02.

Lamb, H. R., & Bachrach, L. L. (2001). Some perspectives on deinstitutionalization. Psychiatric services (Washington, D.C.), 52(8), 1039–1045. https://doi.org/10.1176/appi.ps.52.8.1039.

Mazumder, A. H. (2022). Hazardous drinking and cognition in schizophrenia, schizoaffective disorder and bipolar disorder. (n.d.). Cambridge Cognition. https://cambridgecognition.com/hazardous-drinking-and-cognition-in-schizophrenia-schizoaffective-disorder-and-bipolar-disorder/.

Mental Health Act. (2018). Bangladesh. https://legislativediv.gov.bd/site/page/3c13bbde-76b4-41fc-89cab738dd04a0bb. Retrieved December 12, 2018.

Ministry of Health & Family Welfare. (2021). National Mental Health Survey 2019. http://nimh.gov.bd/wp-content/uploads/2021/11/Mental-Health-Survey-Report.pdf. Retrieved March 29, 2023.

Facility Registry. (2023). Ministry of health and family welfare, Government of people's republic of Bangladesh. http://facilityregistry.dghs.gov.bd/index.php. Retrieved April 04, 2023.

World Health Organization. (2013). *Strengthening primary care to address mental and neurological disorders*. https://www.who.int/publications/i/item/9789290224259. Retrieved November 16, 2023.

World Health Organization. (2021). Bangladesh - WHO Special Initiative for Mental Health Situational Assessment. https://www.who.int/publications/m/item/bangladesh---who-special-initiative-for-mental-health. Retrieved November 16, 2023.

# Chapter 9
# Psychosexual Disorders in Bangladesh: From Bench to Community

**Mohammad Muntasir Maruf, Leuza Mubassara, and Mohammad Shamsul Ahsan**

**Abstract** Psychosexual disorders are common but covert issue in Bangladesh. Due to the lack of community study focusing on these disorders, precise burden of these disorders is yet to be estimated in the country. Various physical and psychiatric disorders are reported both as risk factors and co-morbidities of psychosexual problems. Socio-culture environment, religious proscriptions, poor health literacy are also contributing factors. Besides male and female sexual dysfunctions, dhat syndrome is a common phenomenon in the country. Gender dysphoria, paraphilia, hypersexuality, and pornography addiction are also prevalent, though there is a dearth of scientific researches on these topics. The services for the management of psychosexual disorders are insufficient and uncoordinated, though recently few dedicated psycho-sexual clinics have been established. Due to the lack of awareness and knowledge, help-seeking behavior for these disorders is poor and inappropriate. For raising awareness and capacity building, South Asian Society for Sexual Medicine has become a prominent organization in Bangladesh. Researchers are also becoming interested in exploring various aspects of psychosexual functions and disorders recently. This chapter discusses various aspects of psychosexual disorders and recommendations for strengthening health-care services for these disorders in the country.

**Keywords** Psychosexual disorders · Sexual dysfunctions · Dhat syndrome · Paraphilia · Transgender · Gender identity disorder · Homosexuality · Hijra · Bangladesh

M. M. Maruf (✉)
Department of Addiction Psychiatry, National Institute of Mental Health, Dhaka 1207, Bangladesh
e-mail: marufdmc@gmail.com

L. Mubassara
Department of Child and Adolescent Psychiatry, Bangabandhu Sheikh Mujib Medical University, Dhaka 1000, Bangladesh

M. S. Ahsan
Department of Psychiatry, Bangabandhu Sheikh Mujib Medical University, Dhaka 1000, Bangladesh



S. M. Y. Arafat (ed.), *Mental Health in Bangladesh*,
https://doi.org/10.1007/978-981-97-0610-5_9

## 9.1 Introduction

Psychosexual disorders are complex phenomena with multidimensional facets including biological, psychological, and socio-cultural, psychological component being the predominant factor. Psychiatric disorders and psychotropic medications are factors intimately related with psychosexual disorders. These disorders include sexual dysfunctions as well as paraphilia, problems related to gender identity and sexual orientation, hypersexuality, and other cultural-bound sexual issues (Narang et al., 2016). Though health care services have developed remarkably in Bangladesh over the last few decades, the country still encounters significant challenges regarding the psychosexual disorders. These disorders are prevalent in our society though they are not much discussed openly due to socio-cultural taboo, religious proscriptions, poor health literacy, existent myths and misconceptions, and lack of awareness. As a result, it is difficult to estimate the exact prevalence and extent of impact of these problems. However, despite the lack of systematic studies, there is mounting evidence of economic, symptomatic, humanistic, and other burdens among persons suffering from sexual dysfunctions worldwide (Balon, 2017). Recently, there has been growing interest among the physicians of Bangladesh to deal the bio-psycho-social aspects of sexuality. Effective management strategies of psychosexual disorders warrant sound empirical research studies assessing the exact burden, risk factors, and gaps in several aspects. Against this backdrop, this chapter discusses the prevalence, physical and psychiatric comorbidities and risk factors of sexual dysfunctions, help-seeking behavior of the distressed and management approaches prevailing in the country, legal aspects of psychosexual problems and current researches on sexual dysfunctions and other psychosexual issues including gender identity, paraphilia, and dhat syndrome.

## 9.2 Prevalence and Burden of Psycho-sexual Disorders

There is no community-based study aiming to estimate specifically the prevalence of various types of sexual dysfunctions. Latest National Mental Health Survey found that 0.3% of the adult population of Bangladesh are suffering from sexual dysfunctions, almost all of them from premature ejaculation (Ministry of Health & Family Welfare, 2021a, b). Sexual dysfunctions were reported in 67% of the persons with psychiatric problems seeking help in National Institute of Mental Health (NIMH), Dhaka, where erectile dysfunction (35.1%) and premature ejaculation (26.5%) were the commonest dysfunctions among indoor and outdoor male patients, respectively. For females, sexual interest/arousal disorder was the most common diagnosis for both indoor (34.9%) and outdoor (44.4%) patients (Rony et al., 2017). Prevalence of sexual dysfunctions among other psychiatric population was also high. Hospital-based studies among various female populations (e.g. diabetic, post-menopausal, having gynecological problems etc.) found that more than half of the respondents suffered from sexual dysfunctions. Erectile dysfunction has been reported in 45.3%–60.2% of men with type 2 diabetes mellitus. Premature ejaculation and erectile dysfunction are the commonest types of sexual dysfunctions among the persons seeking help for psychosexual problems (Table 9.1).

## 9.3 Comorbidities of Psychosexual Disorders in Bangladesh

There are a few studies investigating the co-morbidities of sexual dysfunctions in Bangladesh (Table 9.2). Some studies have been conducted to assess erectile dysfunction (ED) in the patients with diabetes mellitus, which is a recognized physical co-morbidity of the sexual dysfunctions (Selim et al., 2015; Asaduzzaman et al., 2020; Mahbub et al., 2019). Regarding co-morbid psychiatric disorders, the prevalence of sexual dysfunctions was determined among the persons with major depressive disorders (MDD), substance use disorders (SUD), and patients having psychosis including schizophrenia, schizophreniform disorder, and mood disorder with psychotic feature (Gofur et al., 2023; Sayed et al., 2021; Kaoser et al., 2019). A study assessed female sexual dysfunctions among post-menopausal women, where the respondents had various physical diseases, like diabetes (29.6%), hypertension (20.4%), bronchial asthma (10.4%), chronic kidney disease (4.2%), polycystic ovarian syndrome (3.5%), cancer (1.5%), and hyperprolactinemia (1.5%), but estimates of co-morbidities between the diseases and sexual dysfunctions were not mentioned (Amin et al., 2022).

## 9.4 Factors Associated with Sexual Dysfunctions in Bangladesh

Researchers globally identified various risk factors for sexual dysfunctions. Age, diabetes mellitus, hypertension, stroke, cancer, penile trauma, anxiety, depression and other psychological factors like poor body image, performance anxiety, taking medications and abusing substances, disturbances in central serotonin activities and post-synaptic 5-HT receptor functioning have been reported as significant risk factors for male sexual dysfunction (Anderson et al., 2022). Regarding female sexual dysfunctions, risk factors found consistently significant were poor physical and mental health, stress, history of abortion, genitourinary problems, genital mutilation, relationship difficulties, and sexual abuse (McCool-Myers et al., 2018).

Same risk factors can be assumed to be responsible for sexual dysfunctions in Bangladesh, though there are very few studies conducted here with sound methodology among the persons with sexual dysfunctions evaluating the risk factors. From clinical experiences and other studies regarding sexual health issues, it can be opined that lack of knowledge and awareness, poor mental health literacy, stigma, and myth

**Table 9.1** Prevalence of psychosexual disorders among various populations

| Study | Study place | Study population | Sample size | Sampling technique | Prevalence of psychosexual disorders/problems |
|---|---|---|---|---|---|
| Gofur et al. (2023) | CTC & CMH, Dhaka | Men with substance use disorders | 400 | Purposive | Sexual dysfunctions—94.2% (PE—54.5%, ED—34.2% Desire disorder—5.5%) |
| Hasan et al. (2023) | Endocrinology OPD of MMCH | Case—women with diabetes Control—women without diabetes | 250 (Case—150 Control—100) | Convenience | Sexual dysfunctions: 79.3% among cases 72% among controls |
| Maruf et al. (2022) | NIMH, Dhaka | Adult male seeking help for sexual concerns | 95 | Convenient | PE—42.1% ED—31.6% |
| Selim et al. (2022) | Department of Endocrinology, BSMMU | Male patients with type 2 diabetes mellitus | 1940 | | Erectile problems—56.3% Decreased libido—27.5% |
| Amin et al. (2022) | Four public and private hospitals in Dhaka and Chattogram | Postmenopausal women | 260 | Multi-stage sampling | Sexual problems—56.9% |
| Das and Malakar (2022) | Psychiatry OPD, Khwaja Yunus Ali Medical College, Sirajgonj | Adult male seeking help for sexual concerns | 100 | Consecutive | ED—31% PE—25% Dhat syndrome—18% ED with PE—17% |

(continued)

**Table 9.1** (continued)

| Study | Study place | Study population | Sample size | Sampling technique | Prevalence of psychosexual disorders/problems |
|---|---|---|---|---|---|
| Sayed et al. (2021) | Sylhet MAG Osmani Medical College | Male patients with MDD | 68 | | Sexual dysfunctions—70.5%<br>(Low sexual drive—35.3%<br>Orgasmic difficulty—35.3%<br>Problem with orgasmic satisfaction—33.8%<br>Difficulty in erection—23.5%<br>Low arousal—16.2%) |
| Rakib et al. (2020) | Department of Internal Medicine, BSMMU, Dhaka | Case—men with hypertension<br>Control—men without hypertension | 150<br>(Case—75<br>Control–75) | Convenience | ED:<br>61.4% among cases<br>37.3% among controls |
| Kaoser et al. (2019) | NIMH, Dhaka | Patients taking antipsychotics | 146 | Convenient | Sexual dysfunctions—52.1%<br>(Disorders of desire, arousal, and orgasm—63.2%<br>Disorders of desire and arousal—23.7%<br>Disorders of desire and orgasm—5.3%<br>Disorders of arousal and orgasm—5.3%<br>Disorders of desire—2.6%) |
| Nahar et al. (2019) | Sex clinic of NIMH, Dhaka | Adult male seeking help for sexual concerns | 280 | Purposive | PE—26.4%<br>(Lifelong—20.3%. Acquired—24.3%,<br>Natural variant—25.7%<br>Premature like ejaculatory dysfunctions—29.7%) |
| Mahbub et al. (2019) | BIRDEM hospital, Dhaka | Male patients with type 2 diabetes mellitus | 508 | | ED—60.2% |

(continued)

**Table 9.1** (continued)

<table>
<tr><th>Study</th><th>Study place</th><th>Study population</th><th>Sample size</th><th>Sampling technique</th><th colspan="4">Prevalence of psychosexual disorders/problems</th></tr>
<tr><td>Chowdhury et al. (2018)</td><td>Unani and Ayurvedic Medical College Hospital, Dhaka</td><td>Unani and Ayurvedic healthcare seeker, both men and women</td><td>220</td><td>Random</td><td colspan="4">PE—26.4%<br>ED—21.8%<br>Low libido—7.7%<br>Loss of libido—4.1%</td></tr>
<tr><td>Salam et al. (2017)</td><td>Psychiatric OPD, BSMMU</td><td>Adult male seeking help for sexual concerns</td><td>142</td><td>Purposive</td><td colspan="4">PE—69.0%<br>ED—23.9%<br>Sexual dysfunctions due to general medical condition—5.6%</td></tr>
<tr><td>Arafat and Ahmed (2017)</td><td>Psychiatric sex clinic of BSMMU, Dhaka</td><td>Both men and women seeking help for sexual concerns</td><td>110 (M-102 F–8)</td><td>Convenient</td><td colspan="4">Misconception—54.4%<br>Commonest male dysfunction: PE (37.3%)<br>Commonest female dysfunction—FSIAD (100%)</td></tr>
<tr><td rowspan="6">Rony et al. (2017)</td><td rowspan="6">NIMH, Dhaka</td><td rowspan="6">Patients with psychiatric complaints in indoor and outdoor</td><td rowspan="6">161</td><td rowspan="6">Purposive</td><td colspan="4">Sexual dysfunctions—67%</td></tr>
<tr><td>Sex</td><td>Dysfunction</td><td>Indoor (%)</td><td>Outdoor (%)</td></tr>
<tr><td rowspan="2">Male</td><td>ED</td><td>35.1</td><td>23.5</td></tr>
<tr><td>PE</td><td>26.3</td><td>26.5</td></tr>
<tr><td rowspan="2">Female</td><td>FSIAD</td><td>34.9</td><td>44.4</td></tr>
<tr><td>Orgasmic disorder</td><td>25.6</td><td>22.2</td></tr>
<tr><td>Ahsan et al. (2016)</td><td>Gynecology, endocrinology, and psychiatry OPD of BSMMU</td><td>Female patients</td><td>173</td><td>Convenient</td><td colspan="4">Sexual problems—56%</td></tr>
</table>

(continued)

**Table 9.1** (continued)

| Study | Study place | Study population | Sample size | Sampling technique | Prevalence of psychosexual disorders/problems |
|---|---|---|---|---|---|
| Rahman et al. (2016) | DMCH | Women with CIN who underwent loop electrosurgical excision procedure | 46 | Purposive | Decrease in sexual desire—13.1%<br>Lower abdominal pain after coitus—10.87%<br>Dyspareunia and vaginal dryness—9%<br>Dissatisfaction to sexual intercourse—6.5% |
| Selim et al. (2015) | OPD of BSMMU, BIRDEM, and 5 diabetic centers, Dhaka | Male patients with type 2 diabetes mellitus | 3790 | | ED—54.0% |
| Asaduzzaman et al. (2020) | Endocrinology OPD of a tertiary care hospital | Male patients with type 2 diabetes mellitus | 150 | Consecutive | ED—45.3%<br>(Mild—14.7%<br>Mild to moderate—18.0%<br>Moderate—6%<br>severe—6.7%) |
| Jahan et al | Gynecology OPD of DMCH and ShSMCH | Women with gynecological problems | 137 | | Sexual problems—51.8%<br>(Among sexual problems—Pain during intercourse—71.8%<br>Reduced desire—54.9% Orgasmic problems—43.66%<br>Arousal problems—32.39%) |
| Mozumder and Rahman (2004) | Sex therapy clinic in Dhaka | Adult male seeking help for sexual concerns | 104 | | PE—47%<br>PE with ED—14%<br>ED—4% |

*Source* Authors

OPD–Outpatient Department, NIMH–National Institute of Mental Health, DMCH–Dhaka Medical College Hospital, BSMMU–Bangabandhu Sheikh Mujib Medical University, ShSMCH–Shahid Suhrawardy Medical College Hospital, MMCH–Mymensingh Medical College Hospital, CMH–Combined Military Hospital, CTC–Central drug addiction Treatment Centre, MDD–Major Depressive Disorder, ED–Erectile Dysfunction, PE–Premature Ejaculation, FSIAD–Female Sexual Interest/Arousal Disorder

**Table 9.2** Physical and psychiatric co-morbidities among the persons with sexual dysfunctions

| Study | Sexual dysfunctions | Physical co-morbidities | Psychiatric co-morbidities |
|---|---|---|---|
| Das and Malakar (2022) | Male sexual dysfunctions | Physical illness—3% | Stress—66%<br>Substance use—14%<br>Other psychiatric disorders—23%<br>(Depression—15%<br>Anxiety disorders—4%<br>Psychosis—2%) |
| Nahar et al. (2017) | Premature ejaculation | | Depression—35.1%<br>Anxiety—12.2%<br>Stress—10.8%<br>Depression + Anxiety + Stress—13.5% |
| Salam et al. (2017) | Male sexual dysfunctions | | Overall psychiatric disorders—59.9%<br>(Depressive disorder—28.8%<br>Anxiety disorder—23.9%<br>Somatization disorder—4.2%<br>Panic disorder without agoraphobia—2.8%) |
| Arafat and Ahmed (2017) | Male and female sexual dysfunctions | Overall physical diseases—15.5%<br>(Infertility—5.5%<br>HTN—2.7%<br>IBS—2.7%<br>Hypothyroidism—1.8%) | Overall psychiatric disorders (Other than SRD)—30.9%<br>(Depressive disorder—13.6%<br>Schizophrenia—3.6%<br>GAD—2.7%)<br>Substance use disorders—8.2% |

(continued)

**Table 9.2** (continued)

| Study | Sexual dysfunctions | Physical co-morbidities | Psychiatric co-morbidities |
|---|---|---|---|
| Ahsan et al. (2016a, b) | Female sexual dysfunctions | Endocrinological—38.2% (Diabetes mellitus—9.3% Hypothyroidism—11.0% Hyperthyroidism—2.3% Polycystic ovarian syndrome—7.5% Hyperprolactinemia—1.7% Sheehan's syndrome—1.7%) Gynecological—37.6% (Pelvic inflammatory disease—5.2% Genitourinary prolapse—1.7% Chronic cervicitis—2.3% Vaginal candidiasis—4.6% Bacterial vaginosis—2.3%) | Overall psychiatric disorders—33.5% (Depressive disorder—14.5% Anxiety disorder—8.1% Bipolar disorder—1.7%) |
| Jahan et al. (2012) | Female sexual dysfunctions | Hypertension—7.0% Sexually transmitted diseases—25.4% Pelvic surgery—11.3% | Mental stress—23.9% |

*Source* Authors

influence sexual functioning and behavior and contribute significantly in developing these disorders.

In Bangladesh, some studies investigated factors associated with one or more types of sexual dysfunctions in a particular subgroup of population, for example—the persons suffering from type 2 diabetes mellitus, postmenopausal women, women with gynecological problems, men with major depressive disorders, help-seeking male with sexual problems (Table 9.3).

## 9.5 Gender and Sexual Diversity-Related Issues in Bangladesh

### *9.5.1 Gender Identity-Related Issues*

In Bangladesh, gender identity issue is one of the most disadvantaged and misunderstood groups. Estimating the prevalence of "transgender" population or the persons with "gender identity disorder" is challenging due to stigma, prejudice, and cultural differences in their definition. However, there has been a slow progress in recent years in overcoming societal prejudices towards transgender persons, which is reflected in

**Table 9.3** Factors associated with sexual dysfunctions

| Study | Study population | Sexual dysfunctions | Associated factors |
|---|---|---|---|
| Hasan et al. (2023) | Case—wmen with diabetes<br>Control—women without diabetes | Female sexual dysfunctions | Duration of diabetes, level of HbA1c, comorbid hypertension, complications of diabetes |
| Amin et al. (2022) | Postmenopausal women | Female sexual dysfunctions | Increasing age, urban population group, multiparous, homemakers, duration of menopause, and postmenopausal women with no hormone therapy<br>(Protective factor—regular physical activity) |
| Sayed et al. (2021) | Men with MDD | Male sexual dysfunctions | Severity of depression |
| Rakib et al. (2020) | Case—men with hypertension<br>Control—men without hypertension | Erectile dysfunctions | Duration and severity of hypertension, older age |
| Mujahid et al. (2020) | Patients taking antipsychotics | Both male and female sexual dysfunctions | Male gender, older age, schizophrenia as a diagnosis, longer duration of illness and treatment, typical antipsychotics and risperidone, higher doses |
| Mahbub et al. (2019) | Men with DM | Erectile dysfunction | Patient's age, housebound bedridden status, sedentary work, diabetes duration, HbA1c level, microvascular complications, IHD, and diuretic drug use<br>Protective factor—moderate physical activity |
| Nahar et al. (2017) | Men attending sex clinic | Premature ejaculation | Increasing age, religion, smoking status, psychiatric comorbidities |
| Selim et al. (2015) | Men with DM | Erectile dysfunction | Age, duration of diabetes, poor glycemic control, type of treatment |

(continued)

**Table 9.3** (continued)

| Study | Study population | Sexual dysfunctions | Associated factors |
|---|---|---|---|
| Asaduzzaman et al. (2020) | Men with DM | Erectile dysfunction | Age, duration of DM, HbA1c, fasting plasma glucose, serum creatinine (independent predictors—duration of DM and serum testosterone) |
| Jahan et al. (2012) | Women attending gynecology outpatient | Female sexual dysfunctions | Parity, history of menstrual regulation, mental stress, and sexual problems of the husband. Age and education (reduced desire)<br>Delivery mode (inhibited desire and arousal problems)<br>(Protective factor—increased frequency of intercourse) |

*Source* Authors

some local media reports on transgender issues. Transgender people consult psychiatrists occasionally in Bangladesh, though many of them suffer from psychiatric illnesses, of which generalized anxiety disorder, depressive disorders, and bipolar disorder are common (Abbasi, 2023). Sometimes, persons with gender dysphoria consult psychiatrists to get the certificate of their conditions to proceed to the next step of management.

### 9.5.2 Sexual Orientation-Related Issues

Being a Muslim-majority country, homosexuality is disapproved and tagged with negative connotations in Bangladesh. Persons with homosexuality encounter stigma and discrimination even from healthcare providers, public humiliation, infidelity of same-sex partner, abandonment from family, pressure from families to get into heterosexual marriage. They become victims of sexual abuse both in childhood and in adulthood. Some suffer internalized homophobia and confusion about sexuality (Alam & Marston, 2023; Mozumder et al., 2016). Compared to heterosexuals, they have poorer mental health having high rate of suicidal ideation, attempt, and self-harm (Mozumder et al., 2023).

### 9.5.3 Hijra—The Intersex Community in Bangladesh

The term "Hijra" cannot be classified as a single category due to stigma, prejudice, and cultural differences. However, according to media statistics, the number of Hijras in Bangladesh can vary between 10,000 and 50,000 out of a total population of 160 million (Al-Mamun et al., 2022). Bangladesh, like many other South Asian countries, has an extended legacy of the Hijra community. The Hijra community has a long history in Hindu civilization, with Hindu holy writings such as the Ramayana and the Mahabharata (Singh, 2017). Hijra individuals in Bangladesh face challenges such as abandonment, lack of basic rights, and social stigma. They often drop out of school at the age of 7–10 years, due to bullying, harassment, and social stigma (Aziz & Azhar, 2020). They struggle to find suitable jobs due to lack of education and skills and often face economic, educational, political, employment, health, and social rights violations.

## 9.6 Other Sexuality Issues

### *9.6.1 Dhat Syndrome—A Culture Bound Syndrome*

Dhat syndrome is a culture bound syndrome, prevalent widely in South Asian culture including Bangladesh. Though it is characterized by various symptoms accompanied primarily with the complaints of semen loss through urine, night emission or masturbation, semen loss through saliva and sweat was also reported in Bangladesh (Arafat et al., 2021; Maruf et al., 2022). Most of the persons with dhat syndrome present in their late adolescence or early adulthood. Common physical symptoms associated with dhat syndrome are physical weakness and vertigo; anxiety and depression being the common psychological and premature ejaculation and erectile dysfunction being the common sexual symptoms (Maruf et al., 2022).

### *9.6.2 Paraphilia*

Exact burden of paraphilia is yet to be estimated precisely in Bangladesh, though there is a strong likelihood of having similar prevalence found in other countries. According to the opinion of local sexual medicine practitioners, pedophilia, exhibitionism, and voyeurism are more frequent here than other types of paraphilia (Arafat, 2019). Pedophilia has been reported in local media of Bangladesh, frotteurism has been observed in public transportation and market places; however, the exact prevalence has yet to be determined. The first case report on paraphilia was published in 2020 in Bangladesh, covering a middle aged men with urophilia who used to be aroused by female urine, collecting urine from them and using it for masturbation (Arafat et al., 2020). In November 2020, the first documented case of necrophilia was identified in a 20-year-old unmarried male working at a Forensic lab. The identical DNA profile had been found in five female deceased bodies delivered to the morgue from various places between 2019 and 2020. Police acquired DNA samples from a discarded cigarette bud in a suspected case of rape on dead victims, charged the individual, arrested him, and brought him to court for prosecution. The proceedings in those cases indicate the ignorance of the mental health issues related to the paraphilia in Bangladesh (Bose et al., 2021).

### 9.6.3 *Pornography Consumption*

Availability of internet created an increased opportunity to explore pornography. According to a survey among students at Jahangirnagar University, Bangladesh, about three-fourths (72%) of the students had consumed pornography at least once in their lives, with around half of them being occasional consumers. Most of them (67%) first came across porn while they were in high school, however, women often did so considerably later (Al Mamun et al., 2019). Another study reported that consumption of pornography was higher among students who spent late evenings with their friends, who frequently quarreled or fought with their friends, played games or joked around with them, and stayed up later than usual (Chowdhury et al., 2018).

### 9.6.4 *Masturbation*

Masturbation is a common practice among men which is reflected in the study regarding dhat syndrome (Maruf et al., 2022). A study among students reported that masturbation is a common occurrence among them (33%) and much more common among males (42.2%). Masturbation rates were higher among students who watched pornography at least once per week or once per month (Chowdhury et al., 2018). A case of childhood masturbation was documented where a 6-year-old girl presented with the history of episodic frictions of the pubic area with the edges of bed, furniture, and other reachable particles for 1.5 years and the typical episode lasting roughly for 5 min. The mother received comprehensive psychoeducation about the disorder and its management methods, including behavior therapy (Arafat, 2019).

### 9.6.5 *Hypersexuality*

Compulsive sexual behavior disorder, sex addiction, or hypersexuality is also a less discussed issue in a sexually conservative nation like Bangladesh. The first case of hypersexuality in the country that has been documented features a young lady who used to engage in sexual activity for 5 to 6 h every day and have five to six orgasms (Arafat et al., 2020). Recently, Bangladesh was included in an international sex survey assessing compulsive sexual behavior disorder (CSBD), where 13.3% of the participants from Bangladesh were found to be at high risk CSBD group (Bőthe et al., 2023).

### *9.6.6 Sex-Related Myths and Misconceptions*

Sex-related myths are highly prevalent (ranging from 37.4% to 93.5%) among the patients in Bangladesh. The common myths and misconceptions are related to size, deformity and elongation of the penis, duration of intercourse, masturbation, night emission, semen loss, and homosexuality (Rabbani et al., 2020). Sex-related misconceptions were highly prevalent (54.4%) also among the help-seeking patients in a sex therapy clinic (Arafat & Ahmed, 2017).

Semen is regarded as a source of vitality which is formed from foods through multistep processes and wasted through masturbation, night emission, and urine, which causes physical and mental illness, sexual problems, and infertility. Dhat syndrome is mistakenly regarded as a disorder of persons from a rural background, which can be treated by changes in dietary habit and sexual behavior (Maruf et al., 2024).

## 9.7 Available Services in Bangladesh for Psychosexual Disorders

### *9.7.1 General Services*

In Bangladesh, health care services are provided by qualified, semi-qualified, and unqualified healthcare providers from allopathy, traditional, and alternative care backgrounds from government, as well as private and informal sector (Ministry of Health & Family Welfare, 2021a, b). Services for psychosexual disorders can also be availed in these systems. In the government-led primary health care settings and private chambers, general practitioners deal with these issues. Among the specialists other than psychiatrists, usually internists, dermatologists, urologists, gynecologists, endocrinologists manage these disorders in hospital settings or their private chambers. But a vast majority receives service from informal unqualified traditional healers or religious healers known as "kabiraj" who typically treat sexual dysfunctions with herbal remedies. As part of their traditional healing methods, they frequently offer various foods such halua, honey, and panipora in addition to talismans. Sometimes they do "jhara-jhari," which involves beating the sufferer with shrubs while uttering religious phrases. They frequently employ appealing phrases like "Kolikata herbal," "VIP herbal," or "Indian herbal" in an effort to draw in more customers (Ghani et al., 2013).

### 9.7.2 *Specialized Services*

In 2010–2011, for the first time, the Department of Psychiatry at Bangabandhu Sheikh Mujib Medical University (BSMMU), Dhaka started a specialized clinic called the Psycho-Sexual Clinic, which was intended to provide one-stop service for patients who need specialized services for their psycho-sexual problems. It has changed its name to Psychiatric Sex Clinic. Since its inception, this clinic has served patients referred from different departments as outpatients. A team consists of psychiatrists, postgraduate residents, and trainee psychologists see clients. After an initial assessment covering predisposing, precipitating and perpetuating and bio-psycho-social aspects, they are offered medication or sex therapy. Male and female sexual disorders, marital discord related to sexuality, gender identity-related issues, and sexual orientation-related problems are addressed (Arafat & Ahmed, 2017).

Following the model of care at BSMMU, PSCs were established in MAG Osmani Medical College, Sylhet (2018), Chattogram Medical College (2020) and Mymensingh Medical College (2022) to serve the patients with psychosexual problems. Currently, these clinics run on a weekly basis for 2 h. Another PSC commenced its journey in 2017 in National Institute of Mental Health, Dhaka, but its activities have been closed since emergence of COVID-19.

The Department of Pediatric Surgery at BSMMU runs a specialized clinic named "Disorder of Sexual Development (DSD) Clinic" to assess patients with incongruous genders. Mostly children and adolescents who are born with ambiguous genitalia, like absence of genitalia, complete sex organs, double gender, or other issues, undergo surgical operations. Prior to surgery, sometimes a team of psychiatrists and endocrinologists' opinions are taken and a management plan is advised.

Despite these specialized services and measures, the majority of patients with sexual problems are dealt with by dermatologists, psychiatrists, urologists, endocrinologists, and gynecologists in their private practices and outpatient services in their respective disciplines in tertiary care hospitals. For an effective change in patient care, the evidence-based knowledge sharing platform (SASSM School Bangladesh) has profound influence on making an effective change by providing bio-psycho-social aspects of sexual dysfunction.

## 9.8 Help-Seeking Behavior for Psychosexual Disorders in Bangladesh

Sexual dysfunction is a prevalent yet often discouraged health issue that affects people all around the world. Since Bangladesh is a largely traditional and patriarchal country, many subjects, including sex education, sexual activity, and homosexuality, are viewed as taboo (Khan 2018). Although schools have sex education programs, the majority of teachers either teach the subject minimally or choose to avoid the chapters on sexuality. Friendship with people of the opposite gender is discouraged, and there are numerous gender segregation schools around the country (Hossain et al., 2022). The network of extended families is highly valued here, which further prevents discussions about sex and sexuality because of awkwardness. As a result, many people are hesitant to seek help for sexual disorders out of embarrassment or shame. Moreover, being a Muslim-dominant nation, religious leaders may have varied interpretations of religious scriptures, which has a significant impact on how individuals understand and handle sexual issues and frequently conflicts with the several well-known therapies available to address sexual dysfunctions (Bhuiyan et al., 2014). Often parents avoid using phrases like "wet dreams" or "penis." Instead, they use indirect terms like "chheleder bepar" or "oisob bepar" [those concerns] to express their discomfort (Camellia et al., 2021). This silence teaches the child that sexual problems should not be discussed, and as a result, when they experience sexual problems, they tend to keep these concerns hidden rather than seeking help.

Media and popular culture frequently mirror irrational standards of sexual performance and appeal, leading persons with sexual dysfunctions to feel ashamed and inadequate. Social judgment can instill a dread of being perceived as different or imperfect, which discourages people from talking about problems or asking for assistance. Furthermore, due to a lack of awareness, sexual dysfunction is viewed as an individual's flaw, which is compounded by a lack of sex education. On top of that, misconceptions and religious dogma continue to perpetuate this stigma.

For years, people in Bangladesh have sought treatment from traditional healers for any health concern. People are more likely to seek Kabiraj's assistance with sexual concerns (Haque et al., 2018). A Bangladeshi study reported that the majority (73%) of the participants with sexual issues initially sought assistance from conventional or spiritual healers, homeopaths, local physicians, herbalists, pharmacists, and canvassers. This trend may be brought on by the accessibility and perceived cost-effectiveness of such treatments. The majority (77%) of participants sought support for their sexual worries from friends, coworkers, and close friends, with married or medically connected people receiving greater attention (Acharjee & Mullick, 2021). Friends and relatives may provide consolation, emotional support, and firsthand experience, but they may not have the expertise to handle complex sexual issues and occasionally may lead the victim misguided (Rao et al., 2018).

Internet is an emerging help-seeking source for the sexual problems in Bangladesh. Most people feel confident to seek help from internet because of anonymity and lack of embarrassment (Courtice et al., 2021). Other sources include books, newspapers, banners, posters, television, and seminars.

Professional assistance is sought at the very end for sexual problems. The majority of individuals who have sexual issues, if intend to get medical treatment, go to general practitioners for assistance. Dermatologists are the specialists who are most frequently consulted by patients. There are also gynecologists, internists, neurologists, and cardiologists among the other specialties. Gynecologists are frequently sought out for female sexual dysfunctions since they are publicly entitled to treat any health issues affecting women (Acharjee & Mullick, 2021). Sexual problems are perceived as physical rather than psychological issues and there is a lack of knowledge regarding seeking psychological help.

It was found that younger and better-educated people seek self-help more. In the aforementioned study, about one-fourths (23%) of the participants sought self-help which is an emerging pattern of help-seeking and thus needs to be addressed in future delivery systems (Acharjee & Mullick, 2021).

## 9.9 Legal Aspects of Sexuality-Related Issues in Bangladesh

During the colonial era, when Bangladesh was subject to English criminal law, the 1860 Penal Code was passed down from the British. After gaining independence, Bangladesh kept the rule in place, and same-sex sexual behavior is still illegal today. The 377 section of the penal code prohibits same-sex sexual behavior in Bangladesh. It makes "carnal intercourse against the order of nature with any man, woman, or animal" a criminal offense. This law only applies to men, and the maximum sentence is a lifetime imprisonment. Despite the fact that Sect. 377 is rarely enacted, there is evidence to suggest that this law is primarily used to harass LGBT individuals (Hossain, 2019). The issue of paraphilia is not officially addressed in the country's legal system though pedophilia is becoming an issue of concern (Bose et al., 2021; Mahmud, 2019). According to Bangladesh's Dissolution of Muslim Marriage Act, Sect. 9.2, a Muslim woman may apply for a divorce on the grounds that her husband was and is still impotent (Chowdhury, 2022).

The Bangladesh government has implemented 'official acknowledgement' to include "Hijra," "other," or "third gender" as a gender identity choice in official identification documents and institutional forms (Haq, 2015). The Department of Immigration and Passports has included a third category of "other" on passport application forms since 2014. However, gender-diverse people continue to confront challenges in the identification process. As a result, in 2022, the Ministry of Social Welfare had revised the definition of "Hijra" and draft is underway to minimize the complexity. Regarding management of gender identity disorder, there is no information available in Bangladesh about the legal status of sex reassignment surgery (SRS) that transgender people often seek as part of their gender transition (Alipour, 2017).

## 9.10 Organizations Working in the Field of Psychosexual Disorders in Bangladesh

Bangladesh, a South Asian nation with diverse cultures and lifestyles, faces challenges like sexual dysfunctions and gender inequality. Despite economic growth, urbanization, and educational advancements, deeply rooted societal structures persist, necessitating the intervention of non-government organizations alongside government initiatives to address these issues. Sexual dysfunctions are often shrouded in silence, affecting individuals and relationships across genders. Key organizations fighting against gender inequality and sexual dysfunctions in Bangladesh include Bangladesh Rehabilitation Assistance Committee (BRAC), Naripokkho, Ain O Shalish Kendra (ASK), Bangladesh Women's Health Coalition (BWHC), and Population Services and Training Center (PSTC). These organizations aim to empower individuals, promote gender equity, and destigmatize sexual health concerns. Their work is not done in isolation, but rather through advocacy and implementation, aiming to create a more inclusive and equitable society.

The South Asian Society for Sexual Medicine (SASSM), being a regional organization formed in 2013 with very eminent sexologists, urologists, and psychiatrists became a leading non-profitable organization working on psychosexual issues in Bangladesh (Krishnappa et al., 2020). Currently, a renowned psychiatrist from Bangladesh is the President of SASSM, indicating the active role of Bangladeshi professionals in the organization. SASSM has launched a collaborative training model to improve the quality of sexual health care. The initiative aims to bridge the knowledge gap between advances in sexual medicine and the clinical expertise of working physicians. The training focuses on improving the professional performance of clinicians, including knowledge, clinical skills, technical skills, and behaviors. SASSM has been organizing three-day foundation courses (SASSM School Bangladesh) on sexual medicine for the physicians of Bangladesh every year since 2017, besides arranging multidisciplinary workshops, seminars, symposiums and international conferences. SASSM School Bangladesh has so far trained 280 + specialists and postgraduate residents and got approval and financial support to run a three-month-long "SASSM School for GPs" to cover more elaborate details and practical aspects of knowledge and skill-based training in sexual medicine.

## 9.11 Current Trend of Researches Regarding Psychosexual Disorders in Bangladesh

In Bangladesh, researches regarding sexual issues have been centered mainly on sexually transmitted diseases. Recently, various aspects of psychosexual functioning and problems are being explored though there is no nationwide epidemiological study and no psychometrically developed instrument. A recent online search on different aspects of sexual medicine in Bangladesh found 72 published articles since 1982, where about three-fifths (58.3%) of the articles are based on original studies, psychiatrist SM Yasir Arafat being the highest contributing author (33%) (Arafat, 2023). Focusing on the recent trends on research, we have found 27 articles published during the last 10 years (2014–2023) based on quantitative and qualitative studies on psychosexual disorders and related issues (Table 9.4).

Some case studies have also been published on not-so-common psychosexual issues including atypical presentation of dhat syndrome, necrophilia, urophilia, hypersexuality, persistent genital arousal disorder, and infantile masturbation (Arafat

**Table 9.4** Studies regarding psychosexual disorders and related issues published in the last 10 years (2014–2023)*

| Study design | Study place | Study population | Sample size | Sampling technique | Investigated issues |
|---|---|---|---|---|---|
| Quantitative: 27<br>(Cross-sectional—24<br>Case—control—2<br>Prospective experimental—1) | BSMMU, Dhaka—7<br>NIMH, Dhaka—5<br>Other single healthcare center/ hospital in Dhaka—5<br>Single healthcare center/hospital outside Dhaka—3<br>Multiple hospitals/ health care centers—5<br>Others—2 | Persons with chronic physical illness (type 2 diabetes mellitus, HTN, gynecological etc.) —10<br>Persons seeking treatment for sexual problems—8<br>Persons seeking treatment for psychiatric problems other than sexual—5<br>Others (students, clinicians, men with homosexuality)—4 | 100 or less: 6<br>>100–500: 17<br>>500: 4 | Probability—2<br>Non-probability—22<br>Not mentioned—3 | Frequency, risk factors/ predictors of sexual dysfunctions/problems—15<br>Comorbidities—5<br>Efficacy of drug—1<br>KAP—1<br>Masturbation and pornography consumption—1<br>Homosexuality—2<br>Sexual history taking competency—1<br>Sexual myths and behavior—1 |
| Qualitative—2 | Dhaka—1<br>BSMMU—1 | Patients with sexual dysfunctions—1<br>LGBTQ + individuals—1 | | Purposive | Gender and sex diversity—1<br>Help-seeking behavior—1 |

* (Hasan et al., 2023; Mozumder et al., 2023; Gofur et al., 2023; Alam & Marston, 2023; Das & Malakar, 2022; Amin et al., 2022; Maruf et al., 2022; Sayed et al., 2021; Acharjee & Mullick, 2021; Nahar et al., 2019; Rakib et al., 2020; Mahbub et al., 2019; Kaoser et al., 2019; Chowdhury et al., 2018; Rony et al., 2017; Arafat & Ahmed, 2017; Sikdar et al., 2017; Salam et al., 2017; Nahar et al., 2017; Ahsan et al., 2016a, b; Rahman et al., 2016; Ahsan et al., 2016a, b; Mozumder et al., 2016; Selim et al., 2015; Asaduzzaman et al., 2020; Miah et al., 2015)

et al., 2021; Bose et al., 2021; Arafat et al., 2020; Arafat & Kar, 2020; Rahman et al., 2016). There is an increasing interest on adapting well-known and widely used instruments in Bangla and validating them on local population. Arizona Sexual Experiences Scale (ASEX), Female Sexual Function Index (FSFI-6), International Index of Erectile Function (IIEF), and Premature Ejaculation Diagnostic Tool have been validated so far (Islam et al., 2021; Mian et al., 2023; Parvez, 2022; Zohra, 2023).

## 9.12 Current Challenges

There are various challenges and obstructing factors in the proper management of psychosexual disorders.

### *9.12.1 Stigma and Cultural Taboos*

Bangladesh is a sexually conservative nation, and as therefore, cultural and societal conventions make talking about sexual health and related issues taboo (Karim et al., 2021). Because sexual health issues are stigmatized, many people are unwilling to ask for information or help.

### *9.12.2 Lack of Awareness and Education*

In schools and communities, there is a substantial lack of awareness and comprehensive sexual education. Teachers frequently feel uncomfortable and hesitant when teaching these issues to children (Khan et al., 2020). As a result of this knowledge gap, there are misconceptions and misinformation concerning sexual health and practices.

### *9.12.3 Limited Access to Healthcare Services*

Access to sexual healthcare services is frequently limited in both urban and rural areas. Furthermore, traditional healers such as kabiraj, homeopaths, herbalists, and pharmacists play an important role in dealing with sexual health issues, which discourages people from obtaining sexual treatment in healthcare settings (Acharjee & Mullick, 2021).

### 9.12.4 Lack of Trained Professionals

There is a shortage of sexual medicine specialists in the medical field. According to a study conducted on a sample of physicians in Bangladesh, 35% were uncomfortable inquiring about sexual history, with 26% expressing discomfort, and 12% concerned about upsetting patients (Ahsan et al., 2016a, b). The vast majority of respondents (95%) agreed that a specialized setup for those suffering from sexual dysfunction should be built. This shortage of specialists may result in poor care for persons with sexual health issues.

### 9.12.5 Lack of Budget and Infrastructure

The Government of Bangladesh is currently investing only 0.44% of its total health budget on mental health (Faruk, 2022), implying that spending on psychosexual health is even lower. People with sexual issues are left with insufficient resources and facilities to deal with sexual dysfunction (Arafat & Ahmed, 2017).

### 9.12.6 Gender Inequality

Gender inequality and discrimination are major driving force for gender violence and have a negative impact on sexual health, including issues of sexual violence, and rights related to reproduction (Jannat et al., 2023).

### 9.12.7 Lack of Research and Data

In Bangladesh, financing for sexuality research is frequently insufficient due to a failure to prioritize sexuality as a major health concern and a failure to recognize sexual dysfunction as a biopsychosocial phenomenon. Sexual health research has primarily focused on sexually transmitted diseases. Multiple aspects of psychosexual functioning and issues have recently been investigated.

## 9.13 Ways Forward

Scientific interest in sexual medicine has grown in the last 20 years as we've gained a better understanding of human sexuality and sexual organ function. However, communication challenges persist, such as imprecise ways for disseminating ideas, a lack of public willingness to address silence, and insufficient education and training opportunities for health professionals. Comprehensive sexual health education must be incorporated into student curricula, and instructors must be trained to overcome their reluctance to teach these issues to children.

Sexual medicine calls for a multidisciplinary team in which each component of sexuality can be addressed by more than one physician if necessary to address the bio-psycho-social aspects of sexuality. Apart from general practitioners, psychiatrists, andrologists, endocrinologists, gynecologists, and dermatologists have been dealing with clients with sexuality-related disorders, but there is a need for liaison services to coordinate the many aspects. Long-term training, such as a one-year fellowship in psychosexual disorders, can be arranged. A 1-to-2-year fellowship or master's degree in a tertiary care teaching hospital like BSMMU or NIMH can create experts. Primary care physicians' education and training in sexual medicine should be prioritized in order to build an effective referral system as well as liaison with other specialties and legislators are required. The Bangladeshi government should allocate more budget on mental health and sexual health. Furthermore, adequate resources and facilities for dealing with sexual dysfunction must be developed. There is a need for mental health services to be integrated into sexual medicine.

An organized communication method should be used to raise awareness about sex-related issues. As religious convictions and cultural norms impact sexual health and help-seeking behavior, advocacy aimed at mitigating sex-related stigma should also take sociocultural and religious factors into consideration. Legal reforms should be initiated for the management of specially gender and sex diversity issues.

More research and data assembling in the field of sexual medicine should be encouraged to better understand the prevalence of sexual health concerns and develop evidence-based ways to address them. Adequate financial support should be given to the authentic researchers for the quality researches.

## 9.14 Conclusion

Despite the lack of community-based study, clinical experiences and other relevant studies indicate that sexual dysfunctions are common in our population. Erectile dysfunction and premature ejaculation are the commonest male dysfunction and sexual interest/arousal disorder is the commonest female dysfunction. Dhat syndrome is also very common among men. Physical and psychiatric co-morbidities are common in the persons with sexual dysfunction. Myths and misconceptions are associated with the dysfunctions, which hinders the help-seeking behavior of the distressed. Moreover, the services for the management of sexual dysfunctions are not adequate and lack co-ordination. For proper management, multidisciplinary approach and measures to build up skilled manpower should be emphasized. Other sex-related issues including gender dysphoria and paraphilia are gaining attention both in the community and in the research arena but legal status reform of these issues is warranted.

## References

Abbasi, N. A. (2023). Psychiatric disorders among adult transgender population in Dhaka city of Bangladesh. (Unpublished FCPS thesis). National Institute of Mental Health, Bangladesh.

Abdullah, A. (2018). Living through resistance: A feminist analysis of Bangladeshi Hijras and gender non-conforming identity representation in media spaces and the documentary films, Call Me Salma (2010) and Are We So Different (2012).

Acharjee, P., & Mullick, M. S. I. (2021). The pattern of help-seeking behavior among patients with sexual dysfunctions attending in psychiatry outpatient department in a tertiary care hospital of Bangladesh. *Sexual Medicine, 9*(4), 100381. https://doi.org/10.1016/j.esxm.2021.100381.

Ahmed, S., & Arafat, S. M. Y. (2017). Taking history to deal with female sexual dysfunctions. *EC Psychology and Psychiatry, 3*(1), 7–9.

Ahsan, M. S., Arafat, S. M. Y., Ali, R., Rahman, S. M. A., Ahmed, S., & Rahman, M. M. (2016a). Sexual history taking competency: A survey among the clinicians in Bangladesh. *International Journal of Psychiatry, 1*(1), 1–4.

Ahsan, M. S., Selim, S., Ahmed, S., Ali, R., Ara, H., Kajol, R. K., Islam, M., & Arafat, S. M. Y. (2016b). Female sexual dysfunction and associated co-morbidities: A cross sectional study with Female Sexual Function Index (FSFI) in a tertiary care hospital of Bangladesh. *Bangladesh Journal of Psychiatry, 30*(2), 27–31.

Alam, P., & Marston, C. (2023). 'Bending' against straightening devices: Queer lived experiences of sexuality and sexual health in Bangladesh. *BMC Public Health, 23*, 173. https://doi.org/10.1186/s12889-023-15085-0.

Alipour, M. (2017). Islamic shari'a law, neotraditionalist Muslim scholars and transgender sex-reassignment surgery: A case study of Ayatollah Khomeini's and Sheikh al-Tantawi's fatwas. *International Journal of Transgenderism, 18*(1), 91–103.

Al-Mamun, M. A., Arafat, S. M. Y., Ambiatunnahar, M., & Griffiths, M. D. (2019). Attitudes and risk factors of pornography consumption among Bangladeshi university students: An exploratory study. *International Journal of Mental Health and Addiction, 17*, 323–335. https://doi.org/10.1007/s11469-018-0021-7

Al-Mamun, M., Hossain, M. J., Alam, M., Parvez, M. S., Dhar, B. K., & Islam, M. R. (2022). Discrimination and social exclusion of third-gender population (Hijra) in Bangladesh: A brief review. *Heliyon, 8*(10), e10840. https://doi.org/10.1016/j.heliyon.2022.e10840.

Amanullah, A. S. M., Abir, T., Husain, T., Lim, D., Osuagwu, U. L., Ahmed, G., Ahmed, S., Nur-A Yazdani, D. M., & Agho, K. E. (2022). Human rights violations and associated factors of the Hijras in Bangladesh-A cross-sectional study. *PLoS ONE, 17*(7), e0269375. https://doi.org/10.1371/journal.pone.0269375.

Amin, M. A., Mozid, N. E., Ahmed, S. B., Sharmin, S., Monju, I. H., Jhumur, S. S., Sarker, W., Dalal, K., & Hawlader, M. D. H. (2022). Status of female sexual dysfunction among postmenopausal women in Bangladesh. *BMC Women's Health, 22*(1), 401. https://doi.org/10.1186/s12905-022-01991-9.

Anderson, D., Laforge, J., Ross, M. M., Vanlangendonck, R., Hasoon, J., Viswanath, O., Kaye, A. D., & Urits, I. (2022). Male sexual dysfunction. *Health psychology research, 10*(3), 37533. https://doi.org/10.52965/001c.37533.

Arafat, S. M. Y. (2019). Paraphilia is an untouched research topic in Bangladesh. *Indian Journal of Health Sexuality and Culture, 5*(2), 104–107. https://doi.org/10.5281/zenodo.3983616.

Arafat, S. M. Y., & Ahmed, S. (2017). Burden of misconception in sexual health care setting: A cross-sectional investigation among the patients attending a psychiatric sex clinic of Bangladesh. *Psychiatry Journal*, 9827083.https://doi.org/10.1155/2017/9827083.

Arafat, S. Y., & Kar, S. K. (2020). Hypersexuality in a Bangladeshi female: A case report. *Journal of Psychosexual Health, 2*(1), 93–95. https://doi.org/10.1177/263183181989893

Arafat, S. Y., & Khan, S. T. (2019). Childhood masturbation: A case report from Bangladesh. *Journal of Psychosexual Health, 1*(3–4), 280–282. https://doi.org/10.1177/2631831819894766

Arafat, S. M. Y., Kar, S. K., & Khan, S. T. (2020). Urophilia associated with obsessive-compulsive disorder in a Bangladeshi male: A rare case report. *Neurology, Psychiatry and Brain Research, 36*, 96–97. https://doi.org/10.1016/j.npbr.2020.04.003.

Arafat, S. M. Y., Mondal, F., & Ghimire, S. (2021). A 47-year-old man passing putrid semen through saliva and sweat: A case of Dhat syndrome. *Journal of General and Family Medicine, 23*(3), 177–179. https://doi.org/10.1002/jgf2.513.

Arafat, S. M. Y. (2023). *Research on Sexual Medicine in Bangladesh: Current Status, Challenges, and Opportunities*. [Conference presentation]. 5th biennial conference 2023 of South Asian Society for Sexual Medicine (SASSM). Dhaka, Bangladesh.

Asaduzzaman, M., Kamrul-Hasan, A. B., Islam, A., Kabir, M. A., Chanda, P. K., Islam, M. A., Sharif, J. M., Ahmed, N., Mandal, T., Ghosh, S., Paul, P. K., Saha, R. K., Hossain, F., Rana, M. S., Alam, K., Kamruzzaman, M., Nandi, A. K., & Siddiqui, N. I. (2020). Frequency and risk factors of erectile dysfunction among Bangladeshi adult men with type 2 diabetes mellitus. *Mymensingh Medical Journal, 29*(1), 66–72.

Aziz, A., & Azhar, S. (2020). Social exclusion and official recognition for Hijra in Bangladesh. *Journal of Research on Women and Gender, 9*(1), 3–19.

Balon, R. (2017). Burden of sexual dysfunction. *Journal of Sex & Marital Therapy, 43*(1), 49–55. https://doi.org/10.1080/0092623X.2015.1113597.

Barua, A., & Khan, S. A. (2023). Addressing violence against transgender people in Bangladesh: A call for policy intervention. *Frontiers in Sociology, 7*, 995448. https://doi.org/10.3389/fsoc.2022.995448.

Bhuiyan, M. K. (2014). Inclusion of sex education in school curriculum of Bangladesh: Parents' attitude. *IOSR Journal of Research & Method in Education, 4*(5), 32–40.

Bose, P. K., Arafat, S. M. Y., Shoib, S., & Reza, A. S. (2021). Necrophilia in a forensic morgue staff in Bangladesh: Forensic psychiatric challenges and implications. *Journal of Affective Disorders Reports, 5*, 100158. https://doi.org/10.1016/j.jadr.2021.100158.

Bőthe, B., Koós, M., Nagy, L., Kraus, S. W., Demetrovics, Z., Potenza, M. N., Michaud, A., Ballester-Arnal, R., Batthyány, D., Bergeron, S., Billieux, J., Briken, P., Burkauskas, J., Cárdenas-López, G., Carvalho, J., Castro-Calvo, J., Chen, L., Ciocca, G., Corazza, O., … Vaillancourt-Morel, M. P. (2023). Compulsive sexual behavior disorder in 42 countries: Insights from the international sex survey and introduction of standardized assessment tools. *Journal of Behavioral Addictions, 12*(2), 393–407. https://doi.org/10.1556/2006.2023.00028.

Camellia, S., Rommes, E., & Jansen, W. (2021). Beyond the talking imperative: The value of silence on sexuality in youth-parent relations in Bangladesh. *Global Public Health, 16*(5), 775–787. https://doi.org/10.1080/17441692.2020.1751862.

Chowdhury, M. S. I., Ahammed, M. M., Taher, M. A., Rahman, M. A., & Ahmed, M. M. (2018). Knowledge, attitude and practice towards use of herbal aphrodisiac among unani & ayurvedic health care seekers in Dhaka city. *Asian Journal of Medical and Biological Research, 4*(4), 400–405. https://doi.org/10.3329/ajmbr.v4i4.40113.

Chowdhury, M. A. (2022). Dissolution of muslim marriage: A critical analysis of laws and procedure related to dissolution of muslim marriage in Bangladesh (Doctoral dissertation, East West University).

Courtice, E. L., Shaughnessy, K., Blom, K., Asrat, Y., Daneback, K., Döring, N., & Byers, E. S. (2021). Young adults' qualitative self-reports of their outcomes of online sexual activities. *European Journal of Investigation in Health, Psychology and Education, 11*(2), 303–320.

Das, A., & Malakar, C. (2022). Prevalence of sexual dysfunctions in male patients of a tertiary hospital. *Archives of NIMH, 5*(2), 34–37.

Faruk, M. O. (2022). Community-based mental health services in Bangladesh: Prospects and challenges. *World Social Psychiatry, 4*(3), 187–192. https://doi.org/10.4103/wsp.wsp_7_22.

Ghani, A. (2013). Present state-of-the art of traditional medicine practice in Bangladesh. *Traditional Medicine and Material Medica, 1*, 59–70.

Gofur, T. B., Hasan, M. K., Bhuiyan, S. M. A. U., & Islam, M. R. (2023). Prevalence of sexual dysfunction among substance use disorder. *Archives of NIMH, 6*(1), 29–34.

Haq, K. (2015). The Hijra comes in from the heat and dust: Notes towards a definition of Bangladeshi writing in English. *Wasafiri, 30*(4), 3–7. https://doi.org/10.1080/02690055.2015.1068982.
Haque, M. I., Chowdhury, A. B. M. A., Shahjahan, M., & Harun, M. G. D. (2018). Traditional healing practices in rural Bangladesh: A qualitative investigation. *BMC Complementary and Alternative Medicine, 18*(1), 62. https://doi.org/10.1186/s12906-018-2129-5.
Hasan, A. B. M. K., Alam, M. S., Zarin, N., Aalpona, F. T. Z., Mustari, M., Akter, F., Jannat, N., Azad, U., Chanda, P. K., Rafi, A., Hasan, M. J., & Selim, S. (2023). Sexual dysfunction in women with type 2 diabetes mellitus: A single-centre cross-sectional study from Bangladesh. *Archives of endocrinology and metabolism, 67*(5), e000635. https://doi.org/10.20945/2359-3997000000635.
Hossain, A. (2017). The paradox of recognition: Hijra, third gender and sexual rights in Bangladesh. *Culture, Health & Sexuality, 19*(12), 1418–1431.
Hossain, B. S., Korishi, R., & Molla, K. (2022). Status of sex education at elementary schools in Bangladesh: A comparative study among few schools in Dhaka. *Britain International of Linguistics Arts and Education Journal, 4*(1), 1–7.
Hossain, A. (2019). Section 377, same-sex sexualities and the struggle for sexual rights in Bangladesh. *Australian journal of Asian law, 20*(1), 115–125. https://ssrn.com/abstract=3516500.
Islam, S. (2019). A theoretical analysis of the legal status of transgender: Bangladesh perspective. *International Journal of Research and Innovation in Social Science, 3*(3), 117–119.
Islam, T., Qusar, M. S., Ahsan, M. S., Morshed, A. S. M., & Haque, S. (2021). Adaptation and validation of Bangla version of premature ejaculation diagnostic tool. *Bangabandhu Sheikh Mujib Medical University Journal, 14*(4), 132–137.
Jabbar, M. (2023). *Gender and property rights: Critical issues in the context of SDG 5 with a focus on Bangladesh*. FriesenPress.
Jahan, M. S., Billah, S. M., Furuya, H., & Watanabe, T. (2012). Female sexual dysfunction: Facts and factors among gynecology outpatients. *The Journal of Obstetrics and Gynaecology Research, 38*(1), 329–335. https://doi.org/10.1111/j.1447-0756.2011.01648.x.
Jannat, S., Sifat, R. I., & Khisa, M. (2023). Sexual and reproductive health conditions of women: Insights from Rohingya Refugee Women in Bangladesh. *Sexuality Research and Social Policy, 20*(3), 855–868.
Jebin, L. (2018). Status of transgender people in Bangladesh: A socio-economic-analysis. *South Asian Journal of Policy and Governance, 42*(1), 49–63.
Kaoser, A. S. M., Mujahid, M. M. A., & Sarkar, A. Z. (2019). Estimates of sexual dysfunction in patients on antipsychotic medications. *Archives of NIMH, 2*(2), 29–31.
Karim, F., Zakaria, M., & Hoque, N. S. (2021). Reproductive health knowledge, attitude, and practice among adolescent girls in urban and rural areas of Bangladesh. *Anthropos, 116*(1), 55–66.
Khan, M. A., & Habiba, U. (2021). Exploring the social status with psychoactive and physical impacts of Hijra community: An evidence based study on Khulna City, Bangladesh. *Asian Journal of Social Sciences and Legal Studies, 3*(1), 1–9.
Khan, S. I., Khan, M. N. M., Hasan, A. M. R., Irfan, S. D., Horng, L. M., Chowdhury, E. I., & Azim, T. (2019). Understanding the reasons for using methamphetamine by sexual minority people in Dhaka, Bangladesh. *The International Journal on Drug Policy, 73*, 64–71. https://doi.org/10.1016/j.drugpo.2019.07.009.
Khan, S. A., Alam, F., Rommes, E., & Rashid, S. F. (2020). Experiencing shame: An affective reading of the sexual and reproductive health and rights classroom in Bangladesh. *Sex Education, 20*(6), 597–611.
Khan, M. N. M., Sarwar, G., Irfan, S. D., Gourab, G., Rana, A. M., & Khan, S. I. (2022). Understanding the barriers of HIV testing services for men who have sex with men and transgender women in Bangladesh: A qualitative study. *Community Health Equity Research & Policy, 42*(3), 309–323.
Khan, T. H. (2018). Young men's experiences and views of sex education in Bangladesh: A Foucauldian discourse analysis.

Khanam, A. (2021). Human rights of Hijras in Bangladesh: An analysis. *Social Science Review, 38*(1), 249–276.

Krishnappa, P., Srini, V. S., Shah, R., Lentz, A. C., Garaffa, G., Martinez-Salamanca, J. I., & Moncada, I. (2020). Cadaveric penile prosthesis workshop training improves surgical confidence levels of urologists: South Asian Society for Sexual Medicine course survey. *International Journal of Urology: Official Journal of the Japanese Urological Association, 27*(11), 1032–1037. https://doi.org/10.1111/iju.14338.

Mahbub, M. I., Kamrul-Hasan, A. B., Selim, S., Mir, A. S., Saifuddin, M., & Pathan, M. F. (2019). Frequency and predictors of erectile dysfunction in Bangladeshi men with type 2 diabetes mellitus: experience from a tertiary center. *Mymensingh Medical Journal, 28*(1), 137–143.

Mahmud, M. E. (2019). Is Paedophilia increasing in Bangladesh? https://www.thedailystar.net/health/news/paedophilia-increasing-bangladesh-1770982.

Maruf, M. M., Khan, M. Z. R., Jahan, N., Ahmed, A. U., Sadiq, M. S., & Ferdush, R. (2022). Sociodemographic profile and co-morbid symptoms among individuals with semen loss. *Bangladesh Journal of Medicine, 33*(1), 64–69. https://doi.org/10.3329/bjm.v33i1.56792.

Maruf, M. M., Saleem, T., & Arafat, S. M. Y. (2024). Dhat syndrome: A fact or myth. In S. K. Kar, S. M. Y. Arafat, V. Menon (Eds.), *Dhat syndrome* (pp). Springer.

Matin, W. M., Fatima, K., Noor, I. K., & Sharmin, S. (2020). Covid-19: Quick survey for community response for TG and Hijra. *Bandhu Social Welfare Society*. https://www.bandhu-bd.org/wp-content/uploads/2020/06/Covid-19-Quick-Survey-for-Community-Response-for-TG-and-Hijra.pdf.

McCool-Myers, M., Theurich, M., Zuelke, A., Knuettel, H., & Apfelbacher, C. (2018). Predictors of female sexual dysfunction: A systematic review and qualitative analysis through gender inequality paradigms. *BMC Women's Health, 18*(1), 108. https://doi.org/10.1186/s12905-018-0602-4.

Miah, M. A. A., Al-Mamun, M. A., Khan, S., & Mozumder, M. K. (2015). Sexual myths and behavior of male patients with psychosexual dysfunction in sexual myths and behavior of male patients with psychosexual dysfunction in Bangladesh. *Dhaka University Journal of Psychology, 39*, 89–100.

Mian, D. M. S., Qusar, M. M. A. S., Hossain, R., Chowdhury, T., & Roy, K. (2023). Cross cultural adaptation and psychometric validation of the Arizona Sexual Experiences Scale (ASEX) into Bangla. *The journal of sexual medicine*, 20 (Suppl 1), qdad060.328. https://doi.org/10.1093/jsxmed/qdad060.328.

Ministry of Health and Family Welfare. (2021). Assessment of healthcare providers in Bangladesh 2021. https://cdn.who.int/media/docs/default-source/searo/bangladesh/assessment-of-healthcare-providers-in-bangladesh-2021.pdf. Retrieved October 29, 2023.

Ministry of Health and Family Welfare. (2021). National mental health survey 2019. http://nimh.gov.bd/wp-content/uploads/2021/11/Mental-Health-Survey-Report.pdf. Retrieved March 29, 2023.

Mozumder, M. K., & Rahman, M. M. (2004). A prevalence study of various male psycho-sexual dysfunctions and problems among individuals attending psychological services in a sex therapy clinic. *Bangladesh Psychological Studies, 14*, 71–88.

Mozumder, M. K., Haque, M. A., Jasmine, U. H., Royal, R. I., & Sharmin, R. (2016). Behavior and experience of male homosexuals in Bangladesh. *Bangladesh Journal of Psychiatry, 30*(2), 41–44.

Mozumder, M. K., Jasmine, U. H., Haque, M. A., & Haque, S. (2023). Mental health and suicide risk among homosexual males in Bangladesh. *PLoS ONE, 18*(8), e0289597. https://doi.org/10.1371/journal.pone.0289597.

Mujahid, M. A., Sarkar, A. A., & Monzur, S. E. (2020). Factors associated with sexual side effects of antipsychotics in patients with psychotic disorders. *Archives of NIMH, 3*(2), 21–24.

Nahar, S., Shaheen, M. M., Islam, T., Alim, S. A. H. M., & Alam, M. F. (2017). Psychosocial factors associated with premature ejaculation among the patients attended in a tertiary level psychiatric hospital, Dhaka, Bangladesh. *Bangladesh Journal of Psychiatry, 31*(2), 27–31.

Nahar, S., Shaheen, M. M., Alam, M. T., & Maruf, M. M. (2019). Premature ejaculation among men attending in the sex clinic of a tertiary level psychiatric hospital. *Archives of NIMH, 2*(1), 20–25.

Narang, T., Garima, & Singh, S. M. (2016). Psychosexual disorders and dermatologists. *Indian Dermatology Online Journal, 7*(3), 149–158.https://doi.org/10.4103/2229-5178.182349.

Parvez, K. H. (2022). Bangla validation of International Index of Erectile Function (Unpublished MD thesis). Bangabandhu Sheikh Mujib Medical University.

Rabbani, M. G., Alim, M. A., Pillai, S., Kabir, R., & Arafat, S. M. Y. (2020). Sexual misconceptions in Bangladesh: Role of digital media. *Indian Journal of Health, Sexuality & Culture, 6*(1), 83–88. https://doi.org/10.5281/zenodo.3929265.

Rahman, S. A., Arafat, S.M.Y., Parveen, S., & Shalahuddin, Q. M. (2016). Persistent genital arousal disorder in perimenopausal woman: A case report. *International Journal of Women's Health Care, 1*(1), 1–3.

Rakib, K. H. B., Alam, A., Rahman, M. A., Al Azad, N., Bahar, A. H., Munna, N. H., ... & Azad, M. A. K. (2020). An evaluation of the frequency and severity of erectile dysfunction in hypertensive married men compared with normotensive married men. *Cardiology and Cardiovascular Research, 4*(3), 85.

Rao, T. S. S., Tandon, A., Manohar, S., & Mathur, S. (2018). Clinical practice guidelines for management of sexual disorders in elderly. *Indian journal of psychiatry, 60*(Suppl 3), S397–S409.https://doi.org/10.4103/0019-5545.224478.

Rony, A. F. M., Alam, M. F., & Khan, M. Z. R. (2017). Sexual dysfunctions among patients in a psychiatric hospital. *Bangladesh Journal of Psychiatry, 31*(2), 43–47. https://doi.org/10.3329/bjpsy.v31i2.45374.

Salam, M. A., Qusar, M. S., Saklain, M. A., Pathan, M. S., Islam, M. M., & Ali, M. (2017). Psychiatric co-morbidity among the male patients with sexual dysfunction in a tertiary hospital of Bangladesh. *Dinajpur Medical College Journal, 10*(2), 278–283.

Selim, S., Chowdhury, S. H., Azad, A. K., Chowdhury, M. A. J., & Rahaman, F. R. (2015). Frequency and risk factors of erectile dysfunction in Bangladeshi diabetic men. *Journal of Endocrinology, Diabetes and Obesity, 3*(3), 1075.

Sema, S. A., & Islam, M. T. (2020). Empowerment state of transgender people in Bangladesh: A study on Savar national memorial based area in Dhaka city. *Asian Journal of Social Sciences and Legal Studies, 2*(1), 1–10.

Sikdar, T. K., Chowdhury, M., Ahsan, M. S., & Ali, R. (2017). Dapoxetine for the management of premature ejaculation. *Bangladesh Journal of Psychiatry, 31*(1), 15–19.

Singh, A. (2017). Debating the contemporary: A study of Mahesh Dattani's plays (Doctoral dissertation).

Syed, M. A., Karim, M. R., Ahmed, K., Royle, R. K. S., Chowdhury, A. R., Uddin, M. M., & Habiba, R. (2021). Pattern of sexual dysfunction in male major depressive disorder patients. *Archives of NIMH, 4*(1), 16–22.

Yunus, M., Forhad, M. A. R., & Islam, R. (2022). Needs assessment of anondomela women entrepreneurs.

Zohra, R. (2023). Bangla validation of Female Sexual Function Index. (Unpublished MD thesis). Bangabandhu Sheikh Mujib Medical University.

# Chapter 10
# Forensic Psychiatry in Bangladesh

**Anis Ahmed, Palash Kumar Bose, and S. M. Yasir Arafat**

**Abstract** Forensic psychiatry, the intersection of psychiatry and the legal system, has gained recognition and importance worldwide. However, it has been a neglected domain in Bangladesh. There is no specialized training in forensic psychiatry in the country even though a high prevalence of mental disorders has been found among the prisoners. There are only 15 inpatient beds in an institute for the whole country. This chapter explores the current status and development of forensic psychiatry services in Bangladesh, a lower middle-income country where the healthcare system undergoing significant transformation. In the context of Bangladesh, the establishment of forensic psychiatry would represent a significant step toward addressing the intricate challenges posed by individuals with mental disorders within the legal framework.

**Keywords** Forensic psychiatry · Law · Mental health act · Bangladesh psychiatry · Mental health · Psychiatric services

## 10.1 Introduction

Forensic psychiatry, the intersection of psychiatry and the legal system, has gained recognition and importance worldwide as societies grapple with the complex interplay of mental health and criminal justice (Arboleda-Flórez, 2006; Niveau & Welle, 2018). In recent years, there has been a growing realization of the need for specialized expertise in this field to address the unique challenges posed by individuals with mental disorders within the legal framework (Niveau & Welle, 2018).

A. Ahmed
Birmingham and Solihull Mental Health NHS Foundation Trust, Aston Medical School, Birmingham, England

P. K. Bose
Department of Forensic Medicine and Toxicology, Enam Medical College, Dhaka, Bangladesh

S. M. Y. Arafat (✉)
Department of Psychiatry, Bangladesh Specialized Hospital Limited, Dhaka, Bangladesh
e-mail: arafatdmc62@gmail.com



S. M. Y. Arafat (ed.), *Mental Health in Bangladesh*,
https://doi.org/10.1007/978-981-97-0610-5_10

Forensic psychiatry involves the application of psychiatric principles, knowledge, and expertise to legal matters. It encompasses a wide range of activities, including the assessment of mental competency, determination of insanity, psychiatric defences, risk assessments, and providing expert testimony in legal proceedings and managing mentally disordered offenders in the community. Forensic psychiatrists bridge the gap between mental health and the legal system, contributing to the fair and just treatment of individuals with mental disorders within legal contexts (Niveau & Welle, 2018).

Forensic psychiatry, by its nature, demands a collaborative approach that goes beyond the boundaries of a single discipline. The intricacies of mental health and legal contexts require the integration of expertise from various fields to ensure comprehensive assessments and effective interventions. Through shared insights, diverse perspectives, and combined skill sets, this multidisciplinary approach in forensic psychiatry fosters a more nuanced evaluation of cases, addresses complex challenges, and contributes to fair and just legal outcomes. The exchange of knowledge and expertise among team members enriches the field, emphasizing the interconnectedness of mental health, law, and societal well-being (Gbadebo-Goyea et al., 2012). This chapter explores the current status and development of forensic psychiatry in Bangladesh, a lower middle-income country where the healthcare system undergoing significant transformation.

## 10.2 Why Forensic Psychiatry is Necessary in Bangladesh?

Forensic psychiatry is indispensable in a civilized society due to its pivotal role in understanding the complex intersection of mental health and offending behaviour that arises out of mental illness. Bangladesh, like many nations, grapples with challenges related to mental health stigma, limited resources, and the need for fair and just legal processes. Forensic psychiatry brings a systematic and evidence-based approach to assess the mental health of individuals entangled in legal matters, ensuring that justice is served while upholding the rights and dignity of those with mental disorders (Balcioglu et al., 2023; Gbadebo-Goyea et al., 2012).

Moreover, the development of forensic psychiatry in Bangladesh is not only crucial for addressing the complexities of mental health in the legal system but also for preventing miscarriages of justice. Without specialized psychiatric assessments, individuals with untreated mental illnesses may remain at a higher risk of being unfairly convicted or receiving inappropriate legal outcomes. Misunderstandings regarding the nature and impact of mental disorders could lead to judgments that fail to account for the individual's mental health needs. Comprehensive package of care, facilitated by forensic psychiatric assessments, not only benefits the individual by improving their mental health but also contributes to the overall well-being of society by rehabilitating mentally disordered offenders. The development of forensic psychiatry in Bangladesh is, therefore, an investment in a fair and effective legal and health system that recognizes the importance of mental health for both individuals and the broader community.

### 10.2.1 Case Study 1

Consider the fictional case of Ahmed, a 28-year-old man in Bangladesh facing legal charges for wounding with intention. Forensic psychiatric assessments reveal that Ahmed has been battling undiagnosed schizophrenia, contributing to his erratic behaviour and impaired decision-making. He has been harbouring persecutory delusional belief that his neighbours have been spying on him and poisoning his food. He started moving homes around the country and ended up homeless. Out of sheer paranoia, he assaulted a stranger on the street believing the stranger was controlling his thoughts and he heard a voice instructing him to assault the stranger. Without this understanding, there is a risk of a miscarriage of justice as the legal system might misinterpret his actions as intentional criminal behaviour rather than a manifestation of untreated mental illness.

The intervention of forensic psychiatry not only sheds light on Ahmed's mental health but also emphasizes the importance of addressing his psychiatric condition in legal proceedings. If he is not assessed for fitness to be interviewed by the police, his statement can lead to a false confession or self-incrimination. If his fitness to plead and to stand trial is not assessed, he could be a victim of a miscarriage of justice. Finally, treatment, including therapy and medication, proves effective in stabilizing Ahmed's mental health, reducing the risk of reoffending, and offering him a chance of rehabilitation. This fictional case illustrates how the absence of forensic psychiatric assessments could lead to misunderstandings, potential injustice, and an increased risk of reoffending, emphasizing the crucial role forensic psychiatry plays in the fair and effective administration of justice in Bangladesh.

### 10.2.2 Case Study 2

Mr. Rahman (anonymous), a British Bangladeshi in his mid-30 s, unfolds tragically within the context of his dual heritage. He was born in Bangladesh and moved to England during his early childhood. Several years ago, the fabric of Mr. Rahman's world began to warp under the weight of paranoia. What initially manifested as unsettling feelings morphed into a chilling belief that a nefarious gang was relentlessly pursuing him. His pleas for understanding within his family fell on deaf ears, cultivating distrust and suspicion. A cruel narrative took root—an insidious conspiracy involving his own family orchestrating his demise. As the grip of paranoia tightens, Mr. Rahman's reality warps further. Delusions of reference contort innocent interactions into signs of betrayal. A simple conversation between his wife and a shopkeeper becomes damning evidence of infidelity, intensifying the torment within his mind. Seeking reprieve, his family embarks on the path to primary care; he was urgently referred to the secondary care mental health team for a comprehensive evaluation.

While awaiting assessment, his family decided to go on holiday to Bangladesh. The change in environment proved disastrous. Dhaka airport, a sea of unfamiliar faces, triggered intense paranoia. Innocent crowds transformed into the ominous gang from his delusions. Fear crescendoed upon reaching his ancestral village, and Mr. Rahman made numerous desperate calls to the British High Commission in Dhaka, pleading for rescue from the imagined threat.

At his home, in the quiet hours of the night, he committed a horrifying act—taking the lives of his own father and wife with a kitchen knife. Local residents acted swiftly, apprehended him in a state of chaos, and eventually, he was remanded in prison with a charge of double murder.

As his mental state deteriorated further, he was seen by a prison doctor who suggested treatment by a psychiatrist, which was not available in the prison. Subsequently, he was granted bail for treatment in a local psychiatric hospital in Bangladesh, and his family members arranged transfer back to England for better treatment. Eventually, he was detained in a medium-secure hospital under the Mental Health Act in England and received treatment with Clozapine.

Upon reaching stability, a poignant twist emerges in Mr. Rahman's story. The weight of the reality he had unknowingly created during a psychotic state becomes an unbearable burden. Suicidal thoughts, born from deep remorse and grief, overshadow his path to recovery. However, the legal repercussions of his actions persist. His criminal case, entangled with the complexities of mental health, justice, and jurisdiction related to dual citizenship dynamics, remains unresolved. Mr. Rahman's story, a poignant exploration of the intersection between mental health and the legal system, unfolds against the unique backdrop of his British Bangladeshi identity, encapsulating the challenges faced in the realm of forensic psychiatry in both Bangladesh and England.

## 10.3 Historical Context

The emergence of forensic psychiatry as a distinct medical specialty took root in the late eighteenth century, although issues intersecting with legal and societal challenges have deep historical roots. Ancient legal systems, such as the Code of Hammurabi in Babylonia, the ancient law of Mesopotamia, had a special section reserved just for dealing with insane criminal defendants. In ancient Hebrew Law, intent played a crucial role in determining the innocence of someone who accidentally caused harm, safeguarding them from avenging relatives. Similarly, in India around 880 BC, leniency was granted in cases of insanity, and special considerations were extended to individuals with intellectual disabilities and children below 15 years of age.

Ancient Greek philosophy, particularly Plato, delved into rational and irrational behaviours, proposing that individuals possess the freedom to choose their actions. In the writings of Macer in 180 AD, during the time of Marcus Aurelius, consequences were imposed on the relatives of a lunatic who, if escaped, caused harm to others. This led to a severe penalty, establishing a unique form of kinship malpractice.

In pre-Norman England, there was no separate criminal code, and the family of an insane murderer was expected to compensate and care for the victim's family.

Insanity, during Norman times, was not a defence but a circumstance that warranted referral to the king for pardon. The ancient Jewish Talmud recommended the execution of a murderer under the influence of alcohol, while Islamic law considered murder by a mentally ill person or a minor as involuntary homicide, subject only to compensation.

The criminal law of England and the United States has long recognized insanity as a mitigating or exculpating factor that exempts the accused from punishment. It is widely believed by lawyers and historians that the "wild beast" test of criminal responsibility, which originated with the English Judge Henry de Bracton in 1256, has been a foundational concept. This principle was gradually evolved and endorsed over the following five centuries, ultimately being formalized by Judge Tracy at the trial of Edward Arnold in 1724 (Platt, 1965).

In the later part of the nineteenth century, Emil Kraepelin contributed theories emphasizing the contextual and naturalistic dependence of mental events relevant to forensic perspectives. The twentieth century saw the organic versus functional distinction and the establishment of organizations such as the American Academy of Psychiatry and the Law (AAPL), bridging the gap between psychiatry and law.

Bangladesh, with its diverse population and a legal system rooted in British colonial history, has faced challenges in adequately addressing mental health concerns within the legal framework. The justice system of Bangladesh is a replicated from the British judicial system (Ashraf et al., 2022). Historically, mental health issues were often stigmatized, and individuals with mental disorders faced marginalization. The recognition of the nexus between mental health and criminal justice has been a relatively recent development, necessitating the establishment of forensic psychiatry as a distinct discipline.

## 10.4 Roles and Responsibilities of Forensic Psychiatrists

Forensic psychiatrists play a pivotal role in bridging the gap between mental health and the legal system (Martone, 2022). Their expertise is essential in conducting comprehensive psychiatric assessments, offering expert testimony, and guiding legal proceedings involving individuals with mental disorders. Following are the standard roles and responsibilities for a forensic psychiatry.

### *10.4.1 Competency Evaluations*

Forensic psychiatrists are tasked with evaluating the mental competency of individuals involved in legal proceedings. This involves assessing a person's ability to understand the charges against them and to participate effectively in criminal justice system. Evaluation of fitness to plead and to stand trial is crucial to ensure a fair trial and proper legal representation.

### *10.4.2 Criminal Responsibility Assessments*

Determining a person's criminal responsibility is a key responsibility of forensic psychiatrists. They assess whether a defendant was mentally sound at the time of the alleged offence, impacting the legal consequences they may face.

### *10.4.3 Risk Assessments*

Forensic psychiatrists are involved in evaluating the risk of future violent behaviour or reoffending. This assessment aids the legal system in making informed decisions about sentencing, parole, or other interventions, with the overarching goal of public safety.

### *10.4.4 Expert Witness Testimony*

Forensic psychiatrists often serve as expert witnesses in court, providing their professional opinion on mental health issues relevant to a case. Their testimony helps judges and juries understand complex psychiatric concepts, contributing to the fair adjudication of legal matters.

### *10.4.5 Prison Psychiatry*

Within the criminal justice system, forensic psychiatrists work in prisons providing mental health treatment to incarcerated individuals. This involves diagnosing and treating mental disorders among inmates, facilitating rehabilitation, and addressing the mental health challenges within the prison environment.

### *10.4.6 Collaboration with Legal Professionals*

Effective communication and collaboration with legal professionals are crucial for forensic psychiatrists. They must convey complex psychiatric findings in a way that is understandable to non-experts, facilitating the integration of mental health considerations into legal decision-making.

### *10.4.7 Research and Advocacy*

Forensic psychiatrists play a crucial role in conducting research that provides valuable insights to both the psychiatric and legal communities. Their contributions are focused on addressing local cultural nuances and resource requirements in alignment with the specific laws and regulations of the region.

## 10.5 Psychiatric Defences in Criminal Courts

In the complex realm of criminal justice, the interplay between mental health and legal culpability is a critical facet addressed by forensic psychiatrists. A range of common psychiatric defences is raised in criminal courts where it is crucial that forensic psychiatrists convey professional and impartial views in accessible language to lay persons.

### *10.5.1 Insanity Defence*

The insanity defence is perhaps the most well-known psychiatric defence, asserting that the defendant, at the time of the alleged crime, was unable to appreciate the wrongfulness of their actions due to a severe mental disorder. Forensic psychiatrists play a crucial role in evaluating the defendant's mental state and providing expert opinions on their capacity for criminal responsibility.

In the medical realm, insanity is primarily a psychiatric diagnosis based on the individual's mental state at the time of the alleged offence. Contrastingly, legal insanity is a construct within the criminal justice system that addresses the defendant's culpability for a crime. It involves whether the defendant, at the time of the offence, had the mental capacity to appreciate the wrongfulness of their actions and to conform their behaviour to the law. Legal standards for insanity may vary across jurisdictions, but they generally incorporate a combination of psychiatric and legal criteria.

The distinction between medical and legal insanity underscores the complex relationship between mental health and legal culpability. Forensic psychiatrists must navigate these nuances carefully, recognizing that while a psychiatric diagnosis may provide insights into an individual's mental state, it is the legal system that ultimately determines the implications for criminal responsibility.

### 10.5.2 Diminished Capacity

Unlike the insanity defence, which focuses on the defendant's inability to understand the wrongfulness of their actions, the diminished capacity defence argues that a mental disorder impaired the defendant's ability to form specific criminal intent. The diminished capacity defence involves the defendant asserting that their mental state at the time of the offence prevented them from forming the specific intent required for the crime. Unlike the insanity defence, the diminished capacity defence does not necessitate the defendant to fulfil the legal standards for insanity. Instead, the defendant must demonstrate a direct correlation between their mental illness and their inability to form the necessary intent for the offence. Forensic psychiatrists assess the extent to which a psychiatric condition influenced the defendant's mental state at the time of the offence.

### 10.5.3 Intoxication as a Mental State

Numerous studies have established a significant correlation between substance abuse and criminal activities, highlighting that a notable proportion of individuals apprehended for serious non-drug-related offences test positive for drug use or alcohol at the time of the offence. Furthermore, it is acknowledged that prolonged and habitual substance abuse can lead to enduring mental disorders that manifest symptoms akin to those arising from organic brain diseases. In cases involving substance abuse, defendants may raise the defence of involuntary intoxication, arguing that the use of drugs or alcohol impaired their mental state to the point where they were incapable of forming criminal intent. Forensic psychiatrists are tasked with evaluating the impact of substance use on the defendant's mental capacity.

### 10.5.4 Automatism

Automatic behaviour is involuntary behaviour and most likely unconscious behaviour. The concept of automatism as a psychiatric defence in criminal court introduces a nuanced distinction between "Non-Insane" and "Insane" automatism. This differentiation is crucial in determining the level of criminal responsibility attributed to the accused based on their mental state at the time of the alleged offence. the distinction is legal, not medical. The defence of automatism asserts that the defendant committed the crime involuntarily without conscious control. Forensic psychiatrists play a pivotal role in examining the defendant's mental state and determining the presence of automatism.

### 10.5.5 Post-traumatic Stress Disorder (PTSD) and Traumatic Brain Injury (TBI)

Individuals who have experienced severe trauma, leading to conditions like PTSD or TBI, may raise these as defences, arguing that their mental health conditions impacted their behaviour during the alleged crime. Forensic psychiatrists in Bangladesh conduct thorough assessments to establish the link between the traumatic experience and the defendant's actions as mitigating factors.

### 10.5.6 Mental Incapacity at Sentencing

Forensic psychiatrists also contribute to the legal process during sentencing by evaluating a defendant's mental health to determine if mitigating factors, such as mental illness, should be considered in sentencing decisions. This involves an assessment of the defendant's capacity for rehabilitation and potential future risk.

## 10.6 Current Status of Forensic Psychiatry Services in Bangladesh

### 10.6.1 Mental Health Act in Bangladesh

After a long debate and demand, Bangladesh has passed "Mental health Act (2018)" in the parliament replacing the inherited colonial law the "Lunacy Act 1912" (Karim & Shaikh, 2021; Mental Health Act, 2018). This law upholds its supremacy over other existing laws. It signifies four major concerns such as setting up and supervision of psychiatric hospitals and rehabilitation centres; assessment, hospitalization and management of psychiatric patients; assessing the mental health capacity and guardianship of the mentally ill person and property of the persons (Karim & Shaikh, 2021; Mental health Act, 2018). It classified hospitalization of mental health patients into three categories mentioned as (a) voluntary admission, (b) non-protesting patient, and (c) unwilling patient (Karim & Shaikh, 2021; Mental Health Act, 2018).

The Mental Health Act of 2018 laid the foundation for the protection of individuals with mental disorders and emphasized the need for expert psychiatric assessment in legal matters (Mental Health Act, 2018). However, the integration of forensic psychiatry into the legal system requires collaborative efforts from mental health professionals, legal practitioners, and policymakers. There are other laws related to Forensic Psychiatry services in Bangladesh that are mentioned in Box 10.1.

**Box 10.1: Laws Related to Forensic Psychiatry Services in Bangladesh (Ashraf et al., 2022)**

I. The Code of Criminal Procedure, 1898
II. The Bangladesh Jail Code, Revised Edition, 2006
III. Penal Code, 1860
IV. The Police Ordinance, 2008 Draft.

### *10.6.2 Forensic Beds*

There are only 15 inpatient beds at National Institute of Mental Health (NIMH), Dhaka for Forensic psychiatry in the whole country (Ashraf et al., 2022).

### *10.6.3 Undergraduate Curriculum*

Forensic psychiatry is not part psychiatry curriculum at the undergraduate level in Bangladesh (BMDC, 2021). It is under Forensic Medicine & Toxicology. There is no available training and courses for Forensic Psychiatry in the country.

### *10.6.4 Prison Mental Health in Bangladesh*

There are 68 establishments of Bangladesh prison. Among them, 13 are central prison and the rest 55 are district prisons. There were 77 203 (September 2023) prisoners in the country with an incarceration rate 44 per 100,000 population (World Prison Brief, 2023). The occupancy rate was 190.4%. Among the prisoners, 75.6% were at pre-trial state, 3.9% were females. There is one prison only for females in the country (Khan et al., 2021) near Dhaka and others have a portion for the female prisoners. There are three child development centres (two for boys; Tongi and Jeshore; One for girls, Konabari) for juvenile delinquent children (Justice Audit Bangladesh, 2023).

There are no formal psychiatric services in the prison of Bangladesh from the Government (Khan et al., 2021). There are some activities from non-government organizations like Dhaka Ahsania Mission (DAM) (Khan et al., 2021; Skuse, 2021). Also, there is no screening system for mental health problems in prisons of Bangladesh (Khan et al., 2021). Psychiatrists or mental health professionals do not visit prisoners. So in any acute or chronic cases, prisoners are escorted to nearby psychiatric setting by two police officers. Both indoor and outdoor services in forensic psychiatry in Bangladesh are provided free of cost (Khan et al., 2021). There are psychotropics like typical antipsychotics, mood stabilizers (Lithium and valproate), benzodiazepines, and amitriptyline are being provided free of cost. Others need to be purchased by the prisoners.

We identified the first study regarding psychiatric disorder among the prisoners that was published in 1998 by Chowdhury and his colleagues. They studied 56 cases referred from Pabna Jail at Pabna Mental Hospital out outpatient department. They found that 51 cases (almost 91%) developed the psychiatric disorder prior to commit crime. The study found 100% of the cases had psychiatric illness (Chowdhury et al., 1998). They made the diagnoses based on the reports from jail doctors and/or jail authority, and history from the patients' guardians. Among the cases, 91% (n = 51) had diminished responsibilities, 23.2% (n = 12) denied their crime, and only 7% (n = 4) were responsible for their crime (Chowdhury et al., 1998). Among the cases 73.2% were under trail, 12.5% were convicted and 14.3% were under safe custody. The majority of the cases were suffering from psychoses (Chowdhury et al., 1998).

We found a similar study from Dhaka Central Jail with 67 male prisoners referred to the Institute of Post-Graduate Medical Education and Research (IPGMR) (Mullick et al., 1998). The study found that 91% of the prisoners had psychiatric disorders according to the International Classification of Diseases (ICD-10) classification. Among the cases 40% were convicted and 60% were under trail (Mullick et al., 1998). This study also identified psychoses as the vital disorder among the cases.

A study was reported from the NIMH, Dhaka assessing 48 admitted patients during 2004–2006. Of them, 87.5% were males. The prevalence of psychiatric disorder was 85.4% (schizophrenia 37.5%) (Hamid et al., 2005). Another recent study found the prevalence of psychiatric disorders was 94.4% (n = 120) among 127 refereed prisoners (Yasmin et al., 2022). Schizophrenia was the commonest diagnosis (34.6%). All the four studies were conducted among the prisoners referred to hospital.

The first study assessing the psychiatric disorders among females and living in Dhaka Central Jail was published in 2004 (Hasan et al., 2004). They interviewed 250 female prisoners by the Structured Clinical Interview for DSM-III-R. The point prevalence was 66.4% (Hasan et al., 2004). This study found neurotic disorders as the major burden (depression 30.4%) (Hasan et al., 2004).

Authors recommended to conduct country-wide epidemiological should be conducted in the prisons along with regular screening system for mental disorders among the prisoners in Bangladesh (Khan et al., 2021).

### *10.6.5 Forensic Psychiatric Assessment Pathway in Bangladesh*

In Bangladesh, forensic psychiatric services are available only in Dhaka at two institutions; i.e. NIMH, prison cell of *Bangabandhu Sheikh Mujib Medical University* (BSMMU). Only the NIMH, Dhaka has a separate forensic psychiatry department and provides both indoor and outdoor services. The BSMMU does not have a dedicated department. However, it provides services through the patients admitted at

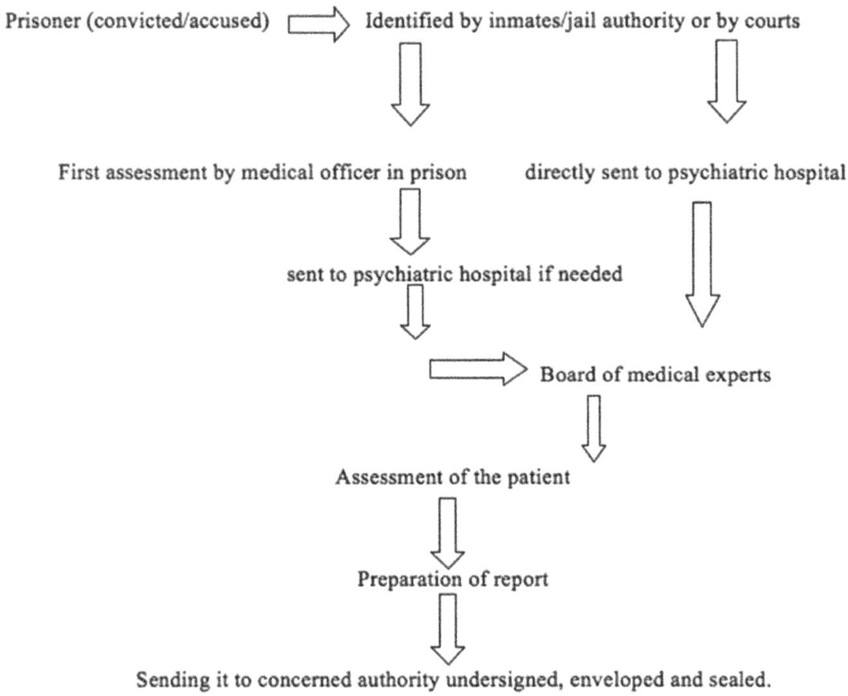


**Fig. 10.1** Forensic psychiatric assessment pathway in Bangladesh

prison cell of the university. The public medical colleges are supposed to provide forensic psychiatry services. Nevertheless, many of them are unable to ensure the services due to lack of human resources and other facilities. Usually suspected mentally ill patients are referred to NIMH under the direction of Court or Jail authority (Ashraf et al., 2022). Therefore, when any behavioural abnormality is suspected among the prisoners by mates or staffs of prison, the person is supposed to refer medical officer for the assessment and subsequent referrals are made if necessary (Fig. 10.1).

### *10.6.6 Forensic Psychiatric Services Spectrum*

The cases that are being referred to the Department of Forensic Psychiatry, NIMH, Dhaka mainly comprise the following four aspects.

#### 10.6.6.1 Liaison with Law Enforcing Authority

The Department of Forensic Psychiatry provides specialist services in Forensic and Other Legal Fields for mentally ill patients or those thought to be mentally ill or having reasonable grounds for suspecting the person to be mentally ill-directed by Honourable Court or equivalent authority. Preparation of assessment reports through the Mental Health Specialist Board (MHSB) for convicts, detainees, or mentally disabled/mentally incapacitated individuals as directed by the Honourable Court equivalent authority has been performed. There may be various issues that are being referred to by the Honourable Court ranging from whether the accused is mentally ill or sound. Whether the accused was mentally sound at the time of the incident? Guardianship and property-related issues when it has been referred to Honourable Court or equivalent authority as per Mental Health Act (2018). Where a dispute arises about whether the person is disabled due to a mental disorder, psychiatric services have been provided. Forensic Psychiatry is also involved in any case where the court is being involved or referred to court.

The Honourable Court seeks a mental assessment report for justice usually in a prescribed form (Bangladesh Form No. 3890) communicating through the appropriate authority where the accused or detainee belongs. The Honourable Court or equivalent authority also mentions the institute name where the mental assessment will be carried on and also mentions the time limit for the submission of the assessment report. Then senior jail super of prison or equivalent authority issues a letter to NIMH for an assessment report countersigned by two assistant surgeons of the prison hospital and a civil surgeon (Medical Officer) of the Prison Hospital. Upon reaching NIMH, the accused or detainee is admitted to the prison cell with security for a minimum of 2 weeks and time is extended if required by communicating to the senior jail super of prison. After preparing the assessment, report is sent to the administrative officer of the judge court or equivalent authority.

The MHSB is an indoor forensic board headed by the head of the Department of Forensic Psychiatry. At least two associate professors and one assistant professor are present on the board. In addition, there are also full-time medical officers and administrative officers to organize the board and prepare the assessment report. The formulation of the board may be customized based on the availability of the psychiatrists. The Director of NIMH presides over the board and by his name all letters are being communicated in black and white. Communication through appropriate authority in black and white is mandatory for any requirement or time extension while preparing this type of assessment report. The usual challenges are a lack of reliable informants and obtaining a personal history.

#### 10.6.6.2 Assessment of Disability Due to Mental Illness

Providing certificates through the Specialist Board under the "Rights and Protection of Disabled Persons Act 2013" is an important service of Forensic Psychiatry in Bangladesh. This is performed in an outdoor board headed by at least two associate professors and two assistant professors, inquiring about the condition very carefully whether the client is disabled due to a serious mental disorder or condition or neurodevelopmental disorder, or intellectual disability. This assessment report is required for getting disability allowance and other facilities provided by the government. The clients need to make an application in a prescribed format with all necessary documents. Then the authority fixes a date when adequate informants are requested to be present on the board.

#### 10.6.6.3 Clinical Services to Mentally Ill Prisoners

Providing psychiatric clinical services to mentally ill patients sent from prison is another aspect of Forensic Psychiatric Services. They may have been suffering from mental disorders during trial or may be diagnosed when being in prison for punishment. They may need admission and then regular follow-up in OPD. They are usually communicated through Senior jail super or equivalent authority with the advice and counter signature of Assistant Surgeon/Medical Officer Prison Hospital.

#### 10.6.6.4 Mental Health-Related Report

Providing mental health-related reports from various government/non-government institutions are supposed to be performed by Forensic Psychiatry. This has been increasing day by day due mental health awareness. It may be requested by the authority, usually autonomous or semi-autonomous institutions. If it is a government institution, then it is usually communicated through the civil surgeon office. Usually, such referrals are sought for assessing the mental fitness for the job extension applications after age of 65 under National University of Bangladesh.

## 10.7 Current Challenges of Forensic Psychiatry in Bangladesh

The development of forensic psychiatry in Bangladesh is not without challenges. Stigma surrounding mental health, limited resources, and the need for specialized training are significant hurdles (Arafat, 2024; Arafat et al., 2024; Ashraf et al., 2022). There is no training facility in Forensic Psychiatry in the country. There is a lack of mental health services facility in the prison. There are some field level challenges while communicating between legal system and Forensic Psychiatry services. Court orders are delayed to reach mental health service, allow inadequate time for psychiatric assessment. There are also gross improper languages (in regards to clinical assessment) mentioned in the order form.

## 10.8 Ways Forward

As Bangladesh takes strides toward integrating forensic psychiatry into its legal system, future directions must be carefully considered. Continued professional development, research initiatives, and ongoing collaboration between mental health and legal professionals will be essential for the sustained growth of forensic psychiatry in the country.

The initiation of fellowship accreditation in forensic psychiatry is a pivotal step in elevating the standards of practice in Bangladesh. Accreditation establishes a benchmark for excellence, ensuring that practitioners meet rigorous criteria and adhere to the highest professional standards. Incorporating regular Continuing Professional Development (CPD) events for faculty development is equally crucial in sustaining the growth of forensic psychiatry in Bangladesh. These events serve as dynamic platforms for faculty members to stay abreast of the latest advancements in the field, share best practices, and engage in collaborative learning.

Moreover, the collaboration between forensic psychiatry education and the judiciary training institution is instrumental in addressing service gaps and fostering a comprehensive understanding of the intersection between mental health and the legal system in Bangladesh. Joint Continuing Professional Development (CPD) events that bring together forensic psychiatrists and legal professionals offer a unique platform for interdisciplinary dialogue and shared learning.

Additionally, there is an urgent need for comprehensive and ongoing training for members of the judiciary on mental health issues. Judges and legal professionals should be equipped with the knowledge and sensitivity required to provide clear, unbiased instructions to mental health experts. This training should emphasize the importance of language in shaping perceptions and encourage the use of neutral and respectful terminology.

Establishment of prison mental health system could be an important initiative in the country. A nation-wide epidemiological study and a regular screening system for the identification of psychiatric disorders among the prisoners are important necessities.

## 10.9 Conclusion

The development of forensic psychiatry in Bangladesh marks a momentous leap forward in addressing the intricate relationship between mental health and the legal system. Bangladesh is on the cusp of a transformative journey, where it confronts challenges with resilience, seizes available opportunities, and nurtures collaborative efforts. Bangladesh is in the early stages of developing specialized services, there is a growing awareness of the need for forensic psychiatric expertise among the smaller southeast Asian countries such as Bhutan, Nepal, and Maldives. Bangladesh can be a role model for these countries in leading service development. Training programs and collaborative initiatives with international organizations contribute to capacity building in these regions.

## References

Arafat, S. M. Y. (2024). Mental health services in Bangladesh. In: S. M. Y. Arafat (Eds.), *Mental health in Bangladesh: From bench to community*. Springer Nature Singapore. https://doi.org/10.1007/978-981-97-0610-5_3

Arafat, S. M. Y., Giasuddin, N. A., & Mazumder, A. H. (2024). Access to mental health care in bangladesh–current status, potential challenges, and ways out. In S. M. Y. Arafat, S. K. Kar (Eds.), *Access to mental health care in South Asia-current status, potential challenges, and ways out*. Springer Nature Singapore. https://doi.org/10.1007/978-981-99-9153-2_3

Arboleda-Flórez, J. (2006). Forensic psychiatry: Contemporary scope, challenges and controversies. *World Psychiatry: Official Journal of the World Psychiatric Association (WPA), 5*(2), 87–91.

Ashraf, S., Amin, Y. M., Sajib, M. S., & Al Azdi, Z. (2022). Situational analysis of forensic mental health in Bangladesh. *Forensic Science International: Mind and Law, 3*, 100074. https://doi.org/10.1016/j.fsiml.2022.100074

Justice Audit Bangladesh. (2023). Child Development Centers (CDC). https://bangladesh.justiceaudit.org/national-data/regional-services/child-development-centers/#:~:text=A%20young%20person%20under%2018,boys%20and%20Konabari%20for%20girls. Retrieved November 23, 23.

Balcioglu, Y. H., Oncu, F., O'Neill, C., Gulati, G., & Scurich, N. (2023). Editorial: Evidence-based frameworks of assessment and treatment in forensic psychiatry practice. *Frontiers in Psychiatry, 14*, 1301759. https://doi.org/10.3389/fpsyt.2023.1301759

BMDC. (2021). MBBS Curriculum Update–2021. https://www.bmdc.org.bd/curriculum-2020. Retrieved August 29, 2023.

Chowdhury, S. H., Rahman, S. M., & Begum, A. (1998). Mentally abnormal offenders a study of refereed patients from jail. *Bangladesh Journal of Psychiatry, 12*(1), 31–37.

Gbadebo-Goyea, E. A., Akpudo, H., Jackson, C. D., Wassef, T., Barker, N. C., Cunningham-Burley, R., Ali, S. A., Jabeen, S., & Bailey, R. K. (2012). Collaboration: The paradigm of practice approach between the forensic psychiatrist and the forensic psychologist. *Frontiers in Psychiatry, 3*, 89. https://doi.org/10.3389/fpsyt.2012.00089

Hamid, M. A., Hossain, M. D., Ahmed, H. U., Rahman, M. M., & Karim, M. E. (2005). Types of psychiatric disorder among patients attended in forensic psychiatry department of National Institute of Mental Health, Dhaka. *Bangladesh Journal of Psychiatry, 19*(2), 51–57.

Hasan, M. K., Jahan, N. A., Khanam, M., & Begum, A. A. (2004). Study on prison population: Psychiatric morbidity among female prisoners. *Bangladesh Journal of Psychiatry., 18*(2), 41–54.

Karim, M. E., & Shaikh, S. (2021). Newly enacted mental health law in Bangladesh. *Bjpsych International, 18*(4), 85–87. https://doi.org/10.1192/bji.2021.1

Khan, A. A., Ryland, H., Pathan, T., Ahmed, H. U., Hussain, A., & Forrester, A. (2021). Mental health services in the prisons of Bangladesh. *Bjpsych International, 18*(4), 88–91. https://doi.org/10.1192/bji.2021.34

Martone, C. (2022). The role of a forensic psychiatrist. *Missouri Medicine, 119*(3), 198–201.

Mental Health Act. (2018). Bangladesh. https://legislativediv.gov.bd/site/page/3c13bbde-76b4-41fc-89cab738dd04a0bb. Retrieved December 12, 2018.

Mullick, M. S. I., Khanam, M., & Nahar, J. S. (1998). Psychiatric Profile of the prisoners referred for psychiatric assessment. *Bangladesh Journal of Psychiatry, 12*(2), 69–75.

Niveau, G., & Welle, I. (2018). Forensic psychiatry, one subspecialty with two ethics? *A Systematic Review. BMC Medical Ethics, 19*(1), 25. https://doi.org/10.1186/s12910-018-0266-5

Platt, A. M. (1965). The origins and development of the "wild beast" concept of mental illness and its relation to theories of criminal responsibility. *Issues in Criminology, 1*(1), 1–18.

Skuse, D. (2021). Current concerns about mental health in Bangladesh. *Bjpsych International, 18*(4), 77–78. https://doi.org/10.1192/bji.2021.43

World Prison Brief. (2023). Bangladesh. https://www.prisonstudies.org/country/bangladesh. Retrieved November 23, 2023.

Yasmin, M., Mamun, A. A., Lopa, A. R., Khaleequzzaman, A. K. M., Sultana, S., & Karim, S. M. S. (2022). Patterns of psychiatric disorders in persons attending the Forensic Psychiatry Department of a tertiary care psychiatric hospital. *Archieves of NIMH, 5*(2), 24–28.

# Chapter 11
# Suicidal Behavior and Suicide Prevention in Bangladesh

**S. M. Yasir Arafat**

**Abstract** Suicide and suicide prevention remains under-prioritized in Bangladesh. Available evidence suggests that the rate of suicide varies widely in estimates from different sources. Reliable good quality data is a challenge in Bangladesh. Females die more than males in the country. Hanging and poisoning are the leading methods of suicide attempts. Young populations especially those below 30 years of age die more in the country. Mental illness, adverse life events, social isolation, unemployment, sexual abuse, substance misuse, past suicide attempts, marital disharmony, and familial discord are the prominent risk factors. A suicide attempt is a criminal offense in Bangladesh. Along with this, there are high stigma and inadequate suicide literacy. Quality of reporting of suicide attempts in print and online newspapers, movies, and drama is low with a high presence of potentially harmful characteristics and an absolute absence of potentially helpful characteristics. Prevention initiatives have been noted albeit they are inadequate, dispersed, and uncoordinated. Nation-wide study, enduring high-quality data, enhanced research, sufficient funds, good governance, adequate political attention, and coordinated efforts are warranted to formulate a national suicide prevention strategy.

**Keywords** Suicide in Bangladesh · Self-harm in Bangladesh · Suicide prevention · Mental health and suicide · Suicide attempt

## 11.1 Introduction

A comprehensive book on suicide *Suicide in Bangladesh* has been published by Springer in 2023. It covers epidemiology and data quality of suicide, forensic aspects of suicide, mental health and suicide, cultural aspects of suicide, media reporting of suicide, family and suicide, crisis trauma and suicide, suicide research, and suicide prevention initiatives in Bangladesh (Arafat & Khan, 2023). There is another chapter

S. M. Y. Arafat (✉)
Department of Psychiatry, Bangladesh Specialized Hospital Limited, Dhaka, Bangladesh
e-mail: arafatdmc62@gmail.com



S. M. Y. Arafat (ed.), *Mental Health in Bangladesh*,
https://doi.org/10.1007/978-981-97-0610-5_11

*Suicidal Behavior in Bangladesh* that has published in 2024 describing the epidemiological aspects of suicidal behavior [thought, plan, attempt (fatal, & non-fatal)], legal status with special attention to declaration of suicide, data sources, suicide stigma and literacy, media reporting, and suicide prevention in Bangladesh (see Arafat & Khan, 2024). It is quite challenging to write a standalone chapter with absolute novel facts and arguments in such short intervals specially in the context of suicidal behavior and suicide prevention in Bangladesh. However, suicide is extremely pertinent to mental health and as the editor and author, I don't feel a mental health book without a chapter on suicide would be complete. In such a circumstance, I would be careful and precise while writing this chapter. At the same time, I mention the important sources in the reference section for detailed exploration.

## 11.2 Epidemiology of Suicidal Behavior in Bangladesh

### *11.2.1 Rate of Suicide*

There are wide variations among the reports estimating the suicide rate in Bangladesh (Arafat, 2019a; Kabir et al., 2023). The latest World Health Organization (WHO) report of 2021 on the suicide rate in 2019 revealed that the age-standardized suicide rate was 3.9, 6, and 1.7 per 100,000 in both sexes, males, and females, respectively (World Health Organization, 2021). These rates are calculated by a modeling approach adopted by WHO. According to that report, about 6000 people died by suicide in 2019 in Bangladesh. The rates are being challenged by several community studies and reports of different organizations (see Kabir et al., 2023). For a detailed review, see our two important chapters discussing the variations of suicide rate in Bangladesh (Arafat & Khan, 2024; Kabir et al., 2023). Secondly, like in other Muslim countries, there are strong chances of under-reporting of suicides in Bangladesh due to several conditions like criminal legal status, high stigma, and enduring culture (Arafat, 2019a). However, at the same time, we do not have any estimate regarding the proportion of under-reporting. So, Bangladesh does not have any reliable suicide data. The primary reason for this lacking is the lack of a national suicide database and surveillance system (Arafat, 2019a; Kabir et al., 2023). Police stations, forensic medicine departments, hospital patients, newspaper reports, and few epidemiological studies are the prominent source of data for suicide research in Bangladesh (Arafat, 2017; Hussain, et al., 2021a, b, c, d, e).

### *11.2.2 Rate of Suicidal Idea, Plan, and Non-fatal Attempt*

The epidemiology of suicidal thought/idea, plan, and non-fatal attempts is understudied. Among the studies, students are the commonest respondents for studies on suicidal behavior perhaps because of their availability and willingness to participate. The latest nationwide epidemiological study assessing suicidal behavior among youths (10–24 years of age) revealed that the prevalence was 4.7%, 1.5%, and 1.5% for suicidal idea, plan, and attempt, respectively (National Institute of Mental Health, 2021). One systematic review and meta-analysis found 12 studies assessing suicidal behavior among students in Bangladesh (Arafat et al., 2023). It revealed the prevalence of suicidal thought was 24%, 13%, and 7% for lifetime, last year, and current time, respectively. The prevalence of suicide plan was 6%, and 8% for lifetime and for last year, respectively. The prevalence of suicide attempt was 9% and 4% for lifetime and last year, respectively. Analysis of secondary data of 2014 from the *Global School-based Student Health Survey (GSHS)* revealed the prevalence of suicidal behavior was 8.9% (thought 4.2%, plan 5.4%, and attempt 4.2%) (Marthoenis & Arafat, 2022). The prevalence of suicidal thought among geriatric population (> 60 years of age) was 23% during the past 2 weeks of interview (Wahlin et al., 2015). One community-based study found the prevalence of non-fatal suicide attempt was 281.8 per 100,000 (Feroz et al., 2012) whilst another community-based study found the lifetime prevalence of suicidal thought among adolescents (14–19 years) was 5% (Begum et al., 2017).

Some studies have been conducted assessing the suicidal behavior among nurses (Arafat et al., 2021a, b, c, 2021d, e), Imams (Arafat et al., 2024), postgraduate residents (Qusar et al., 2020) and sexual minorities (Mozumder et al., 2023). Among the nurses, the prevalence of suicidal ideation was 9.9%, 3.9%, and 2% for lifetime, last year, and last month, respectively (Arafat et al., 2021a, b, c, d, e). Among Imams (Muslim religious leaders), the prevalence of suicidal ideation was 18%, and 7.4% for lifetime and last year, respectively. The prevalence of suicide attempt was 6.2% (Arafat et al., 2024). The prevalence was high among homosexual males in Bangladesh. About one-third (32.4%) of homo-sexual males had history of suicide attempts, about half of them (47.1%) had suicidal thoughts and 40.2% had a history of self-harm (Mozumder et al., 2023). The prevalence of suicidal thought among postgraduate medical students was 20.6%, 10.8%, and 3.9% for lifetime, last year, and last month respectively (Qusar et al., 2020). Among them, 5.9% made plans for suicide attempts, and 2.9% had a history of suicide attempt (Qusar et al., 2020).

### *11.2.3 Gender Distribution*

Suicide is more common among males than females in the world (WHO, 2021). The distribution is opposite in Bangladesh. Although the recent WHO report revealed male dominance, many studies found that females die more than males in Bangladesh (for review see WHO, 2019, Kabir et al., 2023; Arafat, 2019a, b; Khan et al., 2020). There are speculations regarding this female dominance in Bangladesh such as patriarchal social structure, passive gender role, early marriage, inadequate women empowerment, absence of economic and social freedom (Kabir et al., 2023).

### 11.2.4 Life-Stage

Suicides have been noted from 8 to 78 years of age in Bangladesh. However, the majority of the suicides happen before the age of 30. Students and homemakers are the risky groups in Bangladesh (Kabir et al., 2023).

### 11.2.5 Risk Factors

Likewise, the Western countries, risk factors for suicide have distributed in some domains in Bangladesh. Available evidence indicates that psychiatric disorders, previous attempts, adverse life events, social isolation, unemployment, substance abuse, marital disharmony, familial discord, academic failure, and sexual harassment are the prominent risk factors for suicide (Box 11.1; Kabir et al., 2023). The prevalence of mental illness was 61% (depression 44%, personality disorder 14%, substance abuse 9%, and psychosis 1%) in suicide, which is lower than the Western countries (Arafat et al., 2021a, b, c, d, e). The prevalence of mental illness was found 45–65% in non-fatal suicide attempts (Arafat, 2023), which includes depressive disorder, borderline personality disorder, psychosis, conversion disorder, substance abuse, and stress-related disorders. For review see Arafat (2023). Here, social factors play a more prominent role in suicide. The analysis found that about 86% of suicides could be prevented by stopping the life events whilst 50% of suicides could be prevented by reducing the psychiatric illness (Arafat et al., 2021a, b, c, d, e).

**Box 11.1 Major Risk Factor for Suicide in Bangladesh (Kabir et al., 2023)**

1. Psychiatric disorders- depression, personality disorder, Substance (Yaba) abuse
2. Adverse life events-pre-marital affair and marriage, extra-marital affair and sex, pre-marital pregnancy, academic failure, marital discord, familial disharmony
3. Previous suicide attempt
4. Sexual abuse
5. Social isolation
6. Unemployment
7. Domestic violence
8. Academic failure
9. Demanding behavior

### 11.2.6 Methods of Suicide

Hanging and poisoning are the most commonly used methods of suicide in Bangladesh (Arafat et al., 2021a, b, c, d, e; Kabir et al., 2023). Other prominent methods are fall from height, jump in front of running objects (train, bus), firearms, burns, cut injury, and drowning (Kabir et al., 2023). Cut injury and benzodiazepine ingestion are the commonest method of self-harm. Among benzodiazepines, clonazepam is the commonest drug of self-harm.

### 11.2.7 Seasonal Variation of Suicidal Behavior

Studies are inadequate to comment on seasonal variation of suicidal behavior in Bangladesh. However, available evidence suggests that suicide is lower in winter season. One study collected data from newspaper reports and identified the peak of suicidal behavior in March and April, i.e. end of spring and start of summer (Arafat et al., 2018). Another study collected data from the community and identified the peak in summer (Arendse et al., 2021). One study identified the peak of suicides in spring and autumn in *Thakurgaon* district (Arafat & Karmakar, 2019). Further studies are warranted to reveal the seasonality precisely.

## 11.3 Legal Status of Suicidal Behavior in Bangladesh

Bangladesh is a Muslim-majority country and suicide is strictly prohibited in Islam. Suicide attempts, assisting in suicide attempts, and euthanasia (physician-assisted suicide) are illegal in Bangladesh (Suryadevara & Tandon, 2018). According to the law, "whoever attempts to commit suicide and does any act towards the act of commission of such offense, shall be punished with simple imprisonment for a term which may extend to one year, or with fine, or with both" (The Penal Code, 1860). Criminal legal status is an important attributing factor for high stigma. It hinders help-seeking behavior, causes under-reporting suicidal behavior to avoid legal consequences. Due to this criminal status, patients with self-harm and poisoning are avoided by private hospitals and kept in a neglected state in the verandas of public hospitals.

Along with the *International Association for Suicide Prevention (IASP)*, and other organizations, academicians and researchers working in Bangladesh recommend the decriminalization of suicide attempts in Bangladesh (World Health Organization, 2023a, b; International Association for Suicide Prevention, 2020; Bose et al., 2023; United for Global Mental Health, 2021). Among the eight South Asian countries (Afghanistan, Bangladesh, Bhutan, India, Maldives, Nepal, Pakistan, and Sri Lanka), Bangladesh and the Maldives are the countries where suicide is still a criminal offense (Arafat and Kar, 2024; World Health Organization, 2023a, b).

## 11.4 Suicide Literacy and Stigma in Bangladesh

To formulate a national suicide prevention strategy, there needs an acceptable status of suicide literacy and stigma towards suicidal behavior (World Health Organization, 2014). Although suicide literacy and stigma is a newer avenue in Bangladesh there are several studies assessing the statuses among different populations. The first study was published in 2022 validating the two instruments (the *Bangla Literacy of Suicide Scale* (LOSS-B), and the *Bangla Stigma of Suicide Scale* (SOSS-B)) and assessing the statuses among university and medical students (Arafat et al., 2022a, b, c). Subsequent studies are noted among medical students (Arafat et al., 2022a, b, c), doctors (Maruf et al., 2022), and among Imams (Islam et al., 2023). Studies revealed a similar status of suicide literacy among medical students, university students, and Imams raising questions about the association of status with educational attainment. No association between suicide literacy and stigma was found.

## 11.5 Media Reporting of Suicide in Bangladesh

Media reporting of suicide has been measured against the WHO guidelines (World Health Organization, 2017) in multiple studies in Bangladesh (Anik, 2023). The WHO guidelines mention some potentially harmful and some potentially helpful characteristics while reporting suicidal behavior in media and newspapers and recommend reducing potentially harmful characteristics and increasing potentially helpful characteristics (see World Health Organization, 2017, 2023a, b; Anik, 2023). I found two studies assessing printed newspapers (Arafat et al., 2020a, b) and two studies assessing media reports of online news portals (Arafat et al., 2019, 2020c). The studies assessed the quality of newspaper reporting in both the vernacular and English language. However, any comparison between the quality of the two languages was not done yet. The quality of suicide reporting in newspapers was grossly insensible in regard to the WHO reporting guidelines. The reports mentioned high proportions of potentially harmful characteristics like identifying information (name, occupation, location, method) in the headline and body of the news whilst there was an absence of potentially helpful characteristics (helpline, statistics, research findings, services availability).

One study assessed how suicide has been depicted in Bangladesh movies and dramas (Arafat et al., 2022). It revealed a similar picture of epidemiological aspects of suicide in Bangladesh when epidemiology was compared and a similar quality of newspaper reports when quality was assessed against WHO guidelines.

## 11.6 Suicide Research in Bangladesh

A good summary of suicide in Bangladesh has been mentioned by Uddin in 2023. It is great to see that the number of publications on suicide has been increasing since 2016 which indicates academic attention (Uddin, 2023; Arafat et al., 2021a, b, c, d, e). S M Yasir Arafat and M A Mamun are the leading researchers in Bangladesh (Uddin, 2023). *Jahangirnagar University, CHINTA Research Bangladesh, Bangabandhu Sheikh Mujib Medical University (BSMMU), Enam Medical College and Hospital (EMCH),* and *International Centre of Diarrhoeal Disease Research, Bangladesh (ICDDR, B)* are the leading organizations doing suicide research (Uddin, 2023). However, I did not see any nationwide study among adults in Bangladesh assessing various suicidal behaviors. Additionally, there are several untouched domains in suicide research like national burden of suicide, the economic burden of suicide, culture-specific resilient factors, and local interventions for suicidal behavior (Uddin, 2023).

## 11.7 Suicide Prevention in Bangladesh

There are some dispersed and inadequate preventive efforts in Bangladesh (Hoque, 2023). There are two suicide prevention clinical services in BSMMU and EMCH. Among these two clinics, the suicide prevention clinic of BSMMU was ceased during the COVID-19, which is yet to be started (Box 11.2). Another clinic of EMCH has also been ceased in December 2023. There are two hotline services named Kaan Pete Roi and 999 (national emergency service). *SAJIDA Foundation, Society for Voluntary Activities (SOVA),* and *Brighter Tomorrow Foundation (BTF)* are the major non-government organizations (NGOs) in Bangladesh. The *Handicap International (Humanity & Inclusion),* another NGO, did some work on suicide prevention activities in Cox's Bazar among the Rohingya refugees in 2020 (see Hoque, 2023; Arafat & Khan, 2024; Arafat, 2018; Khan et al., 2021). Category I pesticide ban is an important step in suicide prevention in Bangladesh (Chowdhury et al., 2018). The Society for Suicide Prevention Bangladesh (SSPB) was formulated in 2016 with the aim of preventing suicide in the country. However, except for revising their committee, I did not see any activity in favor of suicide prevention. Nothing has been mentioned about suicide prevention in the newly passed Mental Health Act (2018) (Bangladesh Mental Health Act, 2018; Khan et al., 2021).

One study compared the status of WHO proposed 12 criteria for initiating a national suicide prevention strategy which is presented in Table 11.1 (Arafat, 2021; WHO, 2014). Bangladesh needs major attention to initiate a national suicide prevention strategy (see Hoque, 2023; Arafat & Khan, 2024; Arafat, 2018; Khan et al., 2021).

**Table 11.1** Readiness for national suicide prevention strategy (WHO, 2014; Arafat, 2021)

| Serial number | Component | Status of Bangladesh |
|---|---|---|
| 1 | Sensible media reporting | Quality of media reporting is poor. There are no country-specific guidelines |
| 2 | Raising awareness | There are sporadic activities by from NGOs, which are not planned and enduring. No national activity is available |
| 3 | Training and education | Not available, low suicide literacy |
| 4 | Treatment | Inadequate, only two suicide prevention clinics in Dhaka |
| 5 | Economics (funds and political will) | Literally absent |
| 6 | Crisis intervention | Kaan Pete Roi and National emergency service-999 |
| 7 | Oversight and coordination | Absent |
| 8 | Means restriction | Class I pesticides banned |
| 9 | Postvention | Not started yet |
| 10 | Access to services | Not easily accessible |
| 11 | Surveillance | Not started yet |
| 12 | Stigma reduction | High stigma, suicide is a criminal offense |

**Box 11.2 Suicide Prevention Activities (Arafat & Khan, 2024; Hoque, 2023)**

A. Clinical services (Suicide Prevention Clinic)

   i. Bangabandhu Sheikh Mujib Medical University-currently ceased
   ii. Enam Medical College and Hospital-currently ceased

B. Crisis Intervention (Hotline)

   i. Kaan Pete Roi- Several dedicated mobile numbers
   ii. National emergency service-999

C. NGO

   i. SAJIDA Foundation
   ii. Society for Voluntary Activities (SOVA)
   iii. Brighter Tomorrow Foundation (BTF)

iv. Handicap International (humanity & Inclusion)

D. Means Restrictions

i Category I pesticide ban

E. Society for Suicide Prevention, Bangladesh

## 11.8 Ways Forward

Bangladesh needs to move toward the establishment of a national suicide prevention strategy. The establishment of a national surveillance system and national databases for suicidal behavior are immediate priorities to ensure the quality of suicide data. Decriminalization would help to destigmatize and improve help-seeking behavior. Augmented research with multi-sectoral collaboration and funds would facilitate the establishments. Initiatives for improving the quality of media reporting are warranted with facilities of enduring monitoring and collaboration between media and mental health professionals. Universal, selected, and indicated prevention strategies need to be implemented to raise awareness, improve help-seeking, and prevent suicide.

## 11.9 Conclusions

This chapter highlights the basic aspects of suicide and suicide prevention in Bangladesh. Suicide and suicide prevention warrants augmented attention in Bangladesh. We do not know a reliable rate of suicide. There is still a lack of a national suicide surveillance system. Coordinated efforts are warranted to ensure adequate funds and political will, enhanced research, decriminalization, and awareness among community people. Creating additional service avenues and formulating an evidence-based national suicide prevention strategy is necessary.

## References

Anik, A. I. (2023). Media reporting of suicide in Bangladesh. In: S. M. Y. Arafat, M. M. Khan (Eds.), *Suicide in Bangladesh. New perspectives in behavioral & health sciences*. Springer, Singapore. https://doi.org/10.1007/978-981-99-0289-7_5.

Arafat, S. M. Y. (2017). Suicide in Bangladesh: A mini review. *Journal of Behavioral Health, 6*(1), 66–69. https://doi.org/10.5455/jbh.20160904090206.

Arafat, S. (2018). Suicide prevention activities in Bangladesh. *Asian Journal of Psychiatry, 36*, 38. https://doi.org/10.1016/j.ajp.2018.06.009.

Arafat, S. M. Y. (2019b). Females are dying more than males by suicide in Bangladesh. *Asian Journal of Psychiatry, 40*, 124–125. https://doi.org/10.1016/j.ajp.2018.10.014.
Arafat, S. (2021). Formulation of national suicide prevention strategy of Bangladesh: The readiness assessment. *Journal of Public Health (oxford, England), 43*(1), e131–e132. https://doi.org/10.1093/pubmed/fdaa117.
Arafat, S. M. Y., & Karmakar, S. (2019). Seasonality of suicide in Thakurgaon District, Bangladesh, 2014–2018. *Asian Journal of Psychiatry, 44*, 119–120. https://doi.org/10.1016/j.ajp.2019.07.042.
Arafat, S., Mali, B., & Akter, H. (2018). Demography and risk factors of suicidal behavior in Bangladesh: A retrospective online news content analysis. *Asian Journal of Psychiatry, 36*, 96–99. https://doi.org/10.1016/j.ajp.2018.07.008.
Arafat, S. M. Y., Mali, B., & Akter, H. (2019). Quality of online news reporting of suicidal behavior in Bangladesh against world health organization guidelines. *Asian Journal of Psychiatry, 40*, 126–129. https://doi.org/10.1016/j.ajp.2018.10.010.
Arafat, S. M. Y., Khan, M. M., Niederkrotenthaler, T., Ueda, M., & Armstrong, G. (2020a). Assessing the quality of media reporting of suicide deaths in Bangladesh against world health organization guidelines. *Crisis, 41*(1), 47–53. https://doi.org/10.1027/0227-5910/a000603.
Arafat, S. M. Y., Mali, B., & Akter, H. (2020b). Do Bangladeshi newspapers educate public while reporting suicide? A year round observation from content analysis of six national newspapers. *Asian Journal of Psychiatry, 48*, 101920. https://doi.org/10.1016/j.ajp.2019.101920.
Arafat, S. M. Y., Mali, B., & Akter, H. (2020c). Is suicide reporting in Bangla online news portals sensible? A year-round content analysis against world health organization guidelines. *Asian Journal of Psychiatry, 49*, 101943. https://doi.org/10.1016/j.ajp.2020.101943.
Arafat, S. M. Y., Ali, S. A., Menon, V., Hussain, F., Ansari, D. S., Baminiwatta, A., Saleem, T., Singh, R., Varadharajan, N., Biyyala, D., Kar, S. K., & Khan, M. M. (2021a). Suicide methods in South Asia over two decades (2001–2020). *The International Journal of Social Psychiatry, 67*(7), 920–934. https://doi.org/10.1177/00207640211015700.
Arafat, S. M., Laila, Z. D., Akter, H., Mali, B., Chowdhury, M. H., & Morshed, N. M. (2021b). Suicidal behaviors among Bangladeshi nurses: A cross-sectional study in a tertiary care hospital. *Mymensingh Medical Journal: MMJ, 30*(2), 426–431.
Arafat, S., Mohit, M. A., Mullick, M., Kabir, R., & Khan, M. M. (2021c). Risk factors for suicide in Bangladesh: Case-control psychological autopsy study. *Bjpsych Open, 7*(1), e18. https://doi.org/10.1192/bjo.2020.152.
Arafat, S., Khan, M., Knipe, D., & Khan, M. M. (2021d). Population attributable fractions of clinical and social risk factors for suicide in Bangladesh: Finding from a case-control psychological autopsy study. *Brain and Behavior, 11*(12), e2409. https://doi.org/10.1002/brb3.2409.
Arafat, S., Hussain, F., Hossain, M. F., Islam, M. A., & Menon, V. (2022a). Literacy and stigma of suicide in Bangladesh: Scales validation and status assessment among university students. *Brain and Behavior, 12*(1), e2432. https://doi.org/10.1002/brb3.2432.
Arafat, S. M. Y., Maruf, M. M., & Hossain, M. F. (2022b). Literacy and stigma of suicide among medical students of Bangladesh: Status and associated factors. *Bangladesh Medical Research Council Bulletin., 48*(3), 225–230. https://doi.org/10.3329/bmrcb.v48i3.62430.
Arafat, S. M. Y., Baminiwatta, A., Menon, V., Sharma, P., Htay, M. N. N., Akter, H., Marthoenis, M., & Dorji, C. (2023). Prevalence of suicidal behavior among students in South-East Asia: A systematic review and meta-analysis. *Archives of Suicide Research*, 1–21.https://doi.org/10.1080/13811118.2023.2176272.
Arafat, S. M. Y, Kar, S. K. (2024). Epidemiology of psychiatric disorders and overview of access to mental health care in South Asia. In: S. M. Y. Arafat, S. K. Kar (Eds.), *Access to mental health care in South Asia-current status, potential challenges, and ways out*. Springer Nature Singapore. https://doi.org/10.1007/978-981-99-9153-2_1
Arafat, S.M.Y., & Khan, A.R. (2024). Suicidal behavior in Bangladesh. In: S. M. Y. Arafat, M. Rezaeian, M. M. Khan (Eds.), *Suicidal behavior in Muslim majority countries*. Springer Nature.

Arafat, S. M. Y., Hussain, F., Jakaria, K. M., Itu, Z. T., & Islam, M. (2021). Empirical studies on suicide in Bangladesh in a decade (2011–2020). *Global Psychiatry, 4*(1), 109– 122. https://doi.org/10.52095/gp.2021.10692.

Arafat, S. M. Y., Jalil, S. B., Alam, M. S., Sultana, N., Ahmed, M. I. U., Abedin, M. M., & Armstrong, G. (2022). Suicide in bangla movie and drama: A content analysis. *Omega*, 302228221148286. Advance online publication. https://doi.org/10.1177/00302228221148286.

Arafat, S. M. Y., Islam, M. K., Khan, M. A. S., & Amin, R. (2024). The perception of imams (Islamic religious leaders) on the legal status and decriminalization of suicide attempts in Bangladesh: A Cross-sectional study. *Global Psychiatry Achieves*, 7(1), 7–12. https://doi.org/10.52095/gpa.2023.7115.1077.

Arafat, S. M. Y. (2019a). Current challenges of suicide and future directions of management in Bangladesh: a systematic review. *Global Psychiatry, 2*(1), 09–20.https://doi.org/10.2478/gp-2019-0001.

Arafat, S. M. Y. (2023). Mental health and suicide in Bangladesh. In: S. M. Y. Arafat, M. M. Khan (Eds.), *Suicide in Bangladesh.* Springer, Singapore. https://doi.org/10.1007/978-981-99-0289-7_3.

Arafat, S.M.Y., & Khan, M. M. (Eds.). (2023). *Suicide in Bangladesh: Epidemiology, risk factors, and prevention.* Springer Nature. https://doi.org/10.1007/978-981-99-0289-7.

Arendse, N., Khan, A. R., Billah, M., Ratele, K., & Islam, M. Z. (2021). Seasonality of suicide in Jhenaidah District, Bangladesh, 2011–2018. *Journal of Social Health, 4*(1), 64–75.

Bangladesh Mental Health Act. (2018). http://www.mindbank.info/item/6788. Retrieved September 02, 2022.

Begum, A., Rahman, A. F., Rahman, A., Soares, J., Reza Khankeh, H., & Macassa, G. (2017). Prevalence of suicide ideation among adolescentsand young adults in rural Bangladesh. *International Journal of Mental Health, 46*(3), 177–187. https://doi.org/10.1080/00207411.2017.1304074.

Bose, P. K., Kushal, S. A., Arafat, S. M. Y. (2023). Forensic and Legal Aspects of Suicide in Bangladesh. In: S. M. Y. Arafat, M. M. Khan (Eds.), *Suicide in Bangladesh. New perspectives in behavioral & health sciences.* Springer, Singapore. https://doi.org/10.1007/978-981-99-0289-7_2.

Chowdhury, F. R., Dewan, G., Verma, V. R., Knipe, D. W., Isha, I. T., Faiz, M. A., Gunnell, D. J., & Eddleston, M. (2018). Bans of WHO class I pesticides in Bangladesh-suicide prevention without hampering agricultural output. *International Journal of Epidemiology, 47*(1), 175–184. https://doi.org/10.1093/ije/dyx157.

Feroz, A., Islam, S. N., Reza, S., Rahman, A. M., Sen, J., Mowla, M., & Rahman, M. R. (2012). A community survey on the prevalence of suicidal attempts and deaths in a selected rural area of Bangladesh. *Journal of Medicine, 13*(1), 3–9. https://doi.org/10.3329/jom.v13i1.10042.

Hoque, M. B. (2023). Suicide Prevention in Bangladesh: Current status and way forward. In: S. M. Y. Arafat, M. M. Khan (Eds.), *Suicide in Bangladesh. New perspectives in behavioral & health sciences.* Springer, Singapore. https://doi.org/10.1007/978-981-99-0289-7_9.

International Association for Suicide Prevention. The decriminalisation of attempted suicide policy position statement, 2020. Available: https://www.iasp.info/pdf/iasp_decriminalisation_policy_2020.pdf. Retrieved November 01, 2020.

Islam, M. K., Maruf, M. M., Khan, M. A. S., & Arafat, S. M. Y. (2023). Literacy and stigma of suicide among Islamic religious leaders (Imams) in Bangladesh: A cross-sectional study. *International Review of Psychiatry.* https://doi.org/10.1080/09540261.2023.2252507.

Kabir, R., Hasan, M. R., Arafat, S. M. Y. (2023). Epidemiology of suicide and data quality in Bangladesh. In: S. M. Y. Arafat, M. M. Khan (Eds.), *Suicide in Bangladesh. New perspectives in behavioral & health sciences.* Springer, Singapore. https://doi.org/10.1007/978-981-99-0289-7_1.

Khan, A. R., Ratele, K., Arendse, N., Islam, M. Z., & Dery, I. (2020). Suicide and attempted suicide in Jhenaidah District, Bangladesh, 2010–2018. *Crisis, 41*(4), 304–312. https://doi.org/10.1027/0227-5910/a000631.

Khan, A. R., Arendse, N., & Ratele, K. (2021). Suicide prevention in Bangladesh: The current state and the way forward. *Asian Social Work and Policy Review, 15*(1), 15–23. https://doi.org/10.1111/aswp.12214.
Marthoenis, M., & Arafat, S. M. Y. (2022). Rate and associated factors of suicidal behavior among adolescents in Bangladesh and Indonesia: Global school-based student health survey data analysis. *Scientifica, 2022*, 8625345. https://doi.org/10.1155/2022/8625345.
Maruf, M. M., Shormi, F. R., Sajib, M. W. H., Acharjee, P., Ara, H., Roy, S., Ahmed, S., & Arafat, S. M. Y. (2022). Level and associated factors of literacy and stigma of suicide among Bangladeshi Physicians: A cross-sectional assessment. *Mental Illness*, 9914388. https://doi.org/10.1155/2022/9914388.
Mozumder, M. K., Jasmine, U. H., Haque, M. A., & Haque, S. (2023). Mental health and suicide risk among homosexual males in Bangladesh. *PLoS ONE, 18*(8), e0289597. https://doi.org/10.1371/journal.pone.0289597.
National Institute of Mental health. (2021). Epidemiology of suicide and suicidal behavior among youth and adolescents in Bangladesh. (Project Report).
Qusar, M. M. A. S., Parvez, M. K. H., Fariduzzaman, A. M., & Arafat, S. M. Y. (2020). Assessment of suicidality among post graduate medical residents of Bangladesh: A cross sectional study. (Project Report).
Suryadevara, U., & Tandon, R. (2018). Decriminalization of attempted suicide across Asia- It matters! *Asian Journal of Psychiatry, 35*, A2–A3. https://doi.org/10.1016/j.ajp.2018.06.001.
The Penal Code. (1860). Penal Code 1860. Chapter XVI. http://bdlaws.minlaw.gov.bd/act-11/section-3140.html. Retrieved August 24, 2022.
Uddin, M. S. (2023). Suicide research in Bangladesh. In: S. M. Y. Arafat, , M. M. Khan (Eds.), *Suicide in Bangladesh*. Springer, Singapore. https://doi.org/10.1007/978-981-99-0289-7_8.
United for Global Mental Health. (2021). Decriminalising suicide: Saving lives, reducing stigma.
Wahlin, Å., Palmer, K., Sternäng, O., Hamadani, J. D., & Kabir, Z. N. (2015). Prevalence of depressive symptoms and suicidal thoughts among elderly persons in rural Bangladesh. *International Psychogeriatrics, 27*(12), 1999–2008. https://doi.org/10.1017/S104161021500109X.
World Health Organization & International Association for Suicide Prevention. (2017). *Preventing suicide: A resource for media professionals* (2017 update). World Health Organization, WHO IRIS. https://apps.who.int/iris/handle/10665/258814.
World Health Organization. (2014). *Preventing suicide: a global imperative*. WHO: Geneva, Switzerland. https://apps.who.int/iris/handle/10665/131056. Retrieved July 15, 2022.
World Health Organization. (2019). Suicide in the world. Global Health Estimates. https://apps.who.int/iris/bitstream/handle/10665/326948/WHO-MSD-MER-19.3-eng.pdf. Retrieved July 15, 2022.
World Health Organization. (2021). *Suicide worldwide in 2019: Global health estimates*. Retrieved July 28, 2022, https://www.who.int/publications/i/item/9789240026643.
World Health Organization. (2023). WHO Policy Brief on the health aspects of decriminalization of suicide and suicide attempts. https://www.who.int/publications/i/item/9789240078796. Retrieved September 17, 2023.
World Health Organization. (2023). Preventing suicide: a resource for media professionals Update 2023. https://www.who.int/publications/i/item/9789240076846. Retrieved September 17, 2023.

# Chapter 12
# Psychiatric Education and Research System in Bangladesh

**S. M. Yasir Arafat**

**Abstract** Bangladesh is a lower-middle-income country of the Indian Subcontinent with a huge population density. Historically, education and research in mental health have been neglected in this region as well as in the country. Psychiatry is grossly under-prioritized in the undergraduate curriculum in the country. Before, independence mental health professionals were being trained in England. The first mental health specialist course was opened in 1975 named *Diploma in Psychological Medicine* which was ceased later. In 1979 a fellowship course [*Fellow of Bangladesh College of Physicians and Surgeons* (FCPS)] was started under Bangladesh College of Physicians and Surgeons (BCPS). The organization also offers a short-duration membership course. The *Master of Philosophy* (MPhil) in psychiatry was started in 1995 and ceased eventually. The *Doctor of Medicine* (MD) in psychiatry was started in 1995 and revised in 2010 as "Residency Program". The MD in child and adolescent psychiatry was started in 2016 and the FCPS in child and adolescent psychiatry was started in 2022. There are two specialized journals in psychiatry in Bangladesh. In this chapter, I have discussed the education and research system in psychiatry in Bangladesh.

**Keywords** Bangladesh · Education of psychiatry · Research in psychiatry · Mental health · Psychiatry journal

## 12.1 Introduction

Bangladesh is a country in the Indian subcontinent with its emerging economic potential. After getting its independence in 1971, with its huge population Bangladesh achieved remarkable progress in health, especially in reducing maternal and child health. However, mental health and scientific treatment of psychiatric disorders have been neglected the country for many reasons like stigma, low literacy, enduring belief about supernatural causes and healing, poor services development and primarily

S. M. Y. Arafat (✉)
Department of Psychiatry, Bangladesh Specialized Hospital Limited, Dhaka, Bangladesh
e-mail: arafatdmc62@gmail.com



S. M. Y. Arafat (ed.), *Mental Health in Bangladesh*,
https://doi.org/10.1007/978-981-97-0610-5_12

perhaps due to other immediate struggles of life. Therefore, psychiatry is an under-developed branch of medicine in the country, and psychiatric teaching in medical colleges is found inadequate since early days in regards to academic curriculum and human resource (Morning News, 1970). I discuss about the academic and research aspects of psychiatry in Bangladesh in this chapter.

## 12.2 Psychiatric Education in Bangladesh

Psychiatry has been taught in the graduation courses in Bangladesh as a branch of medicine. After graduation, a recognized specialized degree is mandatory to get the registration as a psychiatrist in Bangladesh.

### *12.2.1 Psychiatry in Undergraduate Curriculum*

According to the latest (2021) curriculum of the *Bangladesh Medical and Dental Council (BMDC)*, there are four phases in the undergraduate medical course [called *Bachelor of Medicine, Bachelor of Surgery (MBBS)*] in 5 academic years with an additional one year of internship (BMDC, 2021). The first phase lasts for 1.5 years for anatomy, physiology, and biochemistry followed by a professional examination, the second phase lasts for 1 year for forensic medicine and community medicine followed by a professional exam, the third phase lasts for 1 year for pathology, microbiology, and pharmacology followed by a professional exam, and the last phase lasts for 1.5 years for medicine and allied subjects, surgery and allied subjects, and gynecology (BMDC, 2021). In the total curriculum, there are allocations for psychiatry 20 h for lectures (2 h in the second phase and 18 h in the fourth phase) and 4 weeks of ward placement (2 weeks each for third and fourth phase) (BMDC, 2021). In the 2012 curriculum, the lecture duration was the same 20 h placed in the fourth phase only and the ward placement was only 3 weeks in the fourth phase (BMDC, 2012; Roy & Arafat, 2018). In 2022 curriculum, there were three professional examinations with the same course duration (BMDC, 2002). The lecture duration was 20 h (10 h in the 3rd year, 10 h in the 4th year, no lecture in the 5th year) and clinical placement was allocated for 4 weeks in the 4th year. In summary, in the current MBBS curriculum, there are allocations of 20 h of lectures and 4 weeks of clinical placement (BMDC, 2021). A comparative analysis of undergraduate curriculum of four countries in South Asia (Bangladesh, India, Nepal, and Sri Lanka) revealed that Bangladesh has the lowest time allocation in psychiatry among the four countries (Arafat et al., 2021). Sri Lankan curriculum offers a longer duration in psychiatry and considers psychiatry as a major subject, India has adopted a competency-based curriculum, and Nepal has variations in duration in psychiatry placement (Arafat et al., 2021).

The undergraduate curriculum includes historical perspectives and classificatory systems of psychiatry, communication skills focusing doctor-patient relationship, behavioral science focusing learning process, psychology of memory, personality, and intelligence, analysis of symptoms, mental state examination, neurocognitive disorders (dementia and delirium), child and adolescent psychiatry with autistic disorder, psychosexual dysfunctions, psychopharmacology and electroconvulsive therapy (ECT), substance related disorder and behavioral addictions (gaming, social media, internet and porn), schizophrenia, mania, depression, suicide, self-harm, psychiatric emergency, anxiety disorders including generalized anxiety disorder (GAD), phobic disorders, obsessive–compulsive disorder (OCD), and panic disorder, psychotherapy, somatopsychic disorders including conversion disorder, somatic symptom disorders, personality disorders, stress disorders, movement disorders including extra-pyramidal side effects (EPSE), Parkinson's disease, and tic disorder, seizure disorder, eating disorders, sleep–wake disorders, and psychiatrics disorders related to obstetrics and gynecology. Forensic psychiatry has not been included in the undergraduate curriculum in Bangladesh (BMDC, 2021).

In patient admission, facility would bolster the psychiatry clinical ward placement training and learning during the internship training. In that case, it is important to mention that, psychiatry inpatient services are available in only 10 public medical colleges and other 27 public medical colleges do not have the services (Arafat, 2024; Government of the People's Republic of Bangladesh, 2022). It was available in only four private medical colleges out of 63 (Arafat, 2024; Government of The People's Republic of Bangladesh, 2022). There are even medical colleges without a psychiatry department and a psychiatrist in the country.

### *12.2.2 Specialist Courses in Psychiatry in Bangladesh*

A BMDC-recognized degree is mandatory to do consultancy and teaching in psychiatry in Bangladesh. There are few degrees continuing in the country.

#### 12.2.2.1 Diploma in Psychological Medicine (DPM)

The DMP was the first course for specialization in mental health in Bangladesh. It was started in 1975 under the *Bangabandhu Sheikh Mujib Medical University (BSMMU)* (former *Institute of Postgraduate Medicine and Research* (IPGMR) by Professor Dr. A K M Nazimuddowla Chowdhury (Chowdhury et al., 2024). The course was ceased in 1995 (Arafat et al., 2020).

#### 12.2.2.2 Fellow of Bangladesh College of Physicians and Surgeons (FCPS)

The fellowship in psychiatry was started in 1979 under the *Bangladesh College of Physicians and Surgeons* (BCPS) (Arafat et al., 2020). It was a 4-year duration training in a specified design till January 2020 when it has been increased to 5 years course (Arafat, 2020). The fellows have to pass entrance and exit exams. It is important to mention that the number of seats is not limited in any case. From January 2022, BCPS started a 5-year duration FCPS in Child and Adolescent Psychiatry (BCPS, 2021).

#### 12.2.2.3 Member of the College of Physicians and Surgeons (MCPS)

Along with the fellowships, the BCPS also provides memberships (MCPS) in psychiatry (Arafat, 2020; Arafat et al., 2020). There is no policy of entrance exams for the degree. However, the examinees have to complete at least 4 years after graduation with 1-year training in psychiatry from BCPS recognized institutions (Arafat, 2020). The number of seats is not fixed for the MCPS degree. In February 19, 2022 at the 191st meeting of the BCPS Council (BCPS No. 776/2022/18040), the criteria have been changed (BCPS, 2022). From July 2022 session, the MCPS examinees need a gap of at least years between MBBS completion which was 4 years previously. Additionally, they need a 2-year clinical training, which was 1 year previously. There is no membership course (MCPS) in Child and Adolescent Psychiatry to date. With a membership degree, an individual can practice as a consultant psychiatrist. However, it is not considered for promotions in academic posts like professorship.

#### 12.2.2.4 Master of Philosophy (MPhil)

This specialized degree in psychiatry was started in 1995 after the cessation of the DPM. This course had a 3-year duration. It was carried out by the BSMMU and the *Sylhet MAG Osmani Medical College* (Karim et al., 2006). There was a mandatory criterion to pass a competitive entrance against the limited number of seats. The MPhil was also stopped and the focus was shifted to longer duration courses (Arafat, 2020; Arafat et al., 2020; Mullick, 2007).

#### 12.2.2.5 Doctor of Medicine (MD)

The MD in psychiatry was commenced at BSMMU in 1995. In 2010, a new curriculum "Residency Program", i.e. MD Residency was started. Therefore, the old curriculum (non-residency) had to be stopped (Arafat, 2020). The residency program was extended to other institutes of the country to increase the number of seats from 2014. Till to date the other institutions conducting the course are the NIMH, Dhaka & *MAG Osmani Medical College*, Sylhet. There is a mandatory competitive entrance exam to secure a seat for the MD Residency as the seats are limited in a year and in institutions. The MD is a 5-year duration course consisted of two phases; Phase A for two years and Phase B for 3 years. The MD degree (residency) in child and adolescent psychiatry was commenced at BSMMU in March 2016. To qualify the entrance exam, the candidates have to have a year gap after their internship training.

### *12.2.3 Mental Health and Psychiatric Nursing*

The *National Institute of Advanced Nursing Education and Research (NIANER)* is the leading institute that started master's level (MSc) academic degree in Psychiatric nursing in Bangladesh (National Institute of Advanced Nursing Education and Research, nd; Arafat, 2019). It was started in 20,123 aiming to progress the mental health nursing. The NIANER started a specialized mental health and psychiatric nursing program at the Master's level in July 2016, under BSMMU, which is the first attempt for mental health and psychiatric nursing. This dedicated program develops nurses capable for providing the evidence-based nursing services in clinical setting of psychiatric services care. *Advanced Mental Health and Psychiatric Nursing, Advanced Mental Health Nursing Intervention, Advanced Psychiatric Nursing Practicum for People with Mental Disorders,* and *Advanced Mental Health Nursing Practicum for Vulnerable Population* were the offered courses of the curriculum (National Institute of Advanced Nursing Education and Research, nd). The BSMMU started a specialized mental health and psychiatric nursing program at the Master's level in July 2022. The *Universal Nursing College*, Dhaka also privately started a specialized mental health and psychiatric nursing program at the Master's level in July 2022. Besides this, Diploma in Nursing, Basic and post-basic BSc in Nursing students generally studied psychiatric nursing. The National Institute of Mental Health & Hospital is supposed to start a Diploma in Psychiatric Nursing 1-year program in January 2024. Enam Nursing College has also been offering MSc course in *Mental Health & Psychiatric Nursing* (Enam Nursing, 2023).

## 12.3 Research Systems in Psychiatry in Bangladesh

Research in psychiatry has been grossly neglected and underdeveloped in Bangladesh. Research-based decision-making has not been established in the country yet, researchers have no additional recognition in job, and promotions. According to the WHO-ATLAS Report of 2020, there were only 35 peer-reviewed articles in psychiatry in Bangladesh (World Health Organization, 2022). This status could be attributed to the lack of role model in mental health research in the country, enduring power practice of political influence over academic contribution in posting, overall enduring poor attention of doctors in clinical research in Bangladesh, low investment in mental health research, inadequate, untrained, and poorly motivated researchers, supervisors, and staffs, lack of additional professional gain, rampant professional misconduct in publishing like plagiarism, data fabrication and falsification, guest and ghost authorship (Arafat et al., 2022a). Primarily, strong political attention is warranted to change the status quo in many aspects like increased budget in mental health research, development of mechanism to ensure quality research, and skills among researchers and so on.

### *12.3.1 Specialized Journals in Psychiatry in Bangladesh*

#### 12.3.1.1 Bangladesh Journal of Psychiatry (BJP)

It is the official journal of the *Bangladesh Association of Psychiatrists* (BAP). This is an open-access journal that releases two issues per year (January and July). The latest online available issue was Vol 32 No 2 (2018) (till 14 December 2023). Recently, the journal becomes irregular in uploading published issues online. There is no charge/article processing charge/publication charge in both of the journals.

#### 12.3.1.2 Archives of NIMH (AN)

It is another open access specialized in psychiatry that was started in 2018. It also publishes two issues per year.

There is no open-access publication fee for the authors. However, none of the journals is indexed in DOAJ, PubMed, Scopus, and Web of Science. Perhaps, the journals do not follow a standard peer review system objectively and methodically. None of the journals published any special issues other than their regular cycles and no thematic issue was also noted. BJP uses open journal platform and AN uses personalized website indicating that both journals are published by local publishing facilities.

EIC- Editor-in-Chief; EBM- Editorial Board Member

Here, I reanalyzed the data collected for the assessment of gender distribution of editors in South Asia to see the male–female proportions among the editors of two psychiatry journals (Arafat et al., 2022b, b). There were more than two-third (73%) of the editors were males and all the editor-in-chief positions were occupied by males (Fig. 12.1). In the two journals, there were 58 editorial positions occupied by 53 individual persons. More than 96% of the positions were occupied by psychiatrist, all the 24 positions of BJP were occupied by psychiatrists and only one psychologist and one internist were found in the editorial position of AN. I collected data from websites of the journals regarding the number and types of articles in different volumes and presented in Table 12.1.

The analysis indicates that AN has been publishing more papers both in number and types than BJP even though it is a newer journal.

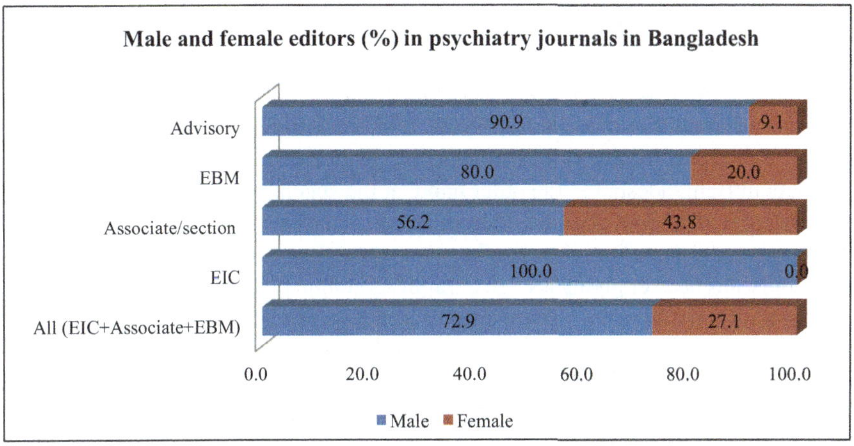


**Fig. 12.1** Proportion of male and female editors in Psychiatry journals in Bangladesh

**Table 12.1** Number and type of articles in psychiatry journals in Bangladesh

| Volume | Number | Original | Review | Case report | Editorial | Total |
|---|---|---|---|---|---|---|
| Archives of NIMH (AN) | | | | | | |
| 2018 | 1 | 3 | 1 | 1 | | 5 |
| 2018 | 2 | 3 | 2 | 1 | | 6 |
| 2019 | 1 | 4 | 1 | 1 | | 6 |
| 2019 | 2 | 4 | 1 | 1 | 1 | 7 |
| 2020 | 1 | 5 | 1 | 1 | 1 | 8 |
| 2020 | 2 | 7 | 1 | 1 | 1 | 10 |
| 2021 | 1 | 6 | 1 | 1 | 1 | 9 |
| 2021 | 2 | 6 | 1 | 1 | 1 | 9 |
| 2022 | 1 | 6 | | | 1 | 7 |
| 2022 | 2 | 7 | | 1 | 1 | 9 |
| Bangladesh journal of psychiatry (BJP) | | | | | | |
| 2018 | 2 | 3 | | 1 | 1 | 5 |
| 2018 | 1 | 3 | | 2 | | 5 |
| 2017 | 2 | 5 | | | | 5 |
| 2017 | 1 | 4 | | 1 | | 5 |
| 2016 | 2 | 5 | | | | 5 |
| 2016 | 1 | 4 | | 1 | | 5 |
| 2015 | 2 | 4 | | 1 | | 5 |
| 2015 | 1 | 8 | 1 | | | 9 |

## 12.4 Conclusions

The current as well as the enduring medical education system and the undergraduate curriculum have little attention to psychiatry. Thus, medical graduates have been found to exhibit inadequate skills in diagnosis, management, and prevention of mental disorders in Bangladesh. On the other hand, at the specialty level, a longer period is required to become a psychiatrist. Moreover, due to the existing stigma on psychiatric disorders, medical graduates are less keen to pursue their careers as a psychiatrist. As the country has been enjoying a stage of rapid economic progress, rapid urbanization, cultural shifting from a low-income to a middle-income country, along with other non-communicable diseases psychiatric disorders are coming at the fore-front day by day. Therefore, gradually, the demand of mental health professional has been mounting, however, the supply of psychiatrist has not been in the same pace of the demand. Bangladesh needs additional attention to the existing research system in psychiatry for the betterment of mental health of the country.

## References


Arafat, S. M. Y. (2019). History of psychiatry in Bangladesh. *Asian Journal of Psychiatry, 46*, 11–12. https://doi.org/10.1016/j.ajp.2019.09.024

Arafat, S. M. Y. (2020). The current status of psychiatric education in Bangladesh. *Asian Journal of Psychiatry, 52*, 102108. https://doi.org/10.1016/j.ajp.2020.102108

Arafat, S. M. Y. (2024). Mental health services in Bangladesh. In S. M. Y. Arafat (Ed.), *Mental health in Bangladesh: From bench to community*. Springer Nature Singapore. https://doi.org/10.1007/978-981-97-0610-5_3

Arafat, S. Y., Ali, S. A. E. Z., Saleem, T., Banerjee, D., Singh, R., Baminiwatta, A., & Shoib, S. (2022a). Academic psychiatry journals in South Asian countries: most from India, none from Afghanistan, Bhutan and the Maldives. *Global Psychiatry Archives*, 5(1), 1–9. https://doi.org/10.52095/gp.2021.4395.1036.

Arafat, S. M. Y., Amin, R., Baminiwatta, A., Hussain, F., Singh, R., Kar, S. K., & Mubashir, A. S. (2022b). Gender distribution of editors in psychiatry journals of South Asia. *Psychiatry Research, 317*, 114819. https://doi.org/10.1016/j.psychres.2022.114819

Arafat, S. M. Y., Kar, S. K., Sharma, P., Marahatta, K., & Baminiwatta, A. K. A. B. (2021). A comparative analysis of psychiatry curriculum at undergraduate level of Bangladesh, India, Nepal, and Sri Lanka. *Indian Journal of Psychiatry, 63*(2), 184–188. https://doi.org/10.4103/psychiatry.IndianJPsychiatry_615_20

Arafat, S. M. Y., Mullick, M. S. I., & Islam, H. (2020). Development of psychiatric services in Bangladesh. *Asian Journal of Psychiatry, 47*, 101870. https://doi.org/10.1016/j.ajp.2019.101870

BCPS .(2021). Notification for introducing new fellowship program in Medical Oncology, Palliative Medicine, Child and Adolescent Psychiatry, Paediatric Endocrinology & Metabolism, Paediatric Critical Care Medicine. Retrieved September 01, 2023, from chrome-extension://efaidnbmnnnibpcajpcglclefindmkaj/http://bcps.edu.bd/bcpscms/upload/Notification_for_introducing_new_fellowship_program_in_Medical_Oncology,_Palliative_Medicine,_Child_and_Adolesent_Psychiatry,_Paediatric_Endocrinology_Metabolism,_Paediatric_Critical_Care_Medicine.pdf.

BCPS. (2022). Notification for counting two years training in MCPS. Retrieved August 30, 2023, from chrome-extension://efaidnbmnnnibpcajpcglclefindmkaj/http://bcps.edu.bd/bcpscms/upload/Notification_for_counting_two_years_training_in_MCPS.pdf.

BMDC. (2002). BM&DC, MBBS Curriculum – 2002. Retrieved 29 August, 2023, from https://www.bmdc.org.bd/curriculum-2002.

BMDC. (2012). MBBS Curriculum Update- 2012. Retrieved 29 August, 2023, from https://www.bmdc.org.bd/curriculum-2012.

BMDC. (2021). MBBS Curriculum Update – 2021. Retrieved 29 August, 2023, from https://www.bmdc.org.bd/curriculum-2020.

Chowdhury, N. F., Fariduzzaman, A. M., & Arafat, S. M. Y. (2024). Prominent figures in psychiatry in Bangladesh. In S. M. Y. Arafat (Ed.) *Mental health in Bangladesh: From bench to community*. Springer Nature Singapore. https://doi.org/10.1007/978-981-97-0610-5_1

Enam Nursing College. (2023). Master of science in nursing. Retrieved September 01, 2023, from https://enc.edu.bd/msc-in-nursing/.

Government of The People's Republic of Bangladesh. (2022). National Mental Health Strategic Plan, 2020–2030. Retrieved May 02, 2023, from https://dghs.gov.bd/sites/default/files/files/dghs.portal.gov.bd/notices/e27171cb_a80b_42d4_99ad_40095adef31b/2022-08-16-08-42-af8622e2c4936593dd45601b84f4920f.pdf.

Karim, M. R., Shaheed, F., & Paul, S. (2006). Psychiatry in Bangladesh. *International Psychiatry: Bulletin of the Board of International Affairs of the Royal College of Psychiatrists, 3*(3), 16–18.

Mullick, M. S. I. (2007). Teaching and training in psychiatry and the need for a new generation of psychiatrists in Bangladesh: Role of the Royal College of Psychiatrists. *International Psychiatry : Bulletin of the Board of International Affairs of the Royal College of Psychiatrists, 4*(2), 29–31.

National Institute of Advanced Nursing Education and Research. (nd). Mental Health & Psychiatric Nursing. http://www.nianer.edu.bd/msn/advanced-specialties/mental-health-psychiatric/.

Morning News. (1970). Mental Health. Published on March 03, 1970.

Roy, S., & Arafat, S. Y. (2018). Recent changes in MBBS curriculum in psychiatry in Bangladesh: A call for attention. *Bangladesh Journal of Psychiatry, 32*(2), 24–25. https://doi.org/10.3329/bjpsy.v32i2.55125

World Health Organization. (2022). Mental Health Atlas 2020 Country Profile: Bangladesh. Retrieved March 30, 2023, from https://www.who.int/publications/m/item/mental-health-atlas-bgd-2020-country-.

# Chapter 13
# Research on Common Mental Disorders in Bangladesh

**Ravi Philip Rajkumar and S. M. Yasir Arafat**

**Abstract** Common mental disorders include depression and anxiety disorders. These conditions are among the leading causes of disability and morbidity worldwide. According to the recent National Mental Health Survey, over 10% of the population of Bangladesh suffers from one of these disorders. In the past decade, there has been a significant increase in the quality and quantity of published research pertaining to CMDs in Bangladesh. The global COVID-19 pandemic provided a further impetus to such efforts. The current chapter reviews the existing research on the epidemiology, pathophysiology, diagnosis, and management of CMDs in Bangladesh, and the ways to surmount them. The quality and quantity of research into CMDs in Bangladesh are also assessed, and the integration of care for CMDs into primary or general health care is discussed.

**Keywords** Research · Evidence · Common mental disorders · Depression · Anxiety disorders · Risk factors · Biomarkers · Bangladesh

## 13.1 Introduction

The term "common mental disorders" (CMD) refers to depressive and anxiety disorders. Depressive disorders include major depression and dysthymia, while anxiety disorders include generalized anxiety disorder, panic disorder with or without agoraphobia, social anxiety disorder, specific phobia, and other anxiety disorders. This term has been introduced to refer to mental disorders commonly seen in community or primary care settings, as opposed to "severe mental disorders"—schizophrenia and bipolar disorder—which are usually diagnosed and treated by mental health professionals in psychiatric settings (Linzer et al., 1996; Steel et al., 2014). CMDs

R. P. Rajkumar (✉)
Department of Psychiatry, Jawaharlal Institute of Postgraduate Medical Education and Research (JIPMER), Puducherry, India
e-mail: ravi.psych@gmail.com

S. M. Y. Arafat
Department of Psychiatry, Bangladesh Specialized Hospital Limited, Dhaka, Bangladesh



S. M. Y. Arafat (ed.), *Mental Health in Bangladesh*,
https://doi.org/10.1007/978-981-97-0610-5_13

are among the leading causes of impaired quality of life, disability, and morbidity worldwide (GBD, 2019 Mental Disorders Collaborators, 2022).

Bangladesh is a South Asian country with a population of over 160 million. It is the eighth most populous country globally, and the third most populous in South Asia. According to GBD data, Bangladesh has the highest estimated prevalence of both depression (4.1%) and anxiety disorders (4.4%) among South Asian countries (World Health Organization, 2017; Ogbo et al., 2018). However, these figures may underestimate the actual burden of CMD in Bangladesh: according to a national survey conducted in 2018–19, the prevalence of depression and anxiety disorders is around 5–7%, National Institute of Mental Health (2021).

Bangladesh is a middle-income country, with a Human Development Index of 0.632 and a gross national income of $4,976 per capita. It is subject to several ecological vulnerabilities, including a high risk of cyclones, floods, and rising temperatures due to climate change (Gros et al., 2019; United Nations Development Programme, 2020). Due to economic inequalities and ongoing sociocultural changes, a significant proportion of the general population experiences a wide range of psychosocial stressors related to education, employment, marriage, health, housing, food security, and economic stability from an early age (Anjum et al., 2022a; Berens et al., 2019). These factors can significantly affect the physical and psychological well-being of the citizens of Bangladesh (Mullick & Karim, 1994; Arobi et al., 2019; Yuan et al., 2022), placing them at an increased risk of common mental disorders (Alam et al., 2021). This risk may be significantly elevated in certain groups, such as women, the elderly, and those from lower socioeconomic strata, as they are exposed to a wider range of chronic stressors and health risks (Alam et al., 2021; Insan et al., 2022). These pre-existing vulnerabilities were compounded by the effects of the COVID-19 pandemic, which caused a significant increase in psychological stress and symptoms of CMD across all strata of society. According to one estimate, at least 47% of the population in Bangladesh had significant symptoms of depression or anxiety because of this pandemic (Hosen et al., 2021; Rathod et al., 2023).

Despite this high burden of common mental disorders, access to mental health care in Bangladesh is often inadequate. This is due to several factors, including low budgetary allocation for mental health, a lack of coordination between levels of mental health care, a concentration of treatment facilities in urban areas, a lack of manpower, cultural attitudes leading to stigmatization of the mentally ill, and poor mental health literacy both in the general population and among health professionals (Koly et al., 2022; Arafat et al., 2024; Arafat, 2024). In such conditions, it is essential to have an accurate estimate of the burden and correlates of CMDs in specific populations, so that limited resources can be used efficiently both in the general population and for specific, high-risk groups (Adams et al., 2023; Shidhaye et al., 2015). Research into the phenomenology of CMDs in Bangladesh, and the appropriate use of screening instruments and rating scales validated in the vernacular, will avoid under-diagnosis or misdiagnosis of patients with these conditions (Faruk et al., 2021). Finally, it is necessary to be aware of existing research on interventions for CMDs in the Bangladeshi context—both pharmacological and psychosocial—so that effective and feasible treatments can be provided more widely (Singla et al., 2017).

It is equally important to understand the possible biological correlates of CMDs, as this may yield valuable information on their pathophysiology and treatment (Iorfino et al., 2016).

This chapter reviews the existing literature on CMDs in Bangladesh under these headings, with the aim of providing a broad and practical overview of the subject for clinicians, researchers, and public health experts. In writing this chapter, relevant papers were retrieved from the PubMed, Scopus, and Bangladesh Journals Online databases of scholarly literature, as well as the Google Scholar search engine. A total of 863 papers were used to obtain relevant data for each of the sections below.

## 13.2 Epidemiology of Common Mental Disorders in Bangladesh

The data on which this section is based was extracted from a total of 152 research studies, though only the key findings are presented here in the interest of clarity. Researchers in Bangladesh have examined the occurrence of CMDs both in the general population, and in specific high-risk groups such as children and adolescents, the elderly, persons with medical illnesses, and those experiencing long-term psychosocial adversity. The break-up of the populations covered by the included studies is provided in Fig. 13.1.

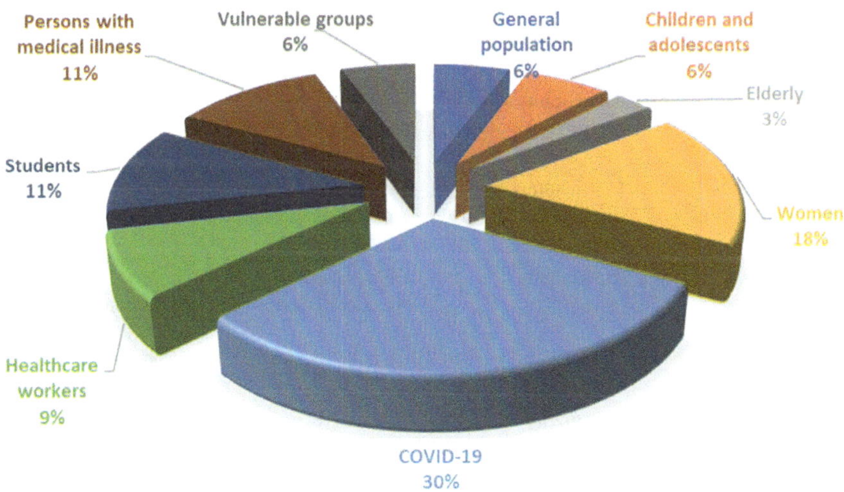


**Fig. 13.1** Populations covered by research on common mental disorders in Bangladesh across 141 research studies

### 13.2.1 Studies Involving the General Population

One of the earliest surveys of the prevalence of CMD in Bangladesh was conducted in 1981 in the rural community of Dasherkandi. Out of 1181 people surveyed, 3.6% suffered from a mental disorder. The most common diagnosis was depression, followed by anxiety disorders. Overall, 2% of this sample fulfilled criteria for a CMD (Chowdhury et al., 1981). Almost three decades later, the Bangladesh National Mental Health Survey found that the prevalence of CMDs in adults was 6.7% for depression and 4.7% for anxiety disorders (Ministry of Health & Family Welfare, 2021). Apart from these two landmark studies, several other epidemiological studies have examined the rates of CMDs in the general population. A summary of these studies is provided in Table 13.1. Taken together, these studies yield an estimated prevalence of 2–8% for depression and 2.7–5% for anxiety disorders, and a higher prevalence of 15–48% for depressive symptoms and 6% for anxiety symptoms. Rates of both disorders were slightly higher in a rural population (Hosain et al., 2007) than in an urban sample (Islam et al., 2003) and depressive symptoms were common in an "urbanizing" community transitioning from a rural to an urban lifestyle (Natasha et al., 2015a). Based on surveys of multiple South Asian countries, depressive symptoms were more common in Bangladesh (48%) than in India (18–40%) or Sri Lanka (11%), and were comparable in frequency to those seen in Nepal (40–49%) (Bishwajit et al., 2017a, b).

**Table 13.1** Frequency of common mental disorders in the general population in Bangladesh

| Study | Population and sample size | Frequency estimates | Risk factors, if identified |
|---|---|---|---|
| Chowdhury et al. (1981) | Rural adults ($n$ = 1181) | Depression and anxiety disorders ≈ 2% (combined) | Female gender |
| Islam et al. (2003) | Urban adults ($n$ = 1145) | Depression 6% Anxiety disorders 2.7% | Female gender, higher income |
| Hosain et al. (2007) | Rural adults ($n$ = 766) | Depression 8% Anxiety disorders 5% | Female gender (depression), male gender (anxiety), large household size (women), low income |
| Natasha et al. (2015a) | Urbanizing adults ($n$ = 2293) | Depressive symptoms 15.3% | Female gender, older age, low education, single status, impaired glucose tolerance |

(continued)

**Table 13.1** (continued)

| Study | Population and sample size | Frequency estimates | Risk factors, if identified |
|---|---|---|---|
| Bishwajit et al. (2017a) | Adults aged ≥ 50 years ($n = 1208$) | Depressive symptoms 47.7% | Female gender, single status, lower education, unemployment, substance use, low physical activity |
| Bishwajit et al. (2017b) | Adults in the general population ($n = 3262$) | Depressive symptoms 39% | Female gender, younger age, single status, lack of formal education, unemployment, substance use, low fruit and vegetable consumption |
| National Institute of Mental Health (2021) | Adults in the general population ($n = 7270$) | Depression 6.7%<br>Anxiety disorders 4.7% | Female gender<br>No consistent association with rural/urban residence or income |
| Wahid et al. (2023) | Adults in the general population ($n = 3606$) | Depressive symptoms 16.3%<br>Anxiety symptoms 6%<br>Both depressive and anxiety symptoms 4.8% | Female gender, older age, lower education, physical disability, rising temperature, exposure to floods |

## *13.2.2 Studies of Specific Populations or Groups*

### 13.2.2.1 Children and Adolescents

The 2019 National Mental Health Survey of Bangladesh, based on data from 2163 children aged 7–17, found an estimated prevalence of 0.4% for depression and 4.7% for anxiety disorders (Ministry of Health & Family Welfare, 2021). Other studies examining the frequency of CMDs or CMD symptoms in children or adolescents are summarized in Table 13.2. Apart from the national survey cited above, all these studies were conducted in older children or adolescents.

In studies examining the presence of a syndromic depressive or anxiety disorder, the estimated prevalence of CMDs was 1.6 to 9% for depression and 4.7–7.8% for anxiety disorders. When symptoms of CMDs were measured without a formal diagnosis, 24.5%–44.5% had depressive symptoms, and 18.1–20.1% had symptoms of anxiety. There was some evidence that anxiety symptoms were more common in

**Table 13.2** Frequency of common mental disorders in children and adolescents in Bangladesh

| Study | Population and sample size | Frequency estimates | Risk factors, if identified |
|---|---|---|---|
| Izutsu et al. (2006) | Children and adolescents (age 11–18) from urban slum and non-slum areas ($n = 602$) | Depression 3.7%<br>Anxiety disorders 5.3% | Female gender, older age, school attendance, being employed, non-slum residence |
| Nasreen et al. (2016) | Adolescents (age 13–19) from rural and urban slum areas ($n = 2440$) | Probable depression 14% | Female gender, urban slum residence, older age, poverty, poor relationship with parents, family history of depression (boys only), reproductive illness (girls only), sexual abuse (girls only) |
| Khan et al. (2017) | Adolescents (age 13–16) attending school ($n = 755$) | Depressive symptoms 25% | Female gender, older age, dissatisfaction with body weight, feeling unsafe at school, low satisfaction with life, poor sleep quality, intake of high-sugar beverages, skipping breakfast |
| Bangladesh National Mental Health Survey (2019) | Children and adolescents (age 7–17) in the general population ($n = 2163$) | Depression 0.4%<br>Anxiety disorders 4.7% | Female gender |
| Khan and Khan (2020) | Children and adolescents (age 11–17) in the general population ($n = 2989$) | Anxiety disorders 4.7% | Female gender, loneliness, bullying, physical abuse, discord with parents, low peer support |
| Mallick and Radwan (2020) | Adolescents (age 14–17) attending school ($n = 276$) | Depression 1.6–9%<br>Specific phobia 2.3–2.7%<br>Social anxiety disorder 2.7–3.4%<br>Panic disorder 0–0.5%<br>Generalized anxiety disorder 2.1–2.3% | Cyberbullying (depression only) |

(continued)

**Table 13.2** (continued)

| Study | Population and sample size | Frequency estimates | Risk factors, if identified |
|---|---|---|---|
| Islam et al. (2021) | Adolescents (age 13–18) attending school ($n = 563$) | Depressive symptoms 26.5% Anxiety symptoms 18.1% | Female gender (depression only), older age, poor sleep quality, smoking, poor peer relationships. Depression predicted anxiety and vice versa |
| Mridha et al. (2021) | Children and adolescents (age 10–17) in the general population ($n = 9856$) | Depressive symptoms 24.5% | Female gender, older age, high maternal education, high paternal education (boys only), Muslim religion (girls only), absence of a younger sibling, small family size (girls only), food insecurity, television viewing, low physical activity, tobacco use (boys only) |
| Anjum et al. (2022b) | Adolescents (age 12–18) attending school ($n = 2313$) | Anxiety symptoms 20.1% | Female gender, older age, smaller family size, urban residence, low physical activity, higher screen time, poor sleep quality, low body weight |
| Salim et al. (2023) | Adolescents (aged 13–19) in a rural community ($n = 339$) | Depressive symptoms 44.5% | Female gender, dropping out of school |

children or adolescents living in urban area, and that both CMDs were slightly more common in non-slum urban areas (Anjum et al., 2022b; Izutsu et al., 2006).

Female gender and older age were both associated with a higher occurrence of CMDs. This is consistent with earlier epidemiological evidence on the increased risk of CMDs during the transition from childhood to adulthood (Rocha et al., 2013). Parental education was associated with depressive symptoms in a single study: maternal education predicted depression in both boys and girls, while paternal education predicted depression in boys (Mridha et al., 2021). Other demographic factors that showed some association with CMD included smaller family size, and the absence of a younger sibling, which was linked to depressive symptoms (Anjum et al., 2022b; Mridha et al., 2021).

A wide range of psychosocial adversities were associated with depression and anxiety in adolescents. These included poor relationships with parents, loneliness and lack of peer support, employment at an early age, physical abuse, food insecurity, experiences of being bullied (including cyberbullying), feeling unsafe at school, and dropping out of school (Izutsu et al., 2006; Khan & Khan, 2020; Mallick & Radwan, 2020; Islam et al., 2021; Mridha et al., 2021; Salim et al., 2023). Similarly, several lifestyle factors were associated with CMDs in youth, including poor sleep quality, higher screen time, tobacco use, and poor dietary practices such as skipping breakfast and consumption of high-sugar beverages (Anjum et al., 2022b; Islam et al., 2021; Khan et al., 2017; Mridha et al., 2021). In contrast, regular physical activity was associated with a lower risk of anxiety (Anjum et al., 2022b). Adolescents' perceptions of their own situation could also influence their mental health: low life satisfaction and dissatisfaction with one's body image were both associated with depression (Khan et al., 2017).

#### 13.2.2.2 Women

CMDs, particularly depressive disorders, are around twice as common in women as in men worldwide. This is due to a variety of biological, psychological, and socioeconomic factors, though their relative importance varies from one country to another. In Bangladesh, women are vulnerable to CMDs because of their exposure to chronic stressors, including discord with spouses or in-laws and intimate partner violence. These difficulties are compounded negative societal attitudes toward mental disorders, leading to stigma and delayed treatment-seeking (Ziaei et al., 2016).

According to the National Mental Health Survey (Ministry of Health & Family Welfare, 2021), the prevalence of CMD in adult women is 7.9% for depression and 5.4% for anxiety disorders. Other researchers have found significant depressive symptoms in 17–20% of women in rural areas and in 30–42% in urban areas (Alam et al., 2020; Esie et al., 2019; Sparling et al., 2020; Sultana et al., 2021). Apart from the National Survey, there are no studies specifically examining the prevalence of anxiety disorders in women in the community.

Both pregnancy and the puerperium are associated with an elevated risk of CMDs in women in Bangladesh. Based on the available research, probable depression is present in 8–33% of pregnant women and 18–57% of women in the postpartum period (Gausia et al., 2009; Insan et al., 2023; Nasreen et al., 2013, 2015). High rates of depressive symptoms have been reported even 12–16 months after birth (Azad et al., 2019; Hossain et al., 2020). There are fewer studies on anxiety disorders, but rates of anxiety symptoms of 26–29% during pregnancy and 59% following a miscarriage have been reported (Nasreen et al., 2010, 2011; Koly et al., 2023).

Marital and pregnancy-related stressors are significantly associated with the occurrence of CMDs in the antepartum and postpartum periods. These include poor relationships with spouses and in-laws, "controlling" behavior on the part of the husband, intimate partner violence, preference of the family for a male child, unplanned pregnancies, gestational diabetes mellitus, adverse pregnancy outcomes such as spontaneous abortion or intrauterine death, poor medical care after such an adverse outcome, and a need to return to work soon after delivery due to financial difficulties (Azad et al., 2019; Gausia et al., 2009; Islam et al., 2017; Nasreen et al., 2011; Natasha et al., 2015b; Tasnim et al., 2022, 2023). More general stressors associated with peripartum CMDs include poverty or financial hardship, poor social support, food insecurity, and chronic stress in general (Hossain et al., 2020; Nasreen et al., 2011; Valdes et al., 2021). The effects of these stressors may be mediated through psychological factors such as low self-esteem and low perceived autonomy

(Islam et al., 2017; Koly et al., 2023). A past history of depression or anxiety may predict the re-emergence of these symptoms during pregnancy or after childbirth (Islam et al., 2017; Nasreen et al., 2015).

#### 13.2.2.3 Elderly Adults

There are relatively few studies of CMDs in the geriatric population, and all of these have focused on depression and not on anxiety disorders. Based on the available results, significant depressive symptoms may be present in 37–45% of elderly adults in the community and in over 80% of those with medical comorbidities. Risk factors for depression in the elderly include older age, lower educational attainment, being single, widowed or separated, lower socioeconomic status, being retired or unemployed, malnutrition, a sedentary lifestyle, and the use of tobacco or caffeine (Disu et al., 2019; Islam et al., 2021; Tabassum et al., 2023; Wahlin et al., 2015). A study of elderly adults in a residential facility also found an association between depression and cognitive impairment (Akter et al., 2023). On the other hand, regular social contacts, participation in religious activities, and involvement in one or more hobbies appear to be protective (Disu et al., 2019).

#### 13.2.2.4 Patients with Medical Illnesses

There is a bidirectional relationship between CMDs and medical illnesses. CMDs can increase the risk of specific medical disorders, such as cardiovascular and neurological illnesses, while chronic medical illnesses can trigger or worsen depression or anxiety disorders (Oosthuizen et al., 2008). This link may be especially strong in the case of non-communicable diseases (NCDs) such as diabetes mellitus, ischemic heart disease, or cancer (Uphoff et al., 2019).

There are several studies examining the frequency of CMDs in patients with a specific medical or surgical condition in Bangladesh. The most frequently studied medical condition in this context is type 2 diabetes mellitus. In patients with this illness, probable depression has been identified in 23–45% and depressive symptoms in 34–36% (Asghar et al., 2007; Roy et al., 2012; Islam et al., 2015a; Lloyd et al., 2018; Kamrul-Hasan et al., 2022a, b, c, d). A clinic-based study found that 14% of patients with diabetes mellitus had generalized anxiety disorder (Sultan-E-Monzur et al., 2015). Correlates of depression in type 2 diabetes mellitus include higher age, female gender, higher body mass index, lower education and income, insufficient physical activity, poor control of diabetes, and past depression. Apart from diabetes, high rates of depressive symptoms have been reported in patients with stroke (Hayee et al., 2001; Islam et al., 2015b), chronic obstructive pulmonary disease (Al Adiluzzaman et al., 2016), chronic renal failure (Rahman et al., 2020) and HIV/AIDS (Rabeya et al., 2023). In these disorders, greater disability or dysfunction was associated with a higher risk of depression.

Infectious diseases other than HIV/AIDS are also associated with an elevated risk of depression. In patients with other sexually transmitted infections, 8% had depression and 11% had anxiety disorders; substance use and sexual dysfunction were associated with higher CMD rates in this population (Mandal et al., 2007). In patients with multi-drug-resistant tuberculosis, almost 34% had comorbid depression, and this rate was higher in those with other medical comorbidities (Huque et al., 2020).

In women, polycystic ovarian syndrome was also associated with symptoms of depression in 60% and anxiety in over 80% of women (Hasan et al., 2022a). High rates of CMDs have also been reported in children and adolescents with medical conditions: 15%–18% of youth with juvenile arthritis had depression (Mullick et al., 2005), and 20–45% of children with epilepsy had depressive or anxiety disorders (Rabin et al., 2013).

#### 13.2.2.5 Healthcare Workers and Students

Healthcare workers, such as doctors, nurses, and allied health professionals, are considered to be at an elevated risk of CMDs due to workplace-related stressors (Dai et al., 2015; Hemmati et al., 2021). Healthcare students also face specific pressures that may lead to elevated rates of anxiety and depression (Pacheco et al., 2017; Tung et al., 2018). Identifying CMDs in these populations is important as they may be associated with poor academic or work performance, medical errors, absenteeism, and even suicide (Pereira-Lima et al., 2019; Ryan et al., 2023). The studies summarized here pertain to the period before the COVID-19 pandemic. CMDs related to the COVID-19 crisis are discussed in Sect. 2.3.

Among undergraduate medical students, 31–43% have depressive symptoms, 53% have anxiety symptoms, and roughly one-fourth screen positive for CMDs (Abbasy et al., 2022; Hasan et al., 2022b; Sultana, 2011, 2021). In a study of dental students: 27% had probable depression and 18% had a probable anxiety disorder (Faruk et al., 2023). Postgraduate medical trainees had depressive symptoms at rates comparable to those of medical undergraduates (Sadiq et al., 2019). Physicians and nurses had high rates of depressive symptoms and 65% of nurses also had significant symptoms of anxiety (Islam et al., 2022a, b; Salma & Hasan, 2020). In a study specifically examining junior doctors—interns and junior medical officers—about 18% screened positive for depression (Mamun et al., 2022a, b). Work-related factors such as the length of working hours, income, and job satisfaction were important predictors of depression in healthcare workers (Salma & Hasan, 2020; Islam et al., 2022a; Mamun et al., 2022a).

#### 13.2.2.6 College and University Students

Recent meta-analyses have found high rates of CMD symptomatology in college students. There are multiple factors involved in the pathogenesis of depression and anxiety in this age group, including life cycle transitions, interpersonal difficulties, and academic stress (Fernandes et al., 2023).

Studies of student mental health in Bangladesh involve surveys of large numbers of students in specific colleges or universities. Formal diagnoses of depression or anxiety disorders were not made, but the frequency of significant symptoms of anxiety or depression was reported. Depressive symptoms were found in 29–83% of students, and anxiety symptoms in 29–95%, with most studies reporting that around 30–60% of students had significant levels of depression (Hossain et al., 2022a; Kamruzzaman et al., 2022; Koly et al., 2021; Mamun et al., 2022b; Rasheduzzaman et al., 2021; Sayeed et al., 2023).

Among the academic factors associated with CMDs in students, dissatisfaction with one's course of study was associated with depression (Koly et al., 2021), academic difficulties were associated with both depression and anxiety (Kamruzzaman et al., 2022; Kundu et al., 2021), and students of science or social science subjects had higher rates of both symptom types (Hossain et al., 2019; Rabby et al., 2023). Some researchers found that depression was more common in the first year of study, while others found that it increased over subsequent years. A longitudinal study found that both depressive and anxiety symptoms increased by over 25% in students followed up for 15 months (Hossain et al., 2019).

### *13.2.3 Studies Specifically Related to the COVID-19 Pandemic*

The occurrence of symptoms of CMDs in relation to the COVID-19 pandemic has been extensively studied by researchers in Bangladesh. For a comprehensive review of this literature, the systematic reviews by Hosen et al. (2021), Hossain et al. (2021a), or Al Mamun et al. (2021) may be consulted. In a comparative review of studies from all South Asian countries, it was found that Bangladesh had the highest rates of anxiety and stress-related problems related to COVID-19 (Kabir et al., 2023). Researchers from Bangladesh have taken an active role in assessing the burden of mental health problems among their country's citizens, and the risk factors associated with them. Out of their large body of work, studies with a specific focus on CMDs are summarized in Table 13.3.

In the general population, depressive symptoms were seen in 21–73% and anxiety symptoms in 25–73%, with higher estimates being obtained as the pandemic progressed (Abir et al., 2021; Das et al., 2021a; Haque et al., 2022; Mamun et al., 2021; Rahman et al., 2021a). Over a fourth of respondents surveyed in one study had symptoms of both CMDs (Al Azdi et al., 2020). Many of the sociodemographic and lifestyle risk factors for both disorders in the community were similar to those seen in pre-COVID studies. This suggests that the stress caused by the COVID-19 pandemic exacerbated pre-existing psychosocial vulnerabilities toward depression and anxiety (Tibber et al., 2023). On the other hand, factors specific to the pandemic also played

**Table 13.3** Frequency of common mental disorders in specific populations in relation to the COVID-19 pandemic in Bangladesh

| Population | Frequency estimates | Risk factors |
|---|---|---|
| General population | Depressive symptoms 21–73%<br>Anxiety symptoms 25–73%<br>Both depression and anxiety ≈ 28% | Female gender, younger age, single marital status, living alone, unemployment, fear of COVID-19, worries about separation from family, financial worries, increased media or social media exposure, smoking, obesity, insomnia, comorbid medical illness, not being immunized |
| Patients with COVID-19 | Acute phase:<br>Depressive symptoms 52–87%<br>Anxiety symptoms 56–64%<br>Post-recovery:<br>Probable CMD 17% | Urban residence, lower education, comorbid physical illness, >3 COVID symptoms, low oxygen saturation at admission |
| Children and adolescents | Depressive symptoms 18%<br>Anxiety symptoms 14%<br>Probable CMD 23% | Female gender, older age, poor parenting, lockdown, food insecurity |
| Students | Depressive symptoms 26–59%<br>Anxiety symptoms 27–69%<br>Both depression and anxiety ≈ 47% | Female gender, low income, nuclear family, later years of study (3rd/4th), fears of being exposed to or having COVID-19, contact with COVID-19, symptoms suggestive of COVID-19, worries about academic performance, delay, and future prospects, insomnia, low physical activity, low involvement in religious practice, recent stressors, loneliness, past history of mental illness |
| Healthcare workers and students | Healthcare workers:<br>Depressive symptoms 27–73%<br>Anxiety symptoms 21–78%<br>Students:<br>Depressive symptoms 59–80% | Female gender, single marital status, rural residence, financial problems, loneliness, family problems, low BMI, substance use, low physical activity, poor self-rated health, difficulty in restricting social media use, emotional abuse, discrimination related to COVID-19, fear of abuse related to COVID-19 work, shortage of protective equipment, overwork, frontline status, early career stage |
| Other specific vulnerable groups | Depressive symptoms 39–66%<br>Anxiety symptoms 35–78% | Low income, low education, single marital status, rural residence, low physical activity, obesity, smoking, financial difficulties, poor self-rated health, loneliness, social isolation, multiple disabilities (in PWD), poor workplace health safety practices, salary reductions, downsizing (in private sector employees) |

**Abbreviations**: BMI, body mass index; CMD, common mental disorder; PWD, persons with disabilities a role in the development of depressive or anxious symptoms in the Bangladeshi general population: these included fear of infection with COVID-19, worries about separation from one's family, and immunization status (Nur et al., 2023).

Patients with acute COVID-19 infection requiring hospitalization or quarantine had high rates of CMD symptoms, with 52–87% reporting depressive symptoms and 56–64% reporting anxiety symptoms. In these patients, illness-related variables such as low oxygen saturation, more severe symptoms, and comorbid medical illnesses were predictive of CMDs (Hasan et al., 2020, 2021; Ripon et al., 2020; Rahman et al., 2021b; Mina et al., 2023). In patients assessed over 6 months after developing COVID-19, 17% fulfilled criteria for a diagnosis of depression or anxiety disorder (Afroze et al., 2023).

CMD symptoms related to COVID-19 were present in 14–23% of children and adolescents in two studies (Haque et al., 2023; Mallik & Radwan, 2021) and were associated with psychosocial adversities such as poor parenting and food insecurity. In a single study of older adults, 40% had symptoms of pandemic-related depression. Elderly adults with socioeconomic difficulties had more severe depressive symptoms (Mistry et al., 2021).

Healthcare workers (HCWs), who were faced with a marked increase in workload and a risk of infection amidst resource scarcity, had high rates of psychological morbidity during this pandemic. Depressive and anxiety symptoms were each present in about 21–78% of HCWs. Work-related factors associated with CMDs in HCWs included early career stage, increased working hours, frontline work, shortage of protective equipment, and fear of infection. (Ali et al., 2021; Chowdhury et al., 2021; Hossain et al., 2021b; Khatun et al., 2021; Repon et al., 2021; Tasnim et al., 2021; Chomon, 2022; Hasan et al., 2022c).

In studies of college and university students affected by the COVID-19 pandemic, 26–59% of students had depressive symptoms and 27–69% had anxiety symptoms (Islam et al., 2020; Shovo et al., 2021; Rahman et al., 2021c; Hossain et al., 2022b; Muzaffar et al., 2022; Rezvi et al., 2022). Comorbidity between depression and anxiety was seen in up to 47% of students (Mehareen et al., 2022; Nahar et al., 2022).

### *13.2.4 Risk Factors for Common Mental Disorders in Bangladesh*

When examining the correlates of common mental disorders, a striking finding is that certain factors were associated with an increased risk of depression or anxiety disorders regardless of the population being studied or the time frame (pre- or post-COVID pandemic). Some of these factors, such as age, gender, and family history of mental illness, can be considered "fixed" and immutable. However, most risk factors for CMDs in Bangladesh are modifiable at least in principle. These modifiable risk factors can be divided into lifestyle and psychosocial factors. Lifestyle

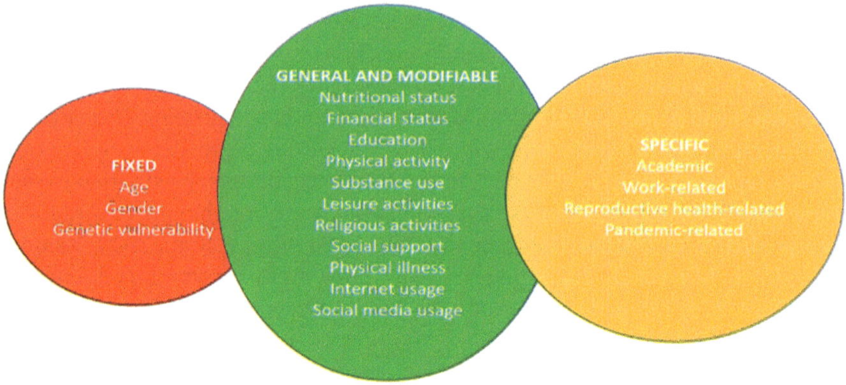


**Fig. 13.2** Risk factors for common mental disorders in Bangladesh

factors associated with CMDs include dietary practices, physical activity, involvement in leisure activities, use of substances such as alcohol, tobacco and sedative-hypnotics, sleep patterns, screen time, and excessive use of the Internet of social media (Bishwajit et al., 2017a, b; Khan et al., 2017; Mridha et al., 2021; Wahid et al., 2023). Psychosocial factors include low educational status, financial difficulties, unemployment, lack of social support, and exposure to chronic stressors (Bishwajit et al., 2017b; Khan & Khan, 2020; Nasreen et al., 2015; Natasha et al., 2015a; Wahid et al., 2023). Apart from these common risk factors, certain variables are specific to the population being studied—for example, pregnancy complications and outcomes in post-partum women, or academic-related stressors in students. These factors are depicted in Fig. 13.2.

A proper understanding of these factors is essential when considering the prevention or treatment of CMDs in the Bangladeshi population. For example, lifestyle factors such as healthy dietary practices, physical activity, and involvement in leisure activities or religious/spiritual activities may be protective in a wide range of settings—in the general population, in adolescents, and in students, for example. Likewise, identification and management of adverse lifestyle factors, such as excessive screen time, unhealthy dietary practices, or the use of alcohol, tobacco, or sedative-hypnotics, may allow individuals in diverse settings to cope better with stress and may reduce the risk of anxiety or depression. At the community level, interventions such as credit-based income generation programs may reduce symptoms of CMDs in people facing economic hardship (Chowdhury and Bhuiya, 2001), while community-based group interventions can address social isolation and a perceived lack of support. On the other hand, when planning or delivering services in a specific setting, such as a college, hospital, or company, an understanding of specific factors is essential, and interventions should be tailored to the realities of each particular situation.

## 13.3 Assessment of CMDs: Psychometric Instruments

When discussing research on CMDs, it is important to distinguish between "depression" and "depressive symptoms," and between "anxiety disorders" and "anxiety symptoms." Depressive and anxiety disorders are diagnosed according to standard diagnostic criteria, usually based on an interview conducted by a mental health professional. On the other hand, "depressive symptoms" and "anxiety symptoms" refer to an individual's scores or responses on a specific rating scale, such as the Patient Health Questionnaire (PHQ-9). Any person who scores above the specified cut-off for a particular tool can be considered to have "symptoms" of CMDs. Not all individuals who screen positive for a CMD actually suffer from the disorder. This was illustrated in the World Mental Health Survey, in which only one-third to one-fifth of those who screened "positive" for depression actually fulfilled the criteria for depressive disorder (Bromet et al., 2011). Similar considerations apply to anxiety disorders. Therefore, when interpreting results such as "72% of a sample had depressive symptoms/screened positive for depression," it is important to recall that the frequency of depression in this sample is actually around 14–24%. This is important when planning and delivering services for CMDs. Wahid et al. (2021) confirmed this in a study of patients from urban slums. Based on latent class analysis of scores on the General Health Questionnaire-12 (GHQ-12), a screening tool for CMDs, they found that individuals fell into three categories: wellness, distress, and severe distress. Some symptoms of depression, such as anhedonia and impaired concentration, were present only in the "severe distress" group. This result suggests that there is a continuum between "CMD symptoms" and "syndromic CMD," with each category requiring a different degree of intervention.

When using screening instruments for CMDs, it is important to ensure that these have been validated for use in the Bangladeshi population. If these instruments are self-rated, they should be translated into Bangla so that they can be easily understood by patients. Several psychometric instruments have been adapted and tested in this manner. For depression, the Patient Health Questionnaire-9 (PHQ-9), Montgomery-Asberg Depression Rating Scale (MADRS), Beck Depression Inventory-II (BDI-II), and World Health Organization-5 Well-Being Index (WHO-5) have been translated and adapted for use in adults in Bangladesh (Soron, 2017; Mostafa Alim et al., 2020; Rahman et al., 2022a). For anxiety, the Generalized Anxiety Disorder 7-item scale (GAD-7) has been validated in young adults (Dhira et al., 2021). For CMDs in general, the Depression, Anxiety, and Stress Scale, 21-item version (DASS-21) has been translated and validated in the local language (Ahmed et al., 2022). Other instruments that have been adapted in this manner include the Edinburgh Postnatal Depression Scale (EPDS) in post-partum women (Gausia et al., 2007), the Geriatric Depression Scale—Short Form for the elderly (Sultana et al., 2022), and the Spence Children's Anxiety Scale and Child and Adolescent Worry Scale for the assessment of anxiety symptoms in children and adolescents (Deeba et al., 2015; Haque, 2022). More recently, researchers from Bangladesh have used machine learning methods to assess depression and suicide risk in students based on self-reported depression rating scores and measures of mobile use (Mahmud et al., 2023; Siraji et al., 2023). This innovative approach may allow patients to report symptoms accurately without fear of stigmatization or cultural taboos.

## 13.4 Phenomenology and Psychopathology

It is also important to understand the way in which culture shapes the phenomenology of depression, influencing local “idioms of distress” and symptom presentations. In an early study, Chowdhury (1979) found that somatic symptoms such as burning pain, gastrointestinal troubles, palpitations, decreased libido, and insomnia were common presentations of depression in Bangladesh. Ideas of guilt and worthlessness were common, but psychomotor retardation was rare. In a qualitative study, Selim (2010) found that the term *bishonnota* (depression) was rarely understood by patients with depression, their caregivers, or members of the general population. When presented with a case vignette of depression, they identified the condition as *chinta rog* (“worry illness”) and placed emphasis on the somatic symptoms experienced in this disorder. Huda et al. (2014) found that a “feeling of fever” without an objective elevation of body temperature was a common presenting symptom of depression or anxiety. Similarly, Qusar et al. (2019) found that depression frequently presented with somatic symptoms such as sensations of heat or burning, headache, body pain, and feelings of “heaviness.” They also noted that in addition to low mood, fear, anger, and suspiciousness were often seen in patients with depression. Wahid et al. (2022) studied idioms of distress in men from urban slums and found that they frequently used terms or metaphors related to the heart, mind, head, body, and mood to describe symptoms of depression or anxiety. The term “tension” was frequently used by these men to denote the above. In women with post-partum depression, Edhborg et al. (2015) found that worry, fear, and guilt (related to inability to adhere to traditional norms regarding childbirth and to care for their child) were common. In men, both depression and anxiety are often associated with concerns regarding semen loss (*dhat* syndrome): in a study of patients with this complaint, 50% had symptoms of anxiety disorder and 39% had features of depression (Maruf et al., 2022).

These results show that CMDs commonly present with somatic symptoms in Bangladesh, and that physicians treating patients with medically unexplained symptoms or concerns regarding sexual functioning should be aware of the possibility of underlying depression or anxiety. Some of these findings also suggest that the boundary between depressive and anxiety symptoms in Bangladesh is “porous,” with many patients experiencing symptoms of both disorders along with somatic symptoms, other negative affects, and significant distress and impairment.

## 13.5 Biomarkers of Common Mental Disorders

In the past two decades, several researchers have examined the physiological and biochemical correlates of depression and anxiety in Bangladesh adults. One of the first studies of this sort found that serum cortisol was elevated in patients with psychiatric disorders in general, indicating dysregulation of the hypothalamic–pituitary–adrenal stress axis (Hossain et al., 2006). Relevant studies in this field are summarized in Table 13.4.

### *13.5.1 Depression*

Depression has been associated with increased peripheral inflammation and oxidative stress in a bidirectional manner. In line with these findings, studies of patients with major depression (MDD) from Bangladesh have found elevated levels of pro-inflammatory cytokines such as interleukin-1 beta (Das et al., 2021a, b), interleukin-3 (Akter et al., 2023), interleukin-8 (Islam et al., 2022a, b), interleukin-10 (Anjum et al.,

**Table 13.4** Biomarkers of common mental disorders identified in patients from Bangladesh

| Disorder | Biomarker | Significance |
|---|---|---|
| Depression | Elevated peripheral IL-1β, IL-3, IL-8, IL-10, MCP-1, TNF-α, resistin<br>Reduced IL-7, lipocalin-2, MCP-4 | Immune-inflammatory dysregulation |
| | Reduced serum BDNF<br>Increased NGF | Altered neural plasticity |
| | Increased IGF-1<br>Reduced adiponectin, relaxin-3 | Impaired glucose and lipid metabolism |
| | Reduced serum Vitamin A, C, D, E<br>Reduced serum methionine, phenylalanine, tryptophan, tyrosine<br>Reduced serum Ca, Mg, Fe, Mn, Se, Zn; increased serum Cu | Vitamin and trace element deficiency |
| | Altered HRV in ECG recordings | Autonomic dysfunction |
| | Increased eveningness | Altered circadian rhythm |
| Anxiety disorder | Increased peripheral IgM (GAD)<br>Reduced peripheral IgG (PD) | Immune-inflammatory dysregulation |
| | Elevated plasma MDA (GAD, PD) | Oxidative stress |
| | Reduced serum Zn (GAD, PD)<br>Reduced serum Cu, Fe, Mn (GAD) | Trace element deficiency |

**Abbreviations**: BDNF, brain-derived neurotrophic factor; ECG, electrocardiogram; HRV, heart rate variability; Ig, immunoglobulin; IGF-1, insulin-like growth factor 1; IL, interleukin; GAD, generalized anxiety disorder; MCP, monocyte chemotactic protein; MDA, malondialdehyde; NGF, nerve growth factor; PD, panic disorder

2020), monocyte chemotactic protein-4 (Nayem et al., 2023), and tumor necrosis factor-alpha (TNF-α) (Das et al., 2021a, b; Nayem et al., 2023). In contrast, levels of monocyte chemotactic protein-1 and interleukin-7 were reduced (Anjum et al., 2020; Proma et al., 2022). Levels of TNF-α were correlated with the severity of MDD (Nayem et al., 2023). In contrast, levels of brain-derived neurotrophic factor (BDNF) were reduced in depression, and BDNF levels were inversely correlated with depressive symptoms, underlining the role of reduced neural plasticity in this disorder (Emon et al., 2020). Levels of nerve growth factor (NGF) were paradoxically elevated in depression, which is unlike studies from other countries (Salsabil et al., 2023; Shi et al., 2020).

Other possible biomarkers of depression identified by researchers from Bangladesh include reduced levels of adiponectin, epidermal growth factor, lipocalin-2, and relaxin-3 (Akter et al., 2023; Ali et al., 2020; Islam et al., 2022a, b; Sohan et al., 2023), and elevated levels of insulin-like growth factor-1 (IGF-1) and resistin (Ali et al., 2020; Rahman et al., 2022a, b). These results highlight the relationship between MDD and impairments in glucose and lipid metabolism. Evidence has also been found for alterations in levels of vitamins and trace elements. These include reduced levels of the amino acids methionine, phenylalanine, tryptophan, and tyrosine (Islam et al., 2020), reduced levels of calcium, magnesium, iron, manganese, selenium, and zinc (Islam et al., 2018), and reduced levels of vitamins A, D, C, and E (Islam et al., 2020; Ria et al., 2022). These findings suggest that nutritional deficiencies may play a role in the pathogenesis of MDD in Bangladesh.

Apart from these biochemical markers, disturbances in physiological parameters have also been observed in Bangladeshi patients with MDD. These include increased eveningness of circadian rhythms (Hasan et al., 2022d), altered heart rate variability on ECG recordings (Jahan et al., 2020), and altered electroencephalographic power spectra (Sakib et al., 2023). In the case of EEG abnormalities, machine learning models were used to distinguish between patients with MDD and controls, and showed good agreement with scores on the PHQ-9. More recently, smartphone tracking of mood and behavior has been used for the digital phenotyping of depression severity (Masud et al., 2020).

### *13.5.2 Anxiety Disorders*

There are relatively fewer studies on biological markers of anxiety disorders in patients from Bangladesh. Evidence of altered trace element levels has been observed in some patient samples, including reduced serum zinc in panic disorder (Nahar et al., 2010), and reduced zinc and increased serum copper, manganese, and iron in generalized anxiety disorder (GAD) (Islam et al., 2013). Two studies found evidence of immune alterations in anxiety disorders: Islam et al. (2014) found elevated levels of immunoglobulin M (IgM) in GAD, while Nahar et al. (2012) found reduced levels of immunoglobulin G (IgG) in panic disorder. Elevated levels of the oxidative stress marker malondialdehyde (MDA) have been seen in both GAD and panic disorder

(Islam et al., 2014; Nahar et al., 2013), and reduced levels of the antioxidant vitamins A and E have been found in panic disorder (Nahar et al., 2013). The available evidence points to a role for trace element alterations, oxidative stress, and altered immune activity in anxiety disorders in patients from Bangladesh, but these results require replication.

## 13.6 Interventional Studies for CMDs in Bangladesh

The management of CMDs involves both pharmacological and psychosocial treatments. As far as pharmacotherapy is concerned, a single study evaluated the role of zinc supplementation of antidepressants in patients with depression; in this study, patients receiving 8 weeks' oral treatment with zinc sulfate along with either sertraline or fluoxetine had a greater reduction in depressive and anxiety symptoms than those who received antidepressant monotherapy (Ghosh et al., 2022). In a study of patients with both diabetes mellitus and depression, treatment with the antidepressant escitalopram was found to improve both depressive symptoms and glycemic control (Israt et al., 2021). These results are notable in light of evidence for reduced serum Zn++ and increased IGF-1 in Bangladeshi patients with depression, as discussed in Sect. 5.1.

There are several studies examining the efficacy of psychosocial interventions or programs in reducing symptoms of CMD in Bangladesh. ASHA, an integrated depression management program that included specific treatments for depression, financial literacy education, and cash transfers, was found to reduce depression and improve hopefulness, self-esteem, and involvement in financial decision-making in women from rural Bangladesh for up to 12 months (Karasz et al., 2015, 2021). This result is similar to that of an earlier study reporting improvement in CMD symptoms after involvement in a micro-credit program (Ahmed & Chowdhury, 2001). Provision of financial assistance in anticipation of floods was associated with reduced depression and suicidal ideation in beneficiaries during the 2017 Bangladesh floods (Gros et al., 2019). These three results suggest that improving patients' socioeconomic conditions is effective in partly alleviating depressive symptoms.

A layperson-led self-management program, involving both physical and mental health components, has been tested in adults from Bangladesh with depression and comorbid medical disorders such as diabetes mellitus, respiratory disorders, cardiovascular disorders, and chronic arthritis. Over a period of four months, this intervention significantly improved depressive symptoms (Griffiths et al., 2005).

A school-based program centered on physical activity has been tested on Bangladeshi adolescents. It was found that those participating in the program experienced a significant reduction in depressive symptoms and greater satisfaction with one's life (Ahmed et al., 2023).

A special education school-based program based on skill-building and counseling by a trained psychologist, administered over 6 months, was implemented for mothers of children with autism spectrum disorder (ASD) who screened positive for depression. This intervention led to a significant improvement in depressive symptoms and quality of life (Naheed et al., 2022a).

Studies of adjunctive music therapy have been conducted in patients with MDD and GAD. In both cases, music therapy based on traditional *ragas* improved cardiac autonomic functioning when compared to pharmacotherapy alone. However, information on whether this treatment improved patients' symptoms was not available (Islam & Ferdousi, 2019; Mallik et al., 2020).

Certain "null" results should also be mentioned. An evaluation of a participatory women's group found that participants had reduced levels of post-partum depressive symptoms compared to controls, but this difference was not statistically significant (Clarke et al., 2014). Similarly, a study of a child-centered nutritional and stimulation program for malnourished children found no significant effect on maternal depressive symptoms (Nahar et al., 2015). These results suggest that to be effective, psychosocial treatments for depression should be patient-centered and target multiple domains of vulnerability to CMDs.

## 13.7 Quality and Quantity of Research on CMDs in Bangladesh

A noteworthy and encouraging trend, meriting discussion in some depth, is the increase in both the quantity and the quality of research into CMDs in Bangladesh. Though it is beyond the scope of this chapter to conduct a complete bibliometric analysis, certain key points are presented below.

Figure 13.3 is an approximate depiction of the quantity of research on depression and anxiety disorders in Bangladesh, based on data obtained from the Scopus database. Three clear phases can be distinguished in this graph. In the first period (1975–2003), the number of annual publications on these topics was less than 10. In the second (2004–2019), a slow but steady upward trend can be discerned, with the annual publication count crossing 25 in 2019. The third phase coincides with the COVID-19 pandemic and its aftermath (2020–). There was a nearly six-fold increase in publications on anxiety and depression in Bangladesh during this period, mostly addressing the mental health impact of COVID-19 in diverse populations. A slight decline was seen in 2023, though the annual number of publications remained high.

The analysis depicts the five indexed journals containing the most publications on depression and anxiety related to Bangladesh. These leading journals were *Heliyon*, *PLoS One*, *BMC Psychiatry*, *BMJ Open*, and the *International Journal of Environmental Research and Public Health*. All these journals are indexed in PubMed, Scopus, and ScienceDirect and are open-access publications which can be easily accessed by readers from low- and middle-income countries. These journals have reasonably high impact factors and citation indices (*Heliyon*: 4.45; *PLoS One*: 3.75; *BMC Psychiatry*: 4.44; *BMJ Open*: 2.97; *IJERPH*: 4.53). It can therefore be

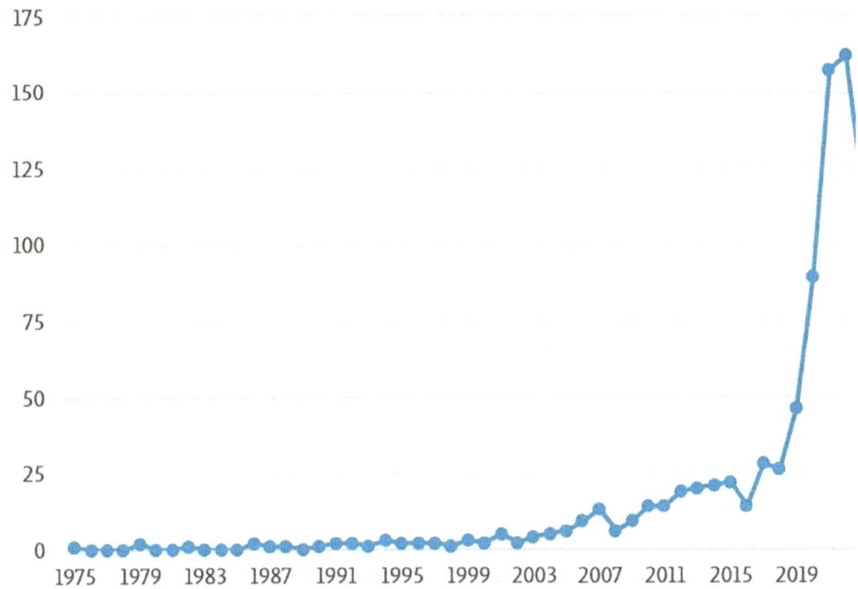


**Fig. 13.3** Research output on common mental disorders in Bangladesh

concluded that research on CMDs in Bangladesh is often published in good quality journals and is in line with the aims of the open-access movement.

While indexing and impact factors are important indicators of publication quality, it should not be forgotten that important research can be published in regional or national journals that have not yet been indexed. Several important studies on the epidemiology, phenomenology, and management of CMDs have been published in journals accessible through the Bangladesh Journals Online database, which is an invaluable resource for researchers.

## 13.8 Summary and Recommendations

The increased availability of research data on the prevalence and determinants of CMDs in Bangladesh is a welcome trend, and represents a significant advance over the earlier research reviewed by Newman (2013) and Hossain et al. (2014). In addition, there are several informative studies on possible biological markers associated with CMDs, trials of pharmacological and psychosocial interventions conducted in naturalistic settings, and explorations of the barriers to effective diagnosis and management of CMDs in Bangladesh. The quality and quantity of this research has increased markedly in the last decade. The existing literature poses challenges to mental health experts and practitioners in Bangladesh in three key domains: research, clinical practice, and public health and policy.

### 13.8.1 Future Directions for Research

How can the existing research into CMDs in Bangladesh be meaningfully extended? In other words, what should the research agenda for CMDs contain over the next decade? Key components of such an agenda could include, but are not limited to:

- Replication of existing findings and results.
- Further research into the prevalence of anxiety disorders, including the comorbidity between these disorders and depression.
- Estimation of the prevalence and determinants of CMDs in certain key populations, such as pre-pubertal children and the elderly.
- Analyses of the bidirectional relationships between CMDs and different groups of medical disorders, including longitudinal studies, exploration of shared biological and psychosocial vulnerabilities, and developing integrated care models for both conditions (Wright et al., 2020).
- Assessing the relationship between CMDs and cognitive impairment or decline in the elderly (Akter et al., 2023).
- Examining the association between environmental factors, such as climate change, soil erosion, flooding and air pollution, and CMDs in the Bangladeshi context (Arobi et al., 2019).
- Strengthening the evidence base on potential protective factors against CMDs in Bangladesh, including social support, cultural and religious beliefs and practices, and dietary patterns.

### 13.8.2 From Research to Clinical Practice

How can the existing research findings be translated into clinical practice? For example, given the high rates of comorbidity between CMDs and NCDs, what steps should clinicians take to screen for and manage depression and anxiety in their patients with conditions such as diabetes mellitus or cardiac disease? How can an effective stepped-care model be developed, so that milder forms of CMD are managed in primary care and more complex presentations handled by mental health specialists? Can treatments that are effective in a research setting be provided in standard clinical contexts in Bangladesh?

Answers to some of these questions can be obtained from the existing literature. For example, patients with diabetes mellitus should be screened and offered pharmacotherapy for depression, as this will improve both their mental health and their glycemic status (Israt et al., 2021). Patients with mild to moderate CMDs who are not responding to pharmacotherapy alone may benefit from lifestyle modifications or nutritional supplements (Ahmed et al., 2023; Ghosh et al., 2022). Patients with NCDs or chronic infectious diseases, such as tuberculosis and HIV, should be screened and offered treatment for depression and anxiety disorders: in some cases, such as ischemic heart disease, this may even improve long-term survival. Treatment packages for CMDs in these patients can be implemented without a high level of expert participation (Griffiths et al., 2005). Likewise, healthcare workers involved in antenatal, postnatal, and early child care should be aware of the frequency and consequences of peripartum depression and its deleterious effects on child health and development (Black et al., 2007, 2009; Khan, 2022; Nasreen et al., 2013). Staff in these settings could be trained in the use of the EPDS and develop an effective liaison model for psychiatric treatment. In summary, it is important that clinicians of all disciplines should be aware of the prevalence of CMDs in the populations they serve, their varied symptom presentations (particularly somatic symptoms), screening methods, treatment options for CMDs at the primary or clinic level, and the indications for referral to a specialist.

### *13.8.3 From Research to Public Health and Policy*

The third and largest challenge involves translating the findings of research on CMDs into actionable policies, plans, and programs in the real-world settings of Bangladesh. Some examples of how this could be done are provided below:

- Data on the prevalence of CMDs in specific regions and settings could be used to guide the allocation of manpower and material resources.
- Replicated results on the risk and protective factors for CMDs in Bangladesh (Fig. 13.2) should be used to develop educational material and locally feasible methods of prevention, early diagnosis, and treatment.
- Information on the distribution of CMDs in specific settings, such as schools, hospitals, and workplaces, can be used to provide basic mental health services in these settings (e.g., counselors in schools) and to provide evidence-based interventions to improve mental health (e.g., physical activity-based programs for school students).
- Information on CMDs in vulnerable populations, such as slum-dwellers or populations affected by natural disasters, can provide a basis for improved coordination between healthcare and social welfare departments. This would provide a firm basis for multidisciplinary interventions to improve both mental health and economic security (e.g., addressing malnutrition in the elderly, or combining psychiatric treatment with financial assistance in disadvantaged populations).
- Evidence on the risk of CMDs following disasters, such as floods or pandemics, could lead to better disaster readiness programs that combine material, psychological, and financial support.

## 13.9 Conclusion

Based on the most recent available data, at least 15–16 million people in Bangladesh suffer from depression or anxiety disorders. A variety of demographic, lifestyle, psychosocial, health-related, and context-specific factors can increase individual vulnerability to CMDs, both in the general population and in high-risk groups. The COVID-19 pandemic has led to a significant increase in symptoms of depression and anxiety in all sections of society. Health professionals in Bangladesh have risen to this challenge by stepping up their investigations into the frequency and correlates of these disorders. This body of evidence provides a multifaceted perspective on common mental disorders in the Bangladeshi context and provides leads toward promising approaches to their prevention and treatment. It is important to ensure that future research on CMDs in Bangladesh receives adequate funding from both the public and private sectors. This would not only improve the prevention, detection, and management of CMDs but also the physical and mental health of families, communities, organizations, and society as a whole.

## References

Abbasy, A. A., Johora, F., Sakin, S. A., Khan, A. A., Nilufar, S., Ferdoush, J., & Salam, A. I. (2022). Prevalence of anxiety and depression among undergraduate medical students in selective medical colleges of Bangladesh. *IAHS Medical Journal, 5*(1), 8–11. https://doi.org/10.3329/iahsmj.v5i1.65693.

Abir, T., Kalimullah, N. A., Osuagwu, U. L., Nur-A Yazdani, D. M., Husain, T., Goson, P. C., Basak, P., Rahman, M. A., Al Mamun, A., Permarupan, P. Y., Khan, M. Y. H., Milton, A. H., & Agho, K. E. (2021). Prevalence and factors associated with mental health impact of COVID-19 pandemic in Bangladesh: A survey-based cross-sectional study. *Annals of Global Health, 87*(1), 43. https://doi.org/10.5334/aogh.3269.

Adams, A. S., Sibeko, G., & Stein, D. J. (2023). Middle-income country perspectives on global mental health. *Current Opinion in Psychiatry, 36*(4), 321–326. https://doi.org/10.1097/YCO.0000000000000877.

Afroze, F., Arafat, S. M., Ahmed, C. M., Alam, B., Banu, S., Islam, M. Z., Mahfuz, M., Parvin, I., Ackhter, M. M., Shormi, I., Islam, F., Sultana, M., Chowdhury, A. N., Ur Rahaman, M. F., Khan, A. H., Hasan, M. N., Ahmed, S., Chisti, M. J., & Ahmed, T. (2023). Features and risk factors of post-COVID-19 syndrome: Findings from a longitudinal study in Bangladesh. *The Lancet Regional Health. Southeast Asia, 11*, 100134. https://doi.org/10.1016/j.lansea.2022.100134.

Ahmed, S. M., & Chowdhury, M. (2001). Micro-credit and emotional well-being: Experience of poor rural women from Matlab, Bangladesh. *World Development, 29*(11), 1957–1966.

Ahmed, O., Faisal, R. A., Alim, S. M. A. H. M., Sharker, T., & Hiramoni, F. A. (2022). The psychometric properties of the depression anxiety stress scale-21 (DASS-21) Bangla version. *Acta Psychologica, 223*, 103509. https://doi.org/10.1016/j.actpsy.2022.103509.

Ahmed, K. R., Horwood, S., & Khan, A. (2023). Effects of a school-based physical activity intervention on adolescents' mental health: A cluster randomized controlled trial. *Journal of Physical Activity & Health, 20*(12), 1102–1108. https://doi.org/10.1123/jpah.2023-0062.

Akter, M. S., Emon, F. A., Nahar, Z., Shalahuddin Qusar, M., Islam, S. M. A., Shahriar, M., Bhuiyan, M. A., & Islam, M. R. (2023). Altered IL-3 and lipocalin-2 levels are associated with the pathophysiology of major depressive disorder: A case-control study. *BMC Psychiatry, 23*(1), 830. https://doi.org/10.1186/s12888-023-05354-y.

Al Adiluzzaman, M.A.-F., Ahmed, S., Islam, M. T., Ferdous, J., Roy, J., Rahim, M. A., Rahman, M. A., & Snigdha, K. S. R. (2016). Prevalence of depression in patients with chronic obstructive pulmonary disease (COPD) attending a tertiary care hospital of Bangladesh. *Chest & Heart Journal, 40*(2), 92–96.

Al Azdi, Z., Islam, K., Chowdhury, A. H., Ahmed, H. U., Alam, R., Hussain, A. H. M. E., & Huque, R. (2020). The magnitude of depression and anxiety during COVID 19: an online survey among adults in Bangladesh. JMIR Preprints, 20576.https://doi.org/10.2196/preprints.20576.

Al Mamun, F., Hosen, I., Misti, J. M., Kaggwa, M. M., & Mamun, M. A. (2021). Mental disorders of bangladeshi students during the COVID-19 pandemic: A systematic review. *Psychology Research and Behavior Management, 14*, 645–654. https://doi.org/10.2147/PRBM.S315961.

Alam, M. M., Ahmed, S., Dipti, R. K., Siddiquee, R., & Hawlader, M. D. H. (2020). The prevalence and associated factors of depression during pre-, peri-, and post-menopausal period among the middle-aged women of Dhaka city. *Asian Journal of Psychiatry, 54*, 102312. https://doi.org/10.1016/j.ajp.2020.102312.

Alam, F., Hossain, R., Ahmed, H. U., Alam, M. T., Sarkar, M., & Halbreich, U. (2021). Stressors and mental health in Bangladesh: Current situation and future hopes. *Bjpsych International, 18*(4), 91–94. https://doi.org/10.1192/bji.2020.57.

Ali, S., Nahar, Z., Rahman, M. R., Islam, S. M. A., Bhuiyan, M. A., & Islam, M. R. (2020). Serum insulin-like growth factor-1 and relaxin-3 are linked with major depressive disorder. *Asian Journal of Psychiatry, 53*, 102164. https://doi.org/10.1016/j.ajp.2020.102164.

Ali, M., Uddin, Z., Ahsan, N. F., Haque, M. Z., Bairagee, M., Khan, S. A., & Hossain, A. (2021). Prevalence of mental health symptoms and its effect on insomnia among healthcare workers who attended hospitals during COVID-19 pandemic: A survey in Dhaka city. *Heliyon, 7*(5), e06985. https://doi.org/10.1016/j.heliyon.2021.e06985.

Anjum, S., Qusar, M. M. A. S., Shahriar, M., Islam, S. M. A., Bhuiyan, M. A., & Islam, M. R. (2020). Altered serum interleukin-7 and interleukin-10 are associated with drug-free major depressive disorder. *Therapeutic Advances in Psychopharmacology, 10*, 2045125320916655. https://doi.org/10.1177/2045125320916655.

Anjum, A., Hossain, S., Hasan, M. T., Christopher, E., Elias Uddin, M., & Tajuddin Sikder, M. (2022a). Stress symptoms and associated factors among adolescents in Dhaka, Bangladesh: Findings from a cross-sectional study. *BMC Psychiatry, 22*, 807. https://doi.org/10.1186/s12888-022-04340-0.

Anjum, A., Hossain, S., Hasan, M. T., Elias Uddin, M., & Tajuddin Sikder, M. (2022b). Anxiety among urban, semi-urban and rural school adolescents in Dhaka, Bangladesh: Investigating prevalence and associated factors. *PLoS ONE, 17*(1), e0262716. https://doi.org/10.1371/journal.pone.0262716.

Arobi, S., Naher, J., & Soron, T. R. (2019). Impact of river bank erosion on mental health and coping capacity in Bangladesh. *Global Psychiatry, 2*(2), 195–200. https://doi.org/10.2478/gp-2019-0011.

Asghar, S., Hussain, A., Ali, S. M. K., Khan, A. K. A., & Magnusson, A. (2007). Prevalence of depression and diabetes: A population-based study from rural Bangladesh. *Diabetic Medicine, 24*, 872–877. https://doi.org/10.1111/j.1464-5491.2007.02136.x.

Azad, R., Fahmi, R., Shrestha, S., Joshi, H., Hasan, M., Khan, A. N. S., Chowdhury, M. A. K., Arifeen, S. E., & Billah, S. M. (2019). Prevalence and risk factors of postpartum depression within one year after birth in urban slums of Dhaka, Bangladesh. *Plos One, 14*(5), e0215735. https://doi.org/10.1371/journal.pone.0215735.

Bangladesh Association of Psychiatrists. (2021). Fact sheets: Bangladesh National Mental Health Survey 2019. https://bapbd.org/factsheet.php.

Berens, A. E., Kumar, S., Tofail, F., Jensen, S. K. G., Alam, M., Haque, R., Kakon, S. H., Petri, W. A., & Nelson, C. A., 3rd. (2019). Cumulative psychosocial risk and early child development:

Validation and use of the childhood psychosocial adversity scale in global health research. *Pediatric Research, 86*(6), 766–775. https://doi.org/10.1038/s41390-019-0431-7.

Bishwajit, G., O'Leary, D. P., Ghosh, S., Yaya, S., Shangfeng, T., & Feng, Z. (2017a). Physical inactivity and self-reported depression among middle- and older-aged population in South Asia: World health survey. *BMC Geriatrics, 17*(1), 100. https://doi.org/10.1186/s12877-017-0489-1.

Bishwajit, G., O'Leary, D. P., Ghosh, S., Sanni, Y., Shangfeng, T., & Zhanchun, F. (2017b). Association between depression and fruit and vegetable consumption among adults in South Asia. *BMC Psychiatry, 17*(1), 15. https://doi.org/10.1186/s12888-017-1198-1.

Black, M. M., Baqui, A. H., Zaman, K., McNary, S. W., Le, K., Arifeen, S. E., Hamadani, J. D., Parveen, M., Yunus, M., & Black, R. E. (2007). Depressive symptoms among rural Bangladeshi mothers: Implications for infant development. *Journal of Child Psychology and Psychiatry, and Allied Disciplines, 48*(8), 764–772. https://doi.org/10.1111/j.1469-7610.2007.01752.x.

Black, M. M., Baqui, A. H., Zaman, K., El Arifeen, S., & Black, R. E. (2009). Maternal depressive symptoms and infant growth in rural Bangladesh. *The American Journal of Clinical Nutrition, 89*(3), 951S-957S. https://doi.org/10.3945/ajcn.2008.26692E.

Bromet, E., Andrade, L. H., Hwang, I., Sampson, N. A., Alonso, J., de Girolamo, G., de Graaf, R., Demyttenaere, K., Hu, C., Iwata, N., Karam, A. N., Kaur, J., Kostyuchenko, S., Lépine, J. P., Levinson, D., Matschinger, H., Mora, M. E., Browne, M. O., Posada-Villa, J., Viana, M. C., … Kessler, R. C. (2011). Crossnational epidemiology of DSM-IV major depressive episode. *BMC Medicine, 9,* 90. https://doi.org/10.1186/1741-7015-9-90

Chomon, R. J. (2022). Depression and suicidal ideation among medical students in a private medical college of Bangladesh. A cross sectional web based survey. *PloS one, 17*(4), e0265367. https://doi.org/10.1371/journal.pone.0265367.

Chowdhury, A. K. (1979). Symptomatology of depressive disorders in Bangladesh. *Bangladesh Medical Research Council Bulletin, 5*(2), 47–59.

Chowdhury, S. R., Sunna, T. C., Das, D. C., Kabir, H., Hossain, A., Mahmud, S., & Ahmed, S. (2021). Mental health symptoms among the nurses of Bangladesh during the COVID-19 pandemic. *Middle East Current Psychiatry, 28*(1), 1–8. https://doi.org/10.1186/s43045-021-00103-x.

Chowdhury, A. K., Alam, M. N., & Ali, S. M. (1981). Dasherkandi project studies. Demography, morbidity and mortality in a rural community of Bangladesh. *Bangladesh Medical Research Council Bulletin, 7*(1), 22–39.

Clarke, K., Azad, K., Kuddus, A., Shaha, S., Nahar, T., Aumon, B. H., Hossen, M. M., Beard, J., Costello, A., Houweling, T. A., Prost, A., & Fottrell, E. (2014). Impact of a participatory intervention with women's groups on psychological distress among mothers in rural Bangladesh: Secondary analysis of a cluster-randomised controlled trial. *PLoS ONE, 9*(10), e110697. https://doi.org/10.1371/journal.pone.0110697.

Dai, Y., Zhang, B., Sun, H., Li, Z., Shen, L., & Liu, Y. (2015). Prevalence and correlates of psychological symptoms in Chinese doctors as measured with the SCL-90-R: A meta-analysis. *Research in Nursing & Health, 38*(5), 369–383. https://doi.org/10.1002/nur.21673.

Das, R., Hasan, M. R., Daria, S., & Islam, M. R. (2021a). Impact of COVID-19 pandemic on mental health among general Bangladeshi population: A cross-sectional study. *British Medical Journal Open, 11*(4), e045727. https://doi.org/10.1136/bmjopen-2020-045727.

Das, R., Emon, M. P. Z., Shahriar, M., Nahar, Z., Islam, S. M. A., Bhuiyan, M. A., Islam, S. N., & Islam, M. R. (2021b). Higher levels of serum IL-1β and TNF-α are associated with an increased probability of major depressive disorder. *Psychiatry Research, 295,* 113568. https://doi.org/10.1016/j.psychres.2020.113568.

Deeba, F., Rapee, R. M., & Prvan, T. (2015). Psychometric properties of two measures of childhood internalizing problems in a Bangladeshi sample. *The British Journal of Clinical Psychology, 54*(2), 214–232. https://doi.org/10.1111/bjc.12071.

Dhira, T. A., Rahman, M. A., Sarker, A. R., & Mehareen, J. (2021). Validity and reliability of the Generalized Anxiety Disorder-7 (GAD-7) among university students of Bangladesh. *PLoS ONE, 16*(12), e0261590. https://doi.org/10.1371/journal.pone.0261590.

Disu, T. R., Anne, N. J., Griffiths, M. D., & Mamun, M. A. (2019). Risk factors of geriatric depression among elderly Bangladeshi people: A pilot interview study. *Asian Journal of Psychiatry, 44*, 163–169. https://doi.org/10.1016/j.ajp.2019.07.050.

Edhborg, M., Nasreen, H. E., & Kabir, Z. N. (2015). I can't stop worrying about everything—experiences of rural Bangladeshi women during the first postpartum months. *International Journal of Qualitative Studies on Health and Well-Being, 10*, 26226. https://doi.org/10.3402/qhw.v10.26226.

Emon, M. P. Z., Das, R., Nishuty, N. L., Qusar, M. M. A. S., Bhuiyan, M. A., & Islam, M. R. (2020). Reduced serum BDNF levels are associated with the increased risk for developing MDD: A case-control study with or without antidepressant therapy. *BMC Research Notes, 13*, 83. https://doi.org/10.1186/s13104-020-04952-3.

Esie, P., Osypuk, T. L., Schuler, S. R., & Bates, L. M. (2019). Intimate partner violence and depression in rural Bangladesh: Accounting for violence severity in a high prevalence setting. *SSM–Population Health, 7*, 100368. https://doi.org/10.1016/j.ssmph.2019.100368.

Faruk, M. O., Alam, F., Chowdhury, K. U. A., & Soron, T. R. (2021). Validation of the Bangla WHO-5 Well-being Index. *Global Mental Health, 8*, e26. https://doi.org/10.1017/gmh.2021.26.

Faruk, M. O., Mamun, M. A., Siddique, A. B., & Griffiths, M. D. (2023). Risk factors for depression and anxiety disorders among Bangladeshi dental students: A cross-sectional survey study. *International Journal of Mental Health and Addiction, 21*, 1501–1514. https://doi.org/10.1007/s11469-021-00603-1.

Fernandes, M. D. S. V., Mendonça, C. R., da Silva, T. M. V., Noll, P. R. E. S., de Abreu, L. C., & Noll, M. (2023). Relationship between depression and quality of life among students: A systematic review and meta-analysis. *Scientific Reports, 13*(1), 6715. https://doi.org/10.1038/s41598-023-33584-3.

Gausia, K., Hamadani, J. D., Islam, M. M., Ali, M., Algin, S., Yunus, M., Fisher, C., & Oosthuizen, J. (2007). Bangla translation, adaptation and piloting of Edinburgh Postnatal Depression Scale. *Bangladesh Medical Research Council Bulletin, 33*(3), 81–87. https://doi.org/10.3329/bmrcb.v33i3.1138.

Gausia, K., Fisher, C., Ali, M., & Oosthuizen, J. (2009). Antenatal depression and suicidal ideation among rural Bangladeshi women: A community-based study. *Archives of Women's Mental Health, 12*(5), 351–358. https://doi.org/10.1007/s00737-009-0080-7.

GBD 2019 Mental Disorders Collaborators. (2022). Global, regional, and national burden of 12 mental disorders in 204 countries and territories, 1990–2019: A systematic analysis for the Global Burden of Disease Study 2019. *The Lancet. Psychiatry, 9*(2), 137–150.https://doi.org/10.1016/S2215-0366(21)00395-3.

Ghosh, S., Ghosh, U. K., Ghosh, M., Rahman, A. K. M. S., & Dewan, Z. F. (2022). Effect of zinc supplementation on depression in selective serotonin reuptake inhibitors-treated major depressive disorder patients. *KYAMC Journal, 13*(1), 18–23. https://doi.org/10.3329/kyamcj.v13i1.59876.

Griffiths, C., Motlib, J., Azad, A., Ramsay, J., Eldridge, S., Feder, G., Khanam, R., Munni, R., Garrett, M., Turner, A., & Barlow, J. (2005). Randomised controlled trial of a lay-led self-management programme for Bangladeshi patients with chronic disease. *The British Journal of General Practice, 55*(520), 831–837.

Gros, C., Bailey, M., Schwager, S., Hassan, A., Zingg, R., Uddin, Mamtaz Uddin, M., Shahjahan, M., Islam, H., Lux, S., Jaime, C., & de Perez, E. C. (2019). Household-level effects of providing forecast-based cash in anticipation of extreme weather events: quasi-experimental evidence from humanitarian interventions in the 2017 floods in Bangladesh. *International Journal of Disaster Risk Reduction, 41*, 101275. https://doi.org/10.1016/j.ijdrr.2019.101275.

Haque, M. (2022). Adaptation of child and adolescent worry scale (CAWS) in Bangla. *Dhaka University Journal of Biological Science, 30*(3), 417–427. https://doi.org/10.3329/dujbs.v30i3.59034.

Haque, M. R., Islam, T., Milton, A. H., & Abir, T. (2022). Mental health status of a population during COVID-19 pandemic in Bangladesh: A cross-sectional study. *Bangladesh Medical Research Council Bulletin, 48*(3), 195–202. https://doi.org/10.3329/bmrcb.v48i3.63811.

Haque, M. A., Anjum, A., Mousum, S., Salwa, M., Ratan, Z. A., Khan, M. M. H., ... & Mamun, M. A. A. (2023). Prevalence of and factors associated with depression, anxiety and stress among adolescents in Bangladesh during the COVID-19 pandemic: A population-based study. *F1000Research, 12*, 730. https://doi.org/10.12688/f1000research.132304.1.

Hasan, M. J., Tabssum, T., Ambia, N. E., Zaman, M. S., Rahman, M., & Khan, A. S. (2021). Mental health of the COVID-19 patients in Bangladesh. *Mymensingh Medical Journal, 30*(1), 189–195.

Hasan, M., Sultana, S., Sohan, M., Parvin, S., Rahman, M. A., Hossain, M. J., Rahman, M. S., & Islam, M. R. (2022a). Prevalence and associated risk factors for mental health problems among patients with polycystic ovary syndrome in Bangladesh: A nationwide cross-Sectional study. *PLoS ONE, 17*(6), e0270102. https://doi.org/10.1371/journal.pone.0270102.

Hasan, M. T., Hossain, S., Gupta, R. D., Podder, V., Mowri, N. A., Ghosh, A., Mahmood, H. R., Ahmmed, F., Khatun, M. S. T. H., Nodi, R. N., Koly, K. N., Yasmeen, S., & Islam, N. (2022b). Depression, sleeping pattern, and suicidal ideation among medical students in Bangladesh: A cross-sectional pilot study. *Journal of Public Health: From Theory to Practice, 30*, 465–473. https://doi.org/10.1007/s10389-020-01304-0.

Hasan, M. T., Anjum, A., Biswas, M. A. A. J., Hossain, S., Alin, S. I., Koly, K. N., Safa, F., Alam, S. F., Rafi, M. A., Podder, V., Hossain, M. M., Trisa, T. I., Azad, D. T., Nodi, R. N., Ashraf, F., Akther, S. M. Q., Ahmed, H. U., & McNaney, R. (2022c). A survey on depressive symptoms and its correlates amongst physicians in Bangladesh during the COVID-19 pandemic. *Frontiers in Psychology, 13*, 846889. https://doi.org/10.3389/fpsyg.2022.846889.

Hasan, M. M., Díaz-Morales, J. F., & Khan, M. H. A. (2022d). Sex differences in the relationship between morningness-eveningness components, mood and well-being among Bangladeshi university students. *Chronobiology International, 39*(5), 725–734. https://doi.org/10.1080/07420528.2022.2032126.

Hasan, M. J., Khan, M. A. S., Rahman, M., Islam, M. S., Debnath, S., & Amin, P. D. M. R. (2020). Sociodemographic profile, clinical characteristics, anxiety, and depression of 74 patients infected with COVID-19: First report from Bangladesh. *Research Square* (preprint). https://doi.org/10.21203/rs.3.rs-32517/v1.

Hayee, M. A., Akhtar, N., Haque, A., & Rabbani, M. G. (2001). Depression after stroke-analysis of 297 stroke patients. *Bangladesh Medical Research Council Bulletin, 27*(3), 96–102.

Hemmati, F., Sarokhani, M., Abdan, Z., Sarokhani, D., Dehkordi, A. H., & Fakhri, M. (2021). The prevalence of depression, anxiety and stress in nurses working in Iranian hospitals: A systematic review and meta-analysis. *Przeglad Epidemiologiczny, 75*(2), 254–262. https://doi.org/10.32394/pe.75.24.

Hosain, G. M., Chatterjee, N., Ara, N., & Islam, T. (2007). Prevalence, pattern and determinants of mental disorders in rural Bangladesh. *Public Health, 121*(1), 18–24. https://doi.org/10.1016/j.puhe.2006.06.018.

Hosen, I., Al-Mamun, F., & Mamun, M. A. (2021). Prevalence and risk factors of the symptoms of depression, anxiety, and stress during the COVID-19 pandemic in Bangladesh: A systematic review and meta-analysis. *Global Mental Health, 8*, e47. https://doi.org/10.1017/gmh.2021.49.

Hossain, M. Z., Latif, S. A., & Khalil, M. (2006). Effects of stresses on serum cortisol level in Bangladeshi people. *Mymensingh Medical Journal, 15*(1), 45–48. https://doi.org/10.3329/mmj.v15i1.16.

Hossain, M. D., Ahmed, H. U., Chowdhury, W. A., Niessen, L. W., & Alam, D. S. (2014). Mental disorders in Bangladesh: A systematic review. *BMC Psychiatry, 14*, 216. https://doi.org/10.1186/s12888-014-0216-9.

Hossain, S., Anjum, A., Uddin, M. E., Rahman, M. A., & Hossain, M. F. (2019). Impacts of socio-cultural environment and lifestyle factors on the psychological health of university students in Bangladesh: A longitudinal study. *Journal of Affective Disorders, 256*, 393–403. https://doi.org/10.1016/j.jad.2019.06.001.

Hossain, S. J., Roy, B. R., Hossain, A. T., Mehrin, F., Tipu, S. M. M. U., Tofail, F., Arifeen, S. E., Tran, T., Fisher, J., & Hamadani, J. (2020). Prevalence of maternal postpartum depression, health-seeking behavior and out of pocket payment for physical illness and cost coping mechanism of the poor families in Bangladesh: A rural community-based study. *International Journal of Environmental Research and Public Health, 17*(13), 4727. https://doi.org/10.3390/ijerph17134727.

Hossain, M. M., Rahman, M., Trisha, N. F., Tasnim, S., Nuzhath, T., Hasan, N. T., Clark, H., Das, A., McKyer, E. L. J., Ahmed, H. U., & Ma, P. (2021a). Prevalence of anxiety and depression in South Asia during COVID-19: A systematic review and meta-analysis. *Heliyon, 7*(4), e06677. https://doi.org/10.1016/j.heliyon.2021.e06677.

Hossain, M. R., Patwary, M. M., Sultana, R., & Browning, M. H. E. M. (2021b). Psychological distress among healthcare professionals during the early stages of the COVID-19 outbreak in low resource settings: A cross-sectional study in Bangladesh. *Frontiers in Public Health, 9*, 701920. https://doi.org/10.3389/fpubh.2021.701920.

Hossain, M. M., Alam, M. A., & Masum, M. H. (2022a). Prevalence of anxiety, depression, and stress among students of Jahangirnagar University in Bangladesh. *Health Science Reports, 5*(2), e559. https://doi.org/10.1002/hsr2.559.

Hossain, M. J., Ahmmed, F., Khandokar, L., Rahman, S. M. A., Hridoy, A., & Ripa, F. A. (2022b). Status of psychological health of students following the extended university closure in Bangladesh: Results from a web-based cross-sectional study. *PLoS Global Public Health, 2*(3), e0000315. https://doi.org/10.1371/journal.pgph.0000315.

Huda, N., Siddiqui, M. N. A., Haque, M. Z., Hoque, M. A., Khan, M. M. R., Rahman, M. K., Islam, M. R., Hussain, A. A., & Haque, J. (2014). Feeling of fever is a feature of psychiatric illness in our patients. *TAJ: Journal of Teachers' Association, 27*(1), 1–3.

Huque, R., Elsey, H., Fieroze, F., Hicks, J. P., Huque, S., Bhawmik, P., Walker, I., & Newell, J. (2020). "Death is a better option than being treated like this": A prevalence survey and qualitative study of depression among multi-drug resistant tuberculosis in-patients. *BMC Public Health, 20*, 848. https://doi.org/10.1186/s12889-020-08986-x.

Insan, N., Weke, A., Forrest, S., & Rankin, J. (2022). Social determinants of antenatal depression and anxiety among women in South Asia: A systematic review & meta-analysis. *PLoS ONE, 17*(2), e0263760. https://doi.org/10.1371/journal.pone.0263760.

Insan, N., Forrest, S., Jaigirdar, A., Islam, R., & Rankin, J. (2023). Social determinants and prevalence of antenatal depression among women in rural Bangladesh: A cross-sectional study. *International Journal of Environmental Research and Public Health, 20*, 2364. https://doi.org/10.3390/ijerph20032364.

Islam, M. R., Ahmed, M. U., Mitu, S. A., Islam, M. S., Rahman, G. K., Qusar, M. M., & Hasnat, A. (2013). Comparative analysis of serum zinc, copper, manganese, iron, calcium, and magnesium level and complexity of interelement relations in generalized anxiety disorder patients. *Biological Trace Element Research, 154*(1), 21–27. https://doi.org/10.1007/s12011-013-9723-7

Islam, S. R., & Ferdousi, S. (2019). Music therapy on non linear assessment of cardiac autonomic function in patients with major depressive disorder. *Journal of the Bangladesh Society of Physiologists, 14*(1), 7–13. https://doi.org/10.3329/jbsp.v14i1.41995.

Islam, M. M., Ali, M., Ferroni, P., Underwood, P., & Alam, M. F. (2003). Prevalence of psychiatric disorders in an urban community in Bangladesh. *General Hospital Psychiatry, 25*(5), 353–357. https://doi.org/10.1016/s0163-8343(03)00067-7.

Islam, M. R., Ahmed, M. U., Islam, M. S., Sayeed, M. S., Sadia, F., Chowdhury, Z. S., Nahar, Z., & Hasnat, A. (2014). Comparative analysis of serum malondialdehyde, antioxidant vitamins and immunoglobulin levels in patients suffering from generalized anxiety disorder. *Drug Research, 64*(8), 406–411. https://doi.org/10.1055/s-0033-1358758.

Islam, S. M. S., Ferrari, U., Seissler, J., Niessen, L., & Lechner, A. (2015a). Association between depression and diabetes among adults in Bangladesh: Hospital-based case-control study. *Journal of Global Health, 5*(2), 020406. https://doi.org/10.7189/jogh.05.020406.

Islam, M. A., Rahman, A., Aleem, M. A., & Islam, S. M. S. (2015b). Prevalence and associated factors of depression among post-stroke patients in Bangladesh. *International Journal of Mental Health and Addiction, 14*, 154–166. https://doi.org/10.1007/s11469-015-9582-x.

Islam, M. J., Broidy, L., Baird, K., & Mazerolle, P. (2017). Intimate partner violence around the time of pregnancy and postpartum depression: The experience of women of Bangladesh. *PLoS ONE, 12*(5), e0176211. https://doi.org/10.1371/journal.pone.0176211.

Islam, M. R., Islam, M. R., Shalahuddin Qusar, M. M. A., Islam, M. S., Kabir, M. H., Mustafizur Rahman, G. K. M., Islam, M. S., & Hasnat, A. (2018). Alterations of serum macro-minerals and trace elements are associated with major depressive disorder: A case-control study. *BMC Psychiatry, 18*(1), 94. https://doi.org/10.1186/s12888-018-1685-z.

Islam, M. R., Ali, S., Karmoker, J. R., Kadir, M. F., Ahmed, M. U., Nahar, Z., Islam, S. M. A., Islam, M. S., Hasnat, A., & Islam, M. S. (2020). Evaluation of serum amino acids and non-enzymatic antioxidants in drug-naïve first-episode major depressive disorder. *BMC Psychiatry, 20*(1), 333. https://doi.org/10.1186/s12888-020-02738-2.

Islam, M. S., Rahman, M. E., Moonajilin, M. S., & van Os, J. (2021). Prevalence of depression, anxiety and associated factors among school going adolescents in Bangladesh: Findings from a cross-sectional study. *PLoS ONE, 16*(4), e0247898. https://doi.org/10.1371/journal.pone.0247898.

Islam, M. N., Dasgupta, D. P., Sultana, N., Yesmine, F., Asaduzzaman, M., Rabeya, M. R., & Ahmed, K. (2022a). Factors associated with depression and determining dimensions of job satisfaction among physicians in Bangladesh. *Heliyon, 8*, e10589. https://doi.org/10.1016/j.heliyon.2022.e10589.

Islam, S., Islam, T., Nahar, Z., Shahriar, M., Islam, S. M. A., Bhuiyan, M. A., & Islam, M. R. (2022b). Altered serum adiponectin and interleukin-8 levels are associated in the pathophysiology of major depressive disorder: A case-control study. *PLoS ONE, 17*(11), e0276619. https://doi.org/10.1371/journal.pone.0276619.

Israt, U. H., Iqbal, M. J. U., Rowshan, M. M., Sultana, S., Ahmed, S., Sultana, N., & Badrudozza, A. S. M. (2021). Efficacy of escitalopram (SSRI) for better glycemic control in the diabetic depressive patients. *Sir Salimullah Medical College Journal, 29*, 100–104.

Izutsu, T., Tsutsumi, A., Islam, A. M., Kato, S., Wakai, S., & Kurita, H. (2006). Mental health, quality of life, and nutritional status of adolescents in Dhaka, Bangladesh: Comparison between an urban slum and a non-slum area. *Social Science & Medicine, 63*(6), 1477–1488. https://doi.org/10.1016/j.socscimed.2006.04.013.

Jahan, C. R., Uddin, M. M., Uddin, M. S., Chowdhury, M. U. H., Wajeunnesa, & Naher, M. Q. (2020). Parasympathetic nerve function status in major depressive disorder patients and its correlation with duration of disease. *Medicine Today, 32*(2), 76–80.https://doi.org/10.3329/medtoday.v32i2.48817.

Kabir, R., Bai, A. C. M., Syed, H. Z., Hasan, M. R., Vinnakota, D., Kar, S. K., Singh, R., Sathian, B., & Arafat, S. M. Y. (2023). The effect of COVID-19 on the mental health of the people in the Indian subcontinent: A scoping review. *Nepal Journal of Epidemiology, 13*(2), 1268–1284. https://doi.org/10.3126/nje.v13i2.52766.

Kamrul-Hasan, A. B. M., Hannan, M. A., Asaduzzaman, M., Rahman, M. M., Alam, M. S., Amin, M. N., Kabir, M. R., Chanda, P. K., Jannat, N., Haque, M. Z., Banik, S. R., Hasan, M. J., & Selim, S. (2022). Prevalence and predictors of diabetes distress among adults with type 2 diabetes mellitus: A facility-based cross-sectional study of Bangladesh. *BMC Endocrine Disorders, 22*, 28. https://doi.org/10.1186/s12902-022-00938-3.

Kamruzzaman, M., Hossain, A., Islam, M. A., Ahmed, M. S., & Kabir, E. (2022). Prevalence of depression, anxiety, stress, and their associated factors among university students in Bangladesh. *ResearchSquare* (preprint). https://doi.org/10.21203/rs.3.rs-1530510/v1.

Karasz, A., Raghavan, S., Patel, V., Zaman, M., Akhter, L., & Kabita, M. (2015). ASHA: Using participatory methods to develop an asset-building mental health intervention for bangladeshi immigrant women. *Progress in Community Health Partnerships: Research, Education, and Action, 9*(4), 501–512. https://doi.org/10.1353/cpr.2015.0080.

Karasz, A., Anne, S., Hamadani, J. D., & Tofail, F. (2021). The ASHA (Hope) project: Testing an integrated depression treatment and economic strengthening intervention in rural Bangladesh: A pilot randomized controlled trial. *International Journal of Environmental Research and Public Health, 18*(1), 279. https://doi.org/10.3390/ijerph18010279.

Khan, A. M. (2022). Maternal mental health and child nutritional status in an urban slum in Bangladesh: A cross-sectional study. *PLoS Global Public Health, 2*(10), e0000871. https://doi.org/10.1371/journal.pgph.0000871.

Khan, M. M. A., & Khan, M. N. (2020). Effects of psychosocial and socio-environmental factors on anxiety disorder among adolescents in Bangladesh. *Brain and Behavior, 10*, e01899. https://doi.org/10.1002/brb3.1899.

Khan, A., Ahmed, R., & Burton, W. (2017). Prevalence and correlates of depressive symptoms in secondary school children in Dhaka city, Bangladesh. *Ethnicity & Health, 25*(1), 34–46. https://doi.org/10.1080/13557858.2017.1398313.

Khatun, M. F., Parvin, M. F., Rashid, M. M., Alam, M. S., Kamrunnahar, M., Talukder, A., Rahman Razu, S., Ward, P. R., & Ali, M. (2021). Mental health of physicians during COVID-19 outbreak in Bangladesh: A web-based cross-sectional survey. *Frontiers in Public Health, 9*, 592058. https://doi.org/10.3389/fpubh.2021.592058.

Koly, K. N., Sultana, S., Iqbal, A., Dunn, J. A., Ryan, G., & Chowdhury, A. B. (2021). Prevalence of depression and its correlates among public university students of Bangladesh. *Journal of Affective Disorders, 282*, 689–694. https://doi.org/10.1016/j.jad.2020.12.137.

Koly, K. N., Christopher, E., Ahmed, S., Baskin, C., Saba, J., Islam, M. S., Tariq, M. R., Alam, S. F., Sultana, M. S., Mushtaq, M., & Ahmed, H. U. (2022). Mental health training needs of physicians in Bangladesh: Views from stakeholders. *SSM–Mental Health, 2*, 100107. https://doi.org/10.1016/j.ssmmh.2022.100107.

Koly, K. N., Saba, J., Billah, M. A., McGirr, A., Sarker, T., Haque, M., Mustary, E., Hanifi, S. M. M. A., & Begum, F. (2023). Depressive symptoms and anxiety among women with a history of abortion living in urban slums of Bangladesh. *BMC Psychology, 11*(1), 197. https://doi.org/10.1186/s40359-023-01224-0

Kundu, S., Bakchi, J., Al Banna, M. H., Sayeed, A., Hasan, M. T., Abid, M. T., Ghosh, S., Sarker, N., & Islam Khan, M. S. (2021). Depressive symptoms associated with loneliness and physical activities among graduate university students in Bangladesh: Findings from a cross-sectional pilot study. *Heliyon, 7*(3), e06401. https://doi.org/10.1016/j.heliyon.2021.e06401.

Linzer, M., Spitzer, R., Kroenke, K., Williams, J. B., Hahn, S., Brody, D., & deGruy, F. (1996). Gender, quality of life, and mental disorders in primary care: Results from the PRIME-MD 1000 study. *The American Journal of Medicine, 101*(5), 526–533. https://doi.org/10.1016/s0002-9343(96)00275-6.

Lloyd, C. E., Nouwen, A., Sartorius, N., Ahmed, H. U., Alvarez, A., Bahendeka, S., Basangwa, D., Bobrov, A. E., Boden, S., Bulgari, V., Burti, L., Chaturvedi, S. K., Cimino, L. C., Gaebel, W., de Girolamo, G., Gondek, T. M., de Braude, M. G., Guntupalli, A., Heinze, M. G., … Xin, Y. (2018). Prevalence and correlates of depressive disorders in people with Type 2 diabetes: Results from the international prevalence and treatment of diabetes and depression (INTERPRET-DD) study, a collaborative study carried out in 14 countries. *Diabetic Medicine, 35*(6), 760–769. https://doi.org/10.1111/dme.13611.

Iorfino, F., Hickie, I. B., Lee, R. S., Lagopoulos, J., & Hermens, D. F. (2016). The underlying neurobiology of key functional domains in young people with mood and anxiety disorders: A systematic review. *BMC psychiatry, 16*, 156. https://doi.org/10.1186/s12888-016-0852-3

Mahmud, S., Mohsin, M., Muyeed, A., Nazneen, S., Abu Sayed, M., Murshed, N., Tonmon, T. T., & Islam, A. (2023). Machine learning approaches for predicting suicidal behaviors among university students in Bangladesh during the COVID-19 pandemic: A cross-sectional study. *Medicine, 102*(28), e34285. https://doi.org/10.1097/MD.0000000000034285.

Mallik, C. I., & Radwan, R. B. (2020). Adolescent victims of cyberbullying in Bangladesh–prevalence and relationship with psychiatric disorders. *Asian Journal of Psychiatry, 48*, 101893. https://doi.org/10.1016/j.ajp.2019.101893.

Mallik, C. I., & Radwan, R. B. (2021). Impact of lockdown due to COVID-19 pandemic in changes of prevalence of predictive psychiatric disorders among children and adolescents in Bangladesh. *Asian Journal of Psychiatry, 56*, 102554. https://doi.org/10.1016/j.ajp.2021.102554.

Mallik, B., Ferdousi, S., & Sultana, S. (2020). Effect of music therapy on heart rate variability in generalized anxiety disorder: A poincare analysis. *Journal of the Bangladesh Society of Physiologists, 15*(1), 39–45. https://doi.org/10.3329/jbsp.v15i1.48113.

Mamun, M. A., Sakib, N., Gozal, D., Bhuiyan, A. I., Hossain, S., Bodrud-Doza, M., Al Mamun, F., Hosen, I., Safiq, M. B., Abdullah, A. H., Sarker, M. A., Rayhan, I., Sikder, M. T., Muhit, M., Lin, C. Y., Griffiths, M. D., & Pakpour, A. H. (2021). The COVID-19 pandemic and serious psychological consequences in Bangladesh: A population-based nationwide study. *Journal of Affective Disorders, 279*, 462–472. https://doi.org/10.1016/j.jad.2020.10.036.

Mamun, M. A., Hossain, M. S., & Griffiths, M. D. (2022b). Mental health problems and associated predictors among Bangladeshi students. *International Journal of Mental Health and Addiction, 20*, 657–671. https://doi.org/10.1007/s11469-019-00144-8.

Mamun, G. M. S., Hassan. M. Z., Khatun, A., Kabir, M. F., Shaima, S. N., Afrin, S., & Seoty, N. R. (2022a). Prevalence and associated factors of depression among junior healthcare professionals of public teaching hospitals of Bangladesh: an analytical cross-sectional study. *medRxiv*, 2022–10. https://doi.org/10.1101/2022.10.23.22281426.

Mandal, M. C., Mullick, S. I., Nahar, J. S., Khanum, M., Lahiry, S., & Islam, M. A. (2007). Prevalence of psychiatric ailments among patients with sexually transmitted disease. *Mymensingh Medical Journal, 16*(2 Suppl.), S23–S27.

Maruf, M. M., Khan, M. Z. R., Jahan, N., Ahmed, A. U., Sadiq, M. S., & Ferdush, R. (2022). Sociodemographic profile and co-morbid symptoms among individuals with semen loss. *Bangladesh Journal of Medicine, 33*, 64–69. https://doi.org/10.3329/bjm.v33i1.56792.

Masud, M. T., Mamun, M. A., Thapa, K., Lee, D. H., Griffiths, M. D., & Yang, S. H. (2020). Unobtrusive monitoring of behavior and movement patterns to detect clinical depression severity level via smartphone. *Journal of Biomedical Informatics, 103*, 103371. https://doi.org/10.1016/j.jbi.2019.103371.

Mehareen, J., Rahman, M. A., Dhira, T. A., & Sarker, A. R. (2022). Prevalence and sociodemographic correlates of depression, anxiety, and co-morbidity during COVID-19: A cross-sectional study among public and private university students of Bangladesh. *Journal of Affective Disorders Reports, 5*, 100179. https://doi.org/10.1016/j.jadr.2021.100179.

Mina, F. B., Billah, M., Karmakar, S., Das, S., Rahman, M. S., Hasan, M. F., & Acharjee, U. K. (2023). An online observational study assessing clinical characteristics and impacts of the COVID-19 pandemic on mental health: A perspective study from Bangladesh. *Journal of Public Health, 31*(2), 319–327. https://doi.org/10.1007/s10389-020-01445-2.

Mistry, S. K., Ali, A. R. M. M., Hossain, M. B., Yadav, U. N., Ghimire, S., Rahman, M. A., Ifran, N. M., & Huque, R. (2021). Exploring depressive symptoms and its associates among Bangladeshi older adults amid COVID-19 pandemic: Findings from a cross-sectional study. *Social Psychiatry and Psychiatric Epidemiology, 56*, 1487–1497. https://doi.org/10.1007/s00127-021-02052-6.

Mostafa Alim, S. M. A. H., Ahmed, M. N., Mullick, M. S. I., Chowdhury, N. F., Akhter, F., & Alam, M. S. (2020). Validation of the Bangla version of beck depression inventory-II. *Brain and Behavior, 10*(3), e01563. https://doi.org/10.1002/brb3.1563.

Mridha, M. K., Hossain, M. M., Khan, M. S. A., Hanif, A. A. M., Hasan, M., Mitra, D., Hossaine, M., Aman Ullah, M., Sarker, S. K., Rahman, S. M. M., Islam Bulbul, M. M., & Shamim, A. A. (2021). Prevalence and associated factors of depression among adolescent boys and girls in Bangladesh: Findings from a nationwide survey. *British Medical Journal Open, 11*, 038954. https://doi.org/10.1136/bmjopen-2020-038954.

Mullick, M. S. I., & Karim, M. E. (1994). Psychosocial stressors in depression. *Bangladesh Journal of Medicine, 5*(2), 49–54.

Mullick, M. S. I., Nahar, J. S., & Haq, S. A. (2005). Psychiatric morbidity, stressors, impact, and burden in juvenile idiopathic arthritis. *Journal of Health, Population and Nutrition, 23*, 142–149.

Muzaffar, R., Koly, K. N., Choudhury, S., Biswas, M. A. A., Kader, S. B., Abdullah, R., Kawser, U., Hasan, M. T., Williams, D., Chowdhury, A. B., & Ahmed, H. U. (2022). Generalized anxiety disorder among Bangladeshi university students during COVID-19 pandemic: Gender specific findings from a cross-sectional study. *Discover Mental Health, 2*, 3. https://doi.org/10.1007/s44192-022-00005-2.

Nahar, Z., Azad, M. A., Rahman, M. A., Rahman, M. A., Bari, W., Islam, S. N., Islam, M. S., & Hasnat, A. (2010). Comparative analysis of serum manganese, zinc, calcium, copper and magnesium level in panic disorder patients. *Biological Trace Element Research, 133*(3), 284–290. https://doi.org/10.1007/s12011-009-8441-7.

Nahar, Z., Khanum, S., Harun, S., Islam, S. N., Sobhan, A., Islam, S., & Hasnat, A. (2012). Immunoglobulin levels in panic disorder patients. *Pakistan Journal of Pharmaceutical Sciences, 25*(1), 149–153.

Nahar, Z., Sarwar, M. S., Safiqul Islam, M., Rahman, A., Nazrul Islam, S., Islam, M. S., & Hasnat, A. (2013). Determination of serum antioxidant vitamins, glutathione and MDA levels in panic disorder patients. *Drug Research, 63*(8), 424–428. https://doi.org/10.1055/s-0033-1343494.

Nahar, Z., Sohan, M., Supti, K. F., Hossain, M. J., Shahriar, M., Bhuiyan, M. A., & Islam, M. R. (2022). Prevalence and associated risk factors for mental health problems among female university students during COVID-19 pandemic: A cross-sectional study findings from Dhaka, Bangladesh. *Heliyon, 8*, e10890. https://doi.org/10.1016/j.heliyon.2022.e10890.

Nahar, B., Hossain, I., Hamadani, J. D., Ahmed, T., Grantham-McGregor, S., & Persson, L. A. (2015). Effect of a food supplementation and psychosocial stimulation trial for severely malnourished children on the level of maternal depressive symptoms in Bangladesh. *Child: Care, Health and Development, 41*(3), 483–493. https://doi.org/10.1111/cch.12176.

Naheed, A., Islam, M. S., Brooks, M. B., Fawzi, M. C. S., Ashraf, M. N., Ahmed, H. U., Uddin, M. M. J., Koly, K. N., Galea, J. T., Akhter, S., Nelson, C., Hossain, S. W., & Munir, K. M. (2022a). Feasibility of a school-based mental health program implementation to improve the status of depression and quality of life of mothers of children with autism spectrum disorders in urban Bangladesh: MENTHOL study. *Global Mental Health, 9*, 146–156. https://doi.org/10.1017/gmh.2022.16.

Naheed, A., Ashraf, M. N., Chakma, N., Jennings, H. M., & Nahar, P. (2022b). Protocol for integrating mental health services into primary healthcare facilities: A qualitative study of the perspectives of patients, family members and healthcare providers in rural Bangladesh. *British Medical Journal Open, 12*(2), e052464. https://doi.org/10.1136/bmjopen-2021-052464.

Nasreen, H. E., Kabir, Z. N., Forsell, Y., & Edhborg, M. (2010). Low birth weight in offspring of women with depressive and anxiety symptoms during pregnancy: Results from a population based study in Bangladesh. *BMC Public Health, 10*, 515. https://doi.org/10.1186/1471-2458-10-515.

Nasreen, H. E., Kabir, Z. N., Forsell, Y., & Edhborg, M. (2011). Prevalence and associated factors of depressive and anxiety symptoms during pregnancy: A population based study in rural Bangladesh. *BMC Women's Health, 11*, 22. https://doi.org/10.1186/1472-6874-11-22.

Nasreen, H. E., Kabir, Z. N., Forsell, Y., & Edhborg, M. (2013). Impact of maternal depressive symptoms and infant temperament on early infant growth and motor development: Results from a population based study in Bangladesh. *Journal of Affective Disorders, 146*(2), 254–261. https://doi.org/10.1016/j.jad.2012.09.013.

Nasreen, H. E., Edhborg, M., Petzold, M., Forsell, Y., & Kabir, Z. N. (2015). Incidence and risk factor of postpartum depressive symptoms in women: A population based prospective cohort study in a rural district in Bangladesh. *Journal of Depression and Anxiety, 4*, 2. https://doi.org/10.4172/2167-1044.1000180.

Nasreen, H. E., Alam, M. A., & Edhborg, M. (2016). Prevalence and associated factors of depressive symptoms among disadvantaged adolescents: Results from a population-based study in Bangladesh. *Journal of Child and Adolescent Psychiatric Nursing: Official Publication of the Association of Child and Adolescent Psychiatric Nurses, Inc, 29*(3), 135–144. https://doi.org/10.1111/jcap.12150

Natasha, K., Hussain, A., Azad Khan, A. K., & Bhowmik, B. (2015a). Prevalence of depression and glucose abnormality in an urbanizing rural population of Bangladesh. *Diabetes & Metabolism Journal, 39*(3), 218–229. https://doi.org/10.4093/dmj.2015.39.3.218.

Natasha, K., Hussain, A., & Khan, A. K. (2015b). Prevalence of depression among subjects with and without gestational diabetes mellitus in Bangladesh: A hospital based study. *Journal of Diabetes and Metabolic Disorders, 14*, 64. https://doi.org/10.1186/s40200-015-0189-3.

National Institute of Mental Health. (2021). National Mental Health Survey 2019. Dhaka: National Institute of Mental Health. https://nimh.gov.bd/english/wp-content/uploads/2021/11/Mental-Health-Survey-Report.pdf.

Nayem, J., Sarker, R., Roknuzzaman, A. S. M., Qusar, M. M. A. S., Raihan, S. Z., Islam, M. R., & Mahmud, Z. A. (2023). Altered serum TNF-α and MCP-4 levels are associated with the pathophysiology of major depressive disorder: A case-control study results. *PLoS ONE, 18*(11), e0294288. https://doi.org/10.1371/journal.pone.0294288.

Newman, M. S. (2013). Review of studies on mental health in Bangladesh, with a focus on depression. *International Journal of Mental Health, 42*(4), 48–77. https://doi.org/10.2753/IMH0020-7411420403.

Nur, M. I., Al-Mamun, F., Yasmin, F., Mohiuddin, M. S., Kaggwa, M. M., Sikder, M. T., & Mamun, M. A. (2023). Psychological benefits of the COVID-19 vaccination: A Bangladeshi comparative study. *Health Science Reports, 6*(7), e1346. https://doi.org/10.1002/hsr2.1346.

Oosthuizen, P., Carey, P., & Emsley, R. A. (2008). Psychiatric disorders and general medical conditions: Implications for the clinician. *African Journal of Psychiatry, 11*(1), 18–22. https://doi.org/10.4314/ajpsy.v11i1.30250.

Pacheco, J. P., Giacomin, H. T., Tam, W. W., Ribeiro, T. B., Arab, C., Bezerra, I. M., & Pinasco, G. C. (2017). Mental health problems among medical students in Brazil: A systematic review and meta-analysis. *Revista Brasileira De Psiquiatria, 39*(4), 369–378. https://doi.org/10.1590/1516-4446-2017-2223.

Pereira-Lima, K., Mata, D. A., Loureiro, S. R., Crippa, J. A., Bolsoni, L. M., & Sen, S. (2019). Association between physician depressive symptoms and medical errors: A systematic review and meta-analysis. *JAMA Network Open, 2*(11), e1916097. https://doi.org/10.1001/jamanetworkopen.2019.16097.

Proma, M. A., Daria, S., Nahar, Z., Ashraful Islam, S. M., Bhuiyan, M. A., & Islam, M. R. (2022). Monocyte chemoattractant protein-1 levels are associated with major depressive disorder. *Journal of Basic and Clinical Physiology and Pharmacology, 33*(6), 735–741. https://doi.org/10.1515/jbcpp-2021-0132.

Qusar, M. S., Arafat, S. M., Chowdhury, M. R., Ahmed, S., Morshed, N. M., & Rahman, W. (2019). Cultural variations in symptom presentations of depression: A cross-sectional observation in a tertiary care hospital of Bangladesh. *Mymensingh Medical Journal, 28*(2), 410–417.

Rabby, M. R., Islam, M. S., Orthy, M. T., Jami, A. T., & Hasan, M. T. (2023). Depression symptoms, anxiety, and stress among undergraduate entrance admission seeking students in Bangladesh: A cross-sectional study. *Frontiers in Public Health, 11*, 1136557. https://doi.org/10.3389/fpubh.2023.1136557.

Rabeya, R., Alam, N., Sonia, Z. F., Mohajon, D. R., Arafat, Y., Hasan, M. K., & Hawlader, M. D. H. (2023). Depressive symptoms and their sociodemographic determinants among people living with HIV/AIDS in Bangladesh: A cross-sectional study. *F1000 Research, 11*, 239. https://doi.org/10.12688/f1000research.108557.3.

Rabin, F., Mullick, S. I., Nahar, J. S., Bhuiyan, S. I., Haque, M. A., Khan, M. H., Khalil, M. I., & Faruki, M. A. (2013). Emotional and behavioral disorders in children with epilepsy. *Mymemsingh Medical Journal, 22*(2), 313–319.

Rahman, A. K. M. S., Ahsan, M. S., Ahsan, M. K., Alam, A. B. M. M., Rahman, T., Mullah, S., Rahman, M. M., Feroz, S., Kaiser, A. M., & Haque, M. S. (2020). Prevalence of depression in pre-dialytic chronic kidney disease patients attending at a tertiary care hospital in Bangladesh. *Journal of Biosciences and Medicines, 8*, 135–148. https://doi.org/10.4236/jbm.2020.812013.

Rahman, M. M., Khan, S. J., Sakib, M. S., Chakma, S., Procheta, N. F., Mamun, Z. A., & Rahman, M. M. (2021a). Assessing the psychological condition among general people of Bangladesh during COVID-19 pandemic. *Journal of Human Behavior in the Social Environment, 31*(1–4), 449–463. https://doi.org/10.1080/10911359.2020.1848688.

Rahman, M. H., Banik, G., Ahmed, A., Arifeen, S. E., Hossain, A. T., Hasan, M. A., & Rahman, A. E. (2021b). Anxiety and depressive symptoms among COVID-19 patients admitted to three isolation facilities in Bangladesh. *Health Psychology Open, 8*(2), 20551029211046104. https://doi.org/10.1177/20551029211046106.

Rahman, M. M., Amin, T., Sultan, S. B., Bithi, M. I., Rahman, F., & Rahman, M. M. (2021c). Depression, anxiety and stress among public university students in Bangladesh during the COVID-19 pandemic. *Journal of Emergency Management, 19*(9), 99–107. https://doi.org/10.5055/jem.0616.

Rahman, M. A., Dhira, T. A., Sarker, A. R., & Mehareen, J. (2022a). Validity and reliability of the Patient Health Questionnaire scale (PHQ-9) among university students of Bangladesh. *PLoS ONE, 17*(6), e0269634. https://doi.org/10.1371/journal.pone.0269634.

Rahman, S., Shanta, A. A., Daria, S., Nahar, Z., Shahriar, M., Qusar, M. S., Islam, S. M. A., Bhuiyan, M. A., & Islam, M. R. (2022b). Increased serum resistin but not G-CSF levels are associated in the pathophysiology of major depressive disorder: Findings from a case-control study. *PLoS ONE, 17*(2), e0264404. https://doi.org/10.1371/journal.pone.0264404.

Rasheduzzaman, M., Al Mamun, F., Faruk, M. O., Hosen, I., & Mamun, M. A. (2021). Depression in Bangladeshi university students: The role of sociodemographic, personal, and familial psychopathological factors. *Perspectives in Psychiatric Care, 57*(4), 1585–1594. https://doi.org/10.1111/ppc.12722.

Rathod, S., Pallikadavath, S., Graves, E., Rahman, M. M., Brooks, A., Rathod, P., Bhargava, R., Irfan, M., Aly, R., Mohammad Saleh Al Gahtani, H., Salam, Z., Chau, S. W. H., Paterson, T. S. E., Turner, B., Gorbunova, V., Klymchuk, V., & Phiri, P. (2023). Effects of cumulative COVID-19 cases on mental health: Evidence from multi-country survey. *World Journal of Psychiatry, 13*(7), 461–477.https://doi.org/10.5498/wjp.v13.i7.461.

Repon, M. A. U., Pakhe, S. A., Quaiyum, S., Das, R., Daria, S., & Islam, M. R. (2021). Effect of COVID-19 pandemic on mental health among Bangladeshi healthcare professionals: A cross-sectional study. *Science Progress, 104*(2), 00368504211026409. https://doi.org/10.1177/00368504211026409.

Rezvi, M. R., Hossain, M. R., & Haque, F. (2022). Prevalence of depression and anxiety among university students during COVID-19 in Bangladesh: A cross sectional study. *Mental Health: Global Challenges, 5*(2), 28–40. https://doi.org/10.56508/mhgcj.v5i2.140.

Ria, N. N., Mohimen, M. A. A., Mahmuda, S., Hussain, A. A., & Ali, M. O. I. (2022). Comparison of vitamin D levels between patients with depressive disorder and apparently healthy individuals attending Rajshahi Medical College Hospital. *TAJ: Journal Of Teachers' Association, 35*(2), 159–168.

Ripon, R. K., Mim, S. S., Puente, A. E., Hossain, S., Babor, M. M. H., Sohan, S. A., & Islam, N. (2020). COVID-19: Psychological effects on a COVID-19 quarantined population in Bangladesh. *Heliyon, 6*(11), e05481. https://doi.org/10.1016/j.heliyon.2020.e05481.

Rocha, T. B., Zeni, C. P., Caetano, S. C., & Kieling, C. (2013). Mood disorders in childhood and adolescence. *Revista Brasileira De Psiquiatria, 35*(Suppl 1), S22–S31. https://doi.org/10.1590/1516-4446-2013-S106.

Roy, T., Lloyd, C. E., Parvin, M., Mohiuddin, K. G. B., & Rahman, M. (2012). Prevalence of co-morbid depression in out-patients with type 2 diabetes mellitus in Bangladesh. *BMC Psychiatry, 12*, 123. https://doi.org/10.1186/1471-244x-12-123.

Ryan, E., Hore, K., Power, J., & Jackson, T. (2023). The relationship between physician burnout and depression, anxiety, suicidality and substance abuse: A mixed methods systematic review. *Frontiers in Public Health, 11*, 1133484. https://doi.org/10.3389/fpubh.2023.1133484.

Sadiq, M. S., Morshed, N. M., Rahman, W., Chowdhury, N. F., Arafat, S. M. Y., & Mullick, M. S. I. (2019). Depression, anxiety, stress among postgraduate medical residents: A cross sectional observation in Bangladesh. *Iranian Journal of Psychiatry, 14*(3), 192–197.

Sakib, N., Islam, M. K., & Faruk, T. (2023). Machine learning model for computer-aided depression screening among young adults using wireless EEG headset. *Computational Intelligence and Neuroscience, 2023*, 1701429. https://doi.org/10.1155/2023/1701429.

Salim, A., Sultana, R., Akhter, S. S., Azim, S. F., Hoshen, M. M., & Islam, M. Z. (2023). Gender disparities in dropping out of high school students and their level of depression. *Eastern Medical College Journal, 8*(1), 1–5.

Salma, U., & Hasan, M. M. (2020). Relationship between job satisfaction and depression, anxiety and stress among the female nurses of Dhaka Medical College and Hospital, Bangladesh. *Public Health Research, 10*(3), 94–102. https://doi.org/10.5923/j.phr.20201003.02.

Salsabil, L., Shahriar, M., Islam, S. M. A., Bhuiyan, M. A., Qusar, M. S., & Islam, M. R. (2023). Higher serum nerve growth factor levels are associated with major depressive disorder pathophysiology: A case-control study. *The Journal of International Medical Research, 51*(4), 3000605231166222. https://doi.org/10.1177/03000605231166222.

Sayeed, A., Hassan, M. N., Rahman, M. H., El Hayek, S., Al Banna, M. H., Mallick, T., & Kundu, S. (2020). Facebook addiction associated with internet activity, depression and behavioral factors among university students of Bangladesh: A cross-sectional study. *Children and Youth Services Review, 118*, 105424. https://doi.org/10.1016/j.childyouth.2020.105424.

Sayeed, A., Rahman, M. H., Hassan, M. N., deSteiguer, A., Kundu, S., Meem, A. E., Hasan, A. R., Mallick, T., Sultana, M. S., Hasanuzzaman, M., Sahrin, S., & Hasan, M. T. (2023). Prevalence and associated factors of depression among Bangladeshi university students: A cross-sectional study. *Journal of American College Health, 71*(5), 1381–1386. https://doi.org/10.1080/07448481.2021.1944168.

Selim, N. (2010). Cultural dimensions of depression in Bangladesh: A qualitative study in two villages of Matlab. *Journal of Health, Population, and Nutrition, 28*(1), 95–106. https://doi.org/10.3329/jhpn.v28i1.4528.

Shi, Y., Luan, D., Song, R., & Zhang, Z. (2020). Value of peripheral neurotrophin levels for the diagnosis of depression and response to treatment: A systematic review and meta-analysis. *European Neuropsychopharmacology: The Journal of the European College of Neuropsychopharmacology, 41*, 40–51. https://doi.org/10.1016/j.euroneuro.2020.09.633

Shidhaye, R., Lund, C., & Chisholm, D. (2015). Closing the treatment gap for mental, neurological and substance use disorders by strengthening existing health care platforms: Strategies for delivery and integration of evidence-based interventions. *International Journal of Mental Health Systems, 9*, 40. https://doi.org/10.1186/s13033-015-0031-9.

Shovo, T., Ahammed, B., Khan, B., Jahan, N., Shohel, T. A., Hossain, M. T., & Islam, M. N. (2021). Determinants of generalized anxiety, depression, and subjective sleep quality among university students during COVID-19 pandemic in Bangladesh. *Dr Sulaiman Al Habib Medical Journal, 3*(1), 27–35. https://doi.org/10.2991/dsahmj.k.210108.001.

Singla, D. R., Kohrt, B. A., Murray, L. K., Anand, A., Chorpita, B. F., & Patel, V. (2017). Psychological treatments for the world: Lessons from low- and middle-income countries. *Annual review of clinical psychology, 13*, 149–181. https://doi.org/10.1146/annurev-clinpsy-032816-045217

Siraji, M. I., Rahman, A. A., Nishat, M. M., Al Mamun, M. A., Faisal, F., Khalid, L. I., & Ahmed, A. (2023). Impact of mobile connectivity on students' wellbeing: Detecting learners' depression using machine learning algorithms. *PLoS ONE, 18*(11), e0294803. https://doi.org/10.1371/journal.pone.0294803.

Sohan, M., Qusar, M. M. A. S., Shahriar, M., Islam, S. M. A., Bhuiyan, M. A., & Islam, M. R. (2023). Association of reduced serum EGF and leptin levels with the pathophysiology of major depressive disorder: A case-control study. *PLoS ONE, 18*(7), e0288159. https://doi.org/10.1371/journal.pone.0288159.

Soron, T. R. (2017). Validation of Bangla montgomery asberg depression rating scale (MADRSB). *Asian Journal of Psychiatry, 28*, 41–46. https://doi.org/10.1016/j.ajp.2017.03.019.

Sparling, T. M., Waid, J. L., Wendt, A. S., & Gabrysch, S. (2020). Depression among women of reproductive age in rural Bangladesh is linked to food security, diets and nutrition. *Public Health Nutrition, 23*(4), 660–673. https://doi.org/10.1017/S1368980019003495.

Steel, Z., Marnane, C., Iranpour, C., Chey, T., Jackson, J. W., Patel, V., & Silove, D. (2014). The global prevalence of common mental disorders: A systematic review and meta-analysis 1980–2013. *International Journal of Epidemiology, 43*(2), 476–493. https://doi.org/10.1093/ije/dyu038.

Sultana, N. (2011). Stress and depression among undergraduate medical students of Bangladesh. *Bangladesh Journal of Medical Education, 2*(1), 6–9.

Sultana, S., Zaman, S., Chowdhury, A. B. M. A., Hasan, I., Haque, M. I., Kamrul Hossain, M., Ahmed, K. R., Chakraborty, P. A., & Hawlader, M. D. H. (2021). Prevalence and factors associated with depression among the mothers of school-going children in Dhaka city, Bangladesh: A multi stage sampling-based study. *Heliyon, 7*, e07493. https://doi.org/10.1016/j.heliyon.2021.e07493.

Sultana, N., Nguyen, T. T. P., Hossain, A., Asaduzzaman, M., Nguyen, M. H., Jahan, I., Nguyen, K. T., & Duong, T. V. (2022). Psychometric properties of the short-form geriatric depression scale (GDS-SF) and its associated factors among the elderly in Bangladesh. *International Journal of Environmental Research and Public Health, 19*(13), 7935. https://doi.org/10.3390/ijerph19137935.

Sultana, A. (2021). Prevalence and associated behavioral factors of depression among private medical students in Bangladesh. *Scholars Journal of Applied Medical Sciences, 9*(1), 54–59. https://doi.org/10.36347/sjams.2021.v09i01.010.

Sultan-e-Monzur, M., Taher, A., Roy, S., Karim, M. E., & Mollah, A. H. (2015). Major depressive disorder and generalized anxiety disorder among the patients with diabetes mellitus. *Bangladesh Journal of Psychiatry, 29*(1), 14–17.

Tabassum, T., Suzuki, T., Iwata, Y., & Ishiguro, H. (2023). Depression and associated factors among the elderly population in an urban tertiary geriatric hospital in Bangladesh. *Gerontology & Geriatric Medicine, 9*, 23337214231178144. https://doi.org/10.1177/23337214231178145.

Tasnim, R., Sujan, M. S. H., Islam, M. S., Ritu, A. H., Siddique, M. A. B., Toma, T. Y., Nowshin, R., Hasan, A., Hossain, S., Nahar, S., Islam, S., Islam, M. S., Potenza, M. N., & van Os, J. (2021). Prevalence and correlates of anxiety and depression in frontline healthcare workers treating people with COVID-19 in Bangladesh. *BMC Psychiatry, 21*(1), 271. https://doi.org/10.1186/s12888-021-03243-w.

Tasnim, S., Auny, F. M., Hassan, Y., Yesmin, R., Ara, I., Mohiuddin, M. S., Kaggwa, M. M., Gozal, D., & Mamun, M. A. (2022). Antenatal depression among women with gestational diabetes mellitus: A pilot study. *Reproductive Health, 19*(1), 71. https://doi.org/10.1186/s12978-022-01374-1.

Tasnim, F., Abedin, S., & Rahman, M. M. (2023). Mediating role of perceived stress on the association between domestic violence and postpartum depression: Cross-sectional study in Bangladesh. *Bjpsych Open, 9*(1), e16. https://doi.org/10.1192/bjo.2022.633.

Tibber, M. S., Milne, G., Fonagy, P., Saunders, R., & Dekker, T. M. (2023). The association between sociodemographic inequalities, COVID-related impacts and mental health. *Journal of Affective Disorders, 325*, 596–603. https://doi.org/10.1016/j.jad.2023.01.037.

Tung, Y. J., Lo, K. K. H., Ho, R. C. M., & Tam, W. S. W. (2018). Prevalence of depression among nursing students: A systematic review and meta-analysis. *Nurse Education Today, 63*, 119–129. https://doi.org/10.1016/j.nedt.2018.01.009.

United Nations Development Programme. (2020). Human Development Report 2020. The next frontier: Human development and the Anthropocene. New York: United Nations Development Programme. https://hdr.undp.org/content/human-development-report-2020.

Uphoff, E. P., Newbould, L., Walker, I., Ashraf, N., Chaturvedi, S., Kandasamy, A., Mazumdar, P., Meader, N., Naheed, A., Rana, R., Wright, J., Wright, J. M., Siddiqi, N., Churchill, R., & NIHR Global Health Research Group – IMPACT. (2019). A systematic review and meta-analysis of the prevalence of common mental disorders in people with non-communicable diseases in

Bangladesh, India, and Pakistan. *Journal of Global Health, 9*(2), 020417. https://doi.org/10.7189/jogh.09.020417.

Valdes, V., Berens, A. E., & Nelson, C. A. (2021). Socioeconomic and psychological correlates of postpartum depression at 6 months in Dhaka, Bangladesh. *International Journal of Psychology, 56*(5), 729–738. https://doi.org/10.1002/ijop.12735.

Wahid, S. S., Sandberg, J., Sarker, M., Arafat, A. S. M. E., Apu, A. R., Rabbani, A., Colón-Ramos, U., & Kohrt, B. A. (2021). A distress-continuum, disorder-threshold model of depression: A mixed-methods, latent class analysis study of slum-dwelling young men in Bangladesh. *BMC Psychiatry, 21*(1), 291. https://doi.org/10.1186/s12888-021-03259-2.

Wahid, S. S., Sarker, M., Arafat, A. S. M. E., Apu, A. R., & Kohrt, B. A. (2022). Tension and other idioms of distress among slum dwelling young men: A qualitative study of depression in Urban Bangladesh. *Culture, Medicine and Psychiatry, 46*(2), 531–563. https://doi.org/10.1007/s11013-021-09735-4.

Wahid, S. S., Raza, W. A., Mahmud, I., & Kohrt, B. A. (2023). Climate-related shocks and other stressors associated with depression and anxiety in Bangladesh: A nationally representative panel study. *The Lancet. Planetary Health, 7*(2), e137–e146. https://doi.org/10.1016/S2542-5196(22)00315-1.

Wahlin, Å., Palmer, K., Sternäng, O., Hamadani, J. D., & Kabir, Z. N. (2015). Prevalence of depressive symptoms and suicidal thoughts among elderly persons in rural Bangladesh. *International Psychogeriatrics, 27*(12), 1999–2008. https://doi.org/10.1017/S104161021500109X.

Williams, A., Sarker, M., & Ferdous, S. T. (2018). Cultural attitudes toward postpartum depression in Dhaka, Bangladesh. *Medical Anthropology, 37*(3), 194–205. https://doi.org/10.1080/01459740.2017.1318875.

World Health Organization. (2017). Depression and Other Common Mental Disorders: Global Health Estimates. Geneva: World Health Organization. https://www.who.int/publications/i/item/depression-global-health-estimates.

Wright, J., Mazumdar, P., Barua, D., Lina, S., Bibi, H., Kanwal, A., Mujeeb, F., Naz, Q., Safi, R., Ul Haq, B., Rana, R. Z., Nahar, P., Jennings, H., Sikander, S., Huque, R., Nizami, A., Jackson, C., & NIHR Global Health Research Group, IMPACT. (2020). Integrating depression care within NCD provision in Bangladesh and Pakistan: A qualitative study. *International Journal of Mental Health Systems, 14,* 63. https://doi.org/10.1186/s13033-020-00399-y

Yuan, D., Gazi, M. A. I., Rahman, M. A., Dhar, B. K., Rahaman, M. A. (2022). Occupational stress and health risk of employees working in the garments sector of Bangladesh: An empirical study. *Front Public Health, 16,* (10), 938248. https://doi.org/10.3389/fpubh.2022.938248. PMID: 36052007; PMCID: PMC9424988.

Zaman, S., Rahim, M. A., Khan, A. H., Habib, S. H., Rahman, M. M., Ahsan, M. S., Afroz, F., Afroze, S. R., Haque, H. F., Ahmed, J. U., Ahmed, A. K. M. S., Hossain, M. D., Rahman, M. R., Musa, A. K. M., & Uddin, K. N. (2014). Prevalence of depression among post-graduate medical trainees: A multi-centre survey. *Birdem Medical Journal, 4*(1), 18–21.

Ziaei, S., Frith, A. L., Ekstrom, E.-C., & Naved, R. T. (2016). Experiencing lifetime domestic violence: Associations with mental health and stress among pregnancy women in rural Bangladesh: The MINIMat randomized trial. *PLoS ONE, 11*(12), e0168103. https://doi.org/10.1371/journal.pone.0168103.

# Chapter 14
# Public Mental Health in Bangladesh

**Ancy Chandrababu Mercy Bai, Sauda Parvin, and Russell Kabir**

**Abstract** Public mental health services is an integral part of health care services to combat with mental health illnesses. The public health plays a fundamental role in promoting mental well-being in a country. This chapter evaluates the current public mental health situation in Bangladesh and reviews the current strategies and practices in place. Improving public mental health will help reduce stigma and discrimination associated with mental health conditions, and ensure that individuals have access to the care and support they need for their mental well-being. Furthermore, improving public mental health will also contribute to the social and economic development of the country.

**Keywords** Public mental health · Bangladesh · Current · Policies · Situation

## 14.1 Introduction

At least 18% of all diseases worldwide are mental disorders, and by 2030, it is estimated that the yearly global costs of these disorders would reach US$6 trillion. Using evidence-based public mental health interventions can be used to reduce mental health-related illnesses and their effects (Campion et al., 2022). Mental health is an integral part of health and promoting mental health is an essential component of public health. Hence, public mental health is not about the investigation and prevention of mental disorders in the population, it includes promotion of mental health by addressing emotional, social, and psychological well-being of the population (Arafat, 2017).

As defined by Campion (2018), public mental health "involves a population approach to mental health and includes treatment of mental disorder, prevention

A. C. M. Bai · R. Kabir (✉)
School of Allied Health, Faculty of Health, Medicine and Social Care, Anglia Ruskin University, Chelmsford, UK
e-mail: russell.kabir@aru.ac.uk

S. Parvin
Department of Nusring and Public Health, University of Sunderland, London, UK

 
S. M. Y. Arafat (ed.), *Mental Health in Bangladesh*,
https://doi.org/10.1007/978-981-97-0610-5_14

of associated impacts, prevention of mental disorder and promotion of mental well-being, including for those people recovering from mental disorder."

Mental health issues have a major role in the development and treatment of chronic illnesses, social injustices, the relationship between physical and mental health, and major causes of disability. On the other hand, mental wellness has numerous positive effects on health and society, such as promoting resilience and illness prevention. Since optimal psychological functioning is the foundation of both social equality and healthy lifestyles, promoting mental wellness can address both of these public health priorities (FPH, 2023). In Bangladesh, poor mental literacy, stigma around mental health issues (Arafat et al., 2024; Arafat, 2024), and lack of empirical mental health research are the major challenges to assess the significance of public mental health situation in the country. The purpose of this chapter is to evaluate the current public mental health situation in Bangladesh and review the current strategies and practices in place.

## 14.2 Public Health Burden of Mental Illness in Bangladesh

Mental illness is a serious public health issue in Bangladesh. The public health impact of mental illness is huge in Bangladesh, affecting people, families, and communities throughout the country, leading to major health, social, and economic problems. Nearly one in five adults and one in eight children in Bangladesh had a mental disorder in 2018–2019. This was based on a survey that visited households across the country and assessed a representative sample of the population using standard criteria for mental disorders (Ministry of Health & Family Welfare, 2021; Islam and Biswas, 2015). Some factors that make women, especially in rural Bangladesh, more likely to have depression are depression and suicidal thoughts during pregnancy, children's poor health and nutrition, violence at home, low education, and low income (Gausia et al., 2009; Nasreen et al., 2011; Ziaei et al., 2016).

The COVID-19 pandemic has had a devastating impact on the mental health of the people in Bangladesh. A study revealed that the adult population now has much higher rates of depressive (57.9%), stress (59.7%), and anxiety (33.7%) symptoms than before the pandemic (Repon et al., 2021). A study also showed that stress (28.5%), anxiety (33.3%), and depressive (46.92%) symptoms were present in more than a quarter of students who were home-quarantined (Islam & Biswas, 2015).

Mental illness not only affects the well-being of individuals but also the economy and productivity. People with mental health problems may have difficulties in keeping or doing well in their jobs. The costs of mental health include healthcare expenses, loss of output, and more burden on caregivers. It is important to deal with the public health problem of mental illness for human rights and sustainable development.

## 14.3 Public Mental Health Programs in Bangladesh

Public mental health programs are essential in Bangladesh for tackling the public health challenge of mental illness, enhancing mental well-being, and making sure that people with mental health problems can get the care and support they require. These programs have the objectives of raising awareness, decreasing stigma, offering treatment and support, and advancing overall mental health outcomes in the nation.

The National Mental Health Policy (NMHP), which started (WHO, 2022), is one of the main initiatives in Bangladesh. The NMHP aims to increase mental health services, make mental health part of primary health care, and improve the ability of healthcare providers to deal with mental health problems (Raisa, 2023). The program wants to make mental health services more accessible, especially in rural areas where there are not many mental health professionals (Raisa, 2023). The NMHP has set up mental health units in hospitals at district and sub-district levels, with mental health professionals who have received training. These units offer outpatient services, such as diagnosis, treatment, and counseling for mental health problems (UNB, 2022). They also help with referrals for more specialized care if needed. This approach helps to reduce the treatment gap and make sure that more people can access mental health services.

The government of Bangladesh has also taken measures to meet the specific mental health needs of groups at risk, such as children and adolescents. The National Adolescent Health Strategy (2017–2030) has plans for mental health improvement, prevention, and treatment services for adolescents (UNB, 2022). The government has also started mental health programs in schools, which try to find and deal with mental health problems among students and give them the support they need.

In addition to these initiatives, other public mental health programs aim to address the mental health needs of the population including:

1. Program that operates in different districts of Bangladesh, intending to provide mental health services at the community level (Government of The People's Republic of Bangladesh, 2022). The program focuses on creating awareness about mental health, detecting mental health disorders early, and providing treatment for mental health disorders. The program also trains community health workers and volunteers to deliver mental health services (Government of The People's Republic of Bangladesh, 2022).
2. Some programs use telemedicine and hotline services to provide mental health support, advice, and counseling to individuals, especially those who live in remote areas where there are few or no mental health professionals (Akon, 2021). These services allow individuals to access mental health care through phone calls, video calls, or online platforms, without having to travel long distances or face stigma.
3. Efforts have been made to integrate mental health services into primary healthcare facilities, such as health centers and clinics. Training programs for primary care workers, such as doctors, nurses, and paramedics, help them to identify and manage common mental health conditions, such as depression, anxiety, and

substance use disorders (Hasan et al., 2021a). This helps to make mental health care more accessible, affordable, and acceptable for the general population.

4. Several campaigns aim to raise awareness about mental health, reduce stigma, and promote understanding and acceptance of mental illnesses within communities (Hasan et al., 2021a). These campaigns use various media, such as radio, television, newspapers, social media, and posters, to disseminate information and messages about mental health. These campaigns also involve community leaders, religious leaders, celebrities, and people with lived experience of mental illness, to share their stories and perspectives on mental health (Hossain et al., 2019).
5. Collaborations between government bodies, non-governmental organizations (NGOs), and international agencies are instrumental in implementing mental health programs, capacity building, and resource allocation (Hasan et al., 2021a). These collaborations help to coordinate and harmonize the efforts and resources of different stakeholders, to ensure the quality and sustainability of mental health programs. These collaborations also help to advocate for the rights and needs of people with mental health conditions and to influence policies and laws related to mental health.

These programs aim to improve access to mental health services, reduce stigma, and enhance mental health literacy among the population. While these initiatives represent significant steps, ongoing efforts and further resources are required to expand these programs, improve accessibility, and meet the mental health needs of the diverse population in Bangladesh.

## 14.4 Current Challenges of Public Mental Health in Bangladesh

Public mental health in Bangladesh is facing many urgent challenges that hinder the effective handling and treatment of mental health problems among the population. Some of the main challenges are:

1. *Stigma and Cultural Beliefs*: There is a strong social stigma around mental health that continues, leading to discrimination and isolation of people with mental illnesses (Akon, 2021). Mental illness stigma remains a major obstacle to getting help and using mental health services (Arafat et al., 2018; Hossain et al., 2019). Many people with mental health problems experience discrimination and isolation, which can make their distress worse and stop them from getting proper care (Hasan et al., 2021a). Cultural beliefs often shape how people view mental health, leading to misunderstandings and unwillingness to get professional help.
2. *Limited Resources and Infrastructure*: There are not enough mental health facilities, trained mental health professionals, and funding to provide complete mental health services (Arafat et al., 2024). This shortage is especially severe in rural

areas, making the gap in access to mental health care between urban and rural areas worse.

3. *Lack of Awareness and Education*: Many people do not know much about mental health, which leads to late recognition and treatment of mental illnesses (Hasan et al., 2021a). People are also not aware of the available services and the importance of getting help as soon as possible, which makes it harder to intervene effectively.
4. *Trauma and Psychosocial Stressors*: Natural disasters, political and social unrest, and economic difficulties cause more stress, trauma, and psychological distress to people (Hossain et al., 2019). However, there are not enough psychosocial support systems and care that are informed by trauma to deal with these issues.
5. *Emergency Mental Health Services*: The availability of emergency mental health services is limited in Bangladesh (Government of The People's Republic of Bangladesh, 2022). During crises, disasters, or emergencies, there is a need for specialized mental health support to address the immediate psychological needs of affected individuals. Strengthening emergency mental health services is crucial to providing timely and appropriate care during such situations.
6. *Integration with Primary Health care*: Although some efforts have been made to make mental health services part of primary care, there is a need for more development and implementation of this approach to ensure that mental health support is available to a large population at the grassroots level (Government of The People's Republic of Bangladesh, 2022).
7. *Scope and Capacity Building*: Training programs for healthcare professionals often do not focus enough on mental health (Government of The People's Republic of Bangladesh, 2022). It is important to improve mental health training for healthcare workers and professionals from different fields to improve early detection and intervention.
8. *Policy and Advocacy*: Mental health policies need to be changed and made consistent with international standards (Government of The People's Republic of Bangladesh, 2022). More advocacy efforts are needed to make mental health a priority on the national healthcare agenda and allocate enough resources for mental health programs.

These challenges need a multifaceted approach that involves different stakeholders. This includes reducing the stigma of mental illness through awareness campaigns, investing in mental health infrastructure and workforce development, making mental health part of primary healthcare systems, creating community support, and advocating for policy changes that prioritize mental health. Improving mental health in Bangladesh should involve collaborations between government agencies, non-governmental organizations, mental health professionals, community leaders, and international partners to create a more supportive and inclusive environment for mental health care and advocacy.

## 14.5 Ways Forward

Public mental health in Bangladesh needs a complete and varied approach that can deal with the current problems and work toward improving the access, awareness, and quality of mental health services. Using universal intervention strategies to target the general population following measures can be introduced:

It is very important to allocate more resources and funding to mental health services. This means investing in mental health infrastructure, such as facilities, equipment, and supplies, training more mental health professionals, such as doctors, nurses, and counselors, and ensuring the availability of essential medications and treatment options, such as antidepressants, psychotherapy, and rehabilitation (Government of The People's Republic of Bangladesh, 2022). More investment will help increase access to quality mental health care nationwide. It is very important to make mental health services more integrated into primary healthcare for early finding, treating, and managing mental health problems (Arafat et al., 2018). This can be done by giving training and support to primary healthcare providers, such as doctors, nurses, and paramedics, and teaching them the necessary knowledge and skills to spot and handle mental health issues effectively. Community-based mental health initiatives (CBMHIs) are effective strategies to address the diverse and complex mental health needs of various communities in Bangladesh. CBMHIs involve the collaboration of community leaders, local organizations, and volunteers to enhance mental health awareness, support, and well-being (Government of The People's Republic of Bangladesh, 2022). By implementing CBMHIs, stigma can be reduced, care can be accessed, and mental health outcomes can be improved at the grassroots level.

To target the the individuals who are at higher risk to suffer from mental health-related problems, the following selective strategies can be followed:

Prevention and early intervention strategies are essential for addressing mental health issues in Bangladesh. Prevention strategies aim to enhance mental health literacy, resilience, and coping skills among the general population. They include promoting mental health education in various settings, such as schools, workplaces, and communities, and implementing mental health promotion programs that foster positive mental health and well-being (Patwary et al., 2022). Early intervention strategies target individuals who are at risk of developing mental health problems or who show signs of distress or suicide. They include providing screening, assessment, referral, and treatment services that are timely, accessible, and culturally appropriate. By focusing on prevention and early intervention strategies, also early communication with mental health professionals—mental health issues can be identified and addressed at an early stage, thereby reducing the impact and severity of mental illness (Arafat et al., 2018).

The following indicated intervention strategies are used for individuals who are already experiencing mental health illness:

Telehealth and digital solutions are innovative ways to overcome geographical barriers and increase access to mental health services in Bangladesh, especially in remote and underserved areas (Akon, 2021). Mental health care services are very rare worldwide and the situation is worse in low- and middle-income countries. Artificial Intelligence (AI) can be used to understand and analyze mental health-related data to guide diagnosis, treatment, and predict outcomes (Kar et al., 2021).

Comprehensive research and data collection on mental health in Bangladesh are essential for evidence-based planning and decision-making. Data-driven approaches enable the identification of priorities, the allocation of resources effectively, and the monitoring and evaluation of the impact of mental health programs.

Collaboration with international organizations, NGOs, and other stakeholders is a key strategy to leverage expertise, resources, and best practices in mental health. Collaboration involves establishing and maintaining partnerships that foster mutual learning, support, and coordination among different actors in the mental health field (Hasan et al., 2021b). Collaboration can facilitate capacity building, which involves enhancing the skills, competencies, and capabilities of individuals, organizations, and systems to deliver quality mental health care and support. Furthermore, collaboration can facilitate the implementation of innovative approaches, which involve developing and testing new and effective ways to address the challenges faced by public mental health in Bangladesh.

These future directions are crucial for improving public mental health in Bangladesh. By implementing these strategies, Bangladesh can significantly improve mental health awareness, care, and support among its population. Improving public mental health will help reduce stigma and discrimination associated with mental health conditions, and ensure that individuals have access to the care and support they need for their mental well-being. Furthermore, improving public mental health will also contribute to the social and economic development of the country, as mental health is closely linked to productivity, education, and human rights. Therefore, Bangladesh must focus on these future directions to address the mental health challenges and opportunities in the country.

## 14.6 Conclusion

Improving the public mental health situation is a challenging task and requires a wider approach that can address the various factors contributing to mental health challenges. Mental health literacy can be improved among the general population by planning and implementing more educational campaigns, and community outreach programs. With the help of religious and community leaders, promote mental health awareness within the community. The local and central government should work along to expand the mental health services and integrate mental health into primary care. By strengthening social support system and through economic empowerment, the wider social determinants of mental health can be addressed in Bangladesh to improve the public mental health situation.

## References


Akon, R. (2021). Mental Health Situation in Bangladesh in 2023. https://newhopepsychology.com/mental-health-situation-in-bangladesh/. Retrieved December 5, 2023.

Arafat, S. (2017). Mental health promotion or public mental health: The time demanded area. *Journal of Behavioral Health, 6*(1), 1. https://doi.org/10.5455/jbh.20161121095655.

Arafat, S. M. Y. (2024) Mental health services in Bangladesh. In S. M. Y. Arafat (Ed.), *Mental health in Bangladesh: From bench to community*. Springer Nature Singapore. https://doi.org/10.1007/978-981-97-0610-5_3

Arafat, S. M. Y, Giasuddin, N. A., & Mazumder, A. H. (2024). Access to mental health care in Bangladesh—Current status, potential challenges, and ways out. In S. M. Y. Arafat, & S. K. Kar (Eds.), *Access to mental health care in South Asia—Current status, potential challenges, and ways out*. Springer Nature Singapore. https://doi.org/10.1007/978-981-99-9153-2_3

Arafat, S. M. Y., Roy, S., & Huq, N. (2018). Integrating mental health into primary health care in Bangladesh: problems and prospects. *Mental Health and Addiction Research, 3*(2). https://doi.org/10.15761/mhar.1000158.

Campion, J. (2018). Public mental health: Key challenges and opportunities. *Bjpsych International, 15*(3), 51–54. https://doi.org/10.1192/bji.2017.11.

Campion, J., Javed, A., Lund, C., Sartorius, N., Saxena, S., Marmot, M., Allan, J., & Udomratn, P. (2022). Public mental health: Required actions to address implementation failure in the context of COVID-19. *The Lancet Psychiatry, 9*(2), 169–182. https://doi.org/10.1016/S2215-0366(21)00199-1.

FPH. (2023). *Why Public Mental Health matters?* https://www.fph.org.uk/policy-advocacy/special-interest-groups/public-mental-health-special-interest-group/better-mental-health-for-all/why-public-mental-health-matters/. Retrieved December 5, 2023.

Gausia, K., Fisher, C., Ali, M., & Oosthuizen, J. (2009). Antenatal depression and suicidal ideation among rural Bangladeshi women: A community-based study. *Archives of Women's Mental Health, 12*(5), 351–358. https://doi.org/10.1007/s00737-009-0080-7.

Government of The People's Republic of Bangladesh. (2022). National Mental Health Strategic Plan, 2020–2030. https://dghs.gov.bd/sites/default/files/files/dghs.portal.gov.bd/notices/e27171cb_a80b_42d4_99ad_40095adef31b/2022-08-16-08-42-af8622e2c4936593dd45601b84f4920f.pdf. Retrieved May 02, 2023.

Hasan, M. T., Anwar, T., Christopher, E., Hossain, S., Hossain, M. M., Koly, K. N., Saif-Ur-Rahman, K. M., Ahmed, H. U., Arman, N., & Hossain, S. W. (2021a). The current state of mental healthcare in Bangladesh: Part 1-an updated country profile. *Bjpsych International, 18*(4), 78–82. https://doi.org/10.1192/bji.2021.41.

Hasan, M. T., Anwar, T., Christopher, E., Hossain, S., Hossain, M. M., Koly, K. N., Saif-Ur-Rahman, K. M., Ahmed, H. U., Arman, N., & Hossain, S. W. (2021b). The current state of mental healthcare in Bangladesh: Part 2 - setting priorities. *Bjpsych International, 18*(4), 82–85. https://doi.org/10.1192/bji.2021.42.

Hossain, M. M., Hasan, M. T., Sultana, A., & Faizah, F. (2019). New mental health act in Bangladesh: Unfinished agendas. *The Lancet Psychiatry, 6*(1), e1. https://doi.org/10.1016/S2215-0366(18)30472-3.

Islam, A., & Biswas, T. (2015). Mental health and the health system in Bangladesh: Situation analysis of a neglected domain. *American Journal of Psychiatry and Neuroscience, 3*(4), 57. https://doi.org/10.11648/j.ajpn.20150304.11.

Kar, S. K., Kabir, R., Menon, V., Arafat, S. M. Y., Prakash, A. J., & Saxena, S. K. (2021). *Artificial Intelligence in Mental Healthcare During COVID-19 Pandemic* (pp. 327–343). https://doi.org/10.1007/978-981-15-7317-0_17.

Ministry of Health & Family Welfare. (2021). National Mental Health Survey 2019. http://nimh.gov.bd/wp-content/uploads/2021/11/Mental-Health-Survey-Report.pdf. Retrieved March 29, 2023.

Nasreen, H. E., Kabir, Z. N., Forsell, Y., & Edhborg, M. (2011). Prevalence and associated factors of depressive and anxiety symptoms during pregnancy: A population based study in rural Bangladesh. *BMC Women's Health, 11*(1), 22. https://doi.org/10.1186/1472-6874-11-22.

Patwary, M. M., Bardhan, M., Disha, A. S., Kabir, M. P., Hossain, Md. R., Alam, M. A., Haque, Md. Z., Billah, S. M., Browning, M. H. E. M., Kabir, R., Swed, S., & Shoib, S. (2022). Mental health status of university students and working professionals during the early stage of COVID-19 in Bangladesh. *International Journal of Environmental Research and Public Health, 19*(11). https://doi.org/10.3390/ijerph19116834.

Raisa, F. Z. A. (2023). Reshaping mental health legislation in Bangladesh. https://www.thedailystar.net/law-our-rights/news/reshaping-mental-health-legislation-bangladesh-3419261. Retrieved December 5, 2023.

Repon, M. A. U., Pakhe, S. A., Quaiyum, S., Das, R., Daria, S., & Islam, M. R. (2021). Effect of COVID-19 pandemic on mental health among Bangladeshi healthcare professionals: A cross-sectional study. *Science Progress, 104*(2), 00368504211026409. https://doi.org/10.1177/00368504211026409.

UNB. (2022). National Mental Health Strategy 2020–2030: Towards ensuring quality mental healthcare. https://unb.com.bd/category/Lifestyle/national-mental-health-strategy-2020-2030-towards-ensuring-quality-mental-healthcare/102276. Retrieved December 5, 2023.

WHO. (2022). Bangladesh WHO Special Initiative for Mental Health. https://www.who.int/initiatives/who-special-initiative-for-mental-health/bangladesh. Retrieved December 5, 2023.

Ziaei, S., Frith, A. L., Ekström, E. -C., & Naved, R. T. (2016). Experiencing lifetime domestic violence: Associations with mental health and stress among pregnant women in rural Bangladesh: The MINIM at randomized trial. *PLOS ONE, 11*(12), e0168103-. https://doi.org/10.1371/journal.pone.0168103.

# Chapter 15
# Climate Change and Mental Health in Bangladesh: Vulnerability, Inequality, and the Crucial Need for Intervention on the Frontlines of the Climate Crisis

**Syed Shabab Wahid, Md. Nurul Islam, and Wameq Azfar Raza**

**Abstract** Climate-vulnerable countries such as Bangladesh will experience disproportionate impacts on health and well-being as climate change continues to worsen over the upcoming decades. The country's unique geographic location and climactic conditions make it highly vulnerable to the effects of climate change—drought, floods, sea water rise, land inundation and salt water intrusion, extreme temperatures and humidity, heatwaves, cyclones, all comprise a constellation of critical risk factors that threaten the mental health and well-being of Bangladeshi populations. There have been observed impacts on depression, anxiety, post-traumatic stress disorder, suicidality, and substance abuse, as a result. Climate change is poised to exacerbate existing vulnerabilities and worsen mental health outcomes for all, but especially for already disadvantaged populations, such as poorer populations, women, and migrants. Community driven solutions are emerging and there has been progress on climate adaptation policies. However, there is a critical need for continued focus on holistic policy, interventions, and research, to fully understand and respond to the issue and safeguard the well-being of millions of Bangladeshi citizens living in precarious conditions on the frontlines of climate change.

**Keywords** Climate change in Bangladesh · Mental health in Bangladesh · Adaptation in Bangladesh · Climate change and mental health

---

S. S. Wahid (✉)
Department of Global Health, School of Health, Georgetown University, Washington, DC, USA
e-mail: ssw64@georgetown.edu

Md. N. Islam
Sajida Foundation, Dhaka, Bangladesh

W. A. Raza
Health, Nutrition and Population Global Practice, The World Bank, Dhaka, Bangladesh

 
S. M. Y. Arafat (ed.), *Mental Health in Bangladesh*,
https://doi.org/10.1007/978-981-97-0610-5_15

## 15.1 Climate Change and Mental Health—An Introduction

Climate change has been described as the "biggest global health threat in the twenty-first century" (Costello et al., 2009). While physical health consequences of climate-related extreme weather have been studied extensively and are well-established (Romanello et al.), emerging research from across the globe is indicating that climate change precipitates a novel constellation of risk factors that pose a serious threat to mental health outcomes across the whole world (Hayes & Poland, 2018).

Climate change profoundly affects mental health by amplifying stress and exposing people to trauma, increasing the likelihood of depressive and anxiety disorders, post-traumatic stress disorder (PTSD), increasing the risk of suicide and suicidality, substance abuse, worsening severe mental health outcomes of those who have schizophrenia or bipolar disorder, among other adverse mental health outcomes (Charlson et al., 2021; Hayes & Poland, 2018; Kabir, 2018). These manifest through a range of interconnected meteorological and sociological pathways. The increased frequency and intensity of extreme weather events, such as hurricanes, cyclones, heatwaves, and floods, directly impact mental health by causing displacement, loss of lives, homes, and livelihoods (Charlson et al., 2021). These events create acute stressors that trigger emotional distress and trauma among affected individuals and communities. Moreover, gradual environmental changes, such as prolonged droughts, habitat loss, land inundation and salinization from increasing sea levels, deforestation, forced migration, and unpredictable weather patterns, generate chronic stress and increased vulnerability to clinical mental disorders, as people struggle with uncertainties about the future including concerns about food security, access to resources, and the sustainability of their way of life (Charlson et al., 2021).

A major pathway through which climate change directly impacts mental health outcomes is via exposure to elevated temperatures. A systematic review of global scientific research indicates that for every 1-degree Celsius increase in ambient temperature, there is a corresponding higher risk of poor mental health, across the spectrum of mental health conditions (Liu et al., 2021). Research indicates that heatwaves can intensify stress levels, leading to irritability, sleep disruptions, and cognitive impairment issues (Chen et al., 2020; Rony & Alamgir, 2023). Moreover, extreme heat can escalate aggression and interpersonal conflicts, further straining mental well-being, especially for women, who are prone to intimate partner violence (Mahendran et al., 2021). Vulnerable populations, including the elderly, children, and individuals with pre-existing mental health conditions, are particularly susceptible to the adverse effects of heat on mental health (Lõhmus, 2018; Rony & Alamgir, 2023). Additionally, heat-related physical health issues, such as heatstroke and dehydration, can indirectly affect mental health. These physical ailments can lead to discomfort, fatigue, and decreased cognitive function, contributing to mood disturbances and overall mental distress (Chen et al., 2020; Lõhmus, 2018; McMorris et al., 2006). While these findings may be indicating a universal vulnerability of human beings to hotter temperature exposure, such outcomes are especially salient for populations residing in hotter tropical climates, as these regions are experiencing increasing frequency and intensity of heatwaves that are projected to worsen as this century unfolds (Im et al., 2017; IPCC, 2021).

While these climate-related risks to mental health and well-being are being experienced around the world, well-resourced countries are substantially better equipped to face the threat of climate change. Populations living in lower income settings, who have contributed the least to the climate problem, will unfortunately face the brunt of its consequences (Bathiany, Dakos, Scheffer, & Lenton), reflecting deep inequality and injustice elements intertwined with the climate change crisis (King & Harrington, 2018). Adverse impacts on mental health reflect a substantial component of such outcomes. In this way, the state of things reflects deep global inequity that is only amplified by the reality that mental health services in low- and middle-income nations of the world are already plagued by weak infrastructure and capacity (Aguilar-Gaxiola et al., 2018), and need considerable investment to address this additional climate threat to mental health and well-being of affected populations.

In this chapter, the connection between climate change and mental health is examined in Bangladesh, a lower middle-income country in South Asia, and one of the world's most vulnerable countries to climate change. The range and role of climate-related stressors is examined along with the consequent impacts on mental health for the population of Bangladesh. Direct and indirect pathways of this connection are presented and illustrated via salient case studies. Current approaches for adaptation to the mental health crisis, in terms of care provision and models of service delivery to address these issues, are discussed in the context of Bangladesh. The chapter concludes by discussing major gaps and future directions for research and practice to address this complex challenge affecting the well-being of millions of Bangladeshi citizens.

## 15.2 Vulnerability of Bangladesh to Climate Change

In 2021, the Global Climate Risk Index ranked Bangladesh as the seventh most climate vulnerable country (Eckstein, 2021). The sixth report of the Intergovernmental Panel on Climate Change indicated that Bangladesh is at heightened risk from climate change, and predicted that its economy is likely to receive severe shocks in the coming decade (IPCC, 2021). Bangladesh has received significant attention in the sixth IPCC assessment with over 430 mentions in the entire report. Under the current emissions scenario, the country is likely to face extreme heat and humidity, increased in precipitation and continued rise of sea level resulting in agriculture output reduction, depletion of fisheries stocks, fresh water contamination by salinity and arsenic, displacement, increase in flood hazards, increase in water born disease and compromised societal stability (IPCC, 2021). The IPCC report further elaborates on the precarious position of Bangladesh in the face of climate change. From 2050 to 2100 Bangladesh could lose 2 to 9 percent of its gross domestic production due to climate change. Agricultural output in part of the country could be reduced by 31 to 40 percent due to sea level rise alone. Sea level rise could also displace up to

4 million people from coastal areas. Overall rice production could be declined by 12-17 percent. IPCC has projected a significant reduction in fresh water coverage in coastal regions of the country from 40 percent to as low 17 percent by the middle of the twenty-first century (IPCC, 2021).

Located in one of the world's largest deltas consisting of the Ganges, Brahmaputra, and Meghna rivers, more than 60 percent of Bangladesh's landmass is just five meters above sea level. This leaves the country highly vulnerable to flood hazards. Additionally, around one-third of the country belongs to the coastal region that is highly susceptible to tidal flooding, sea level rise, cyclone, related storm surges, and salinity intrusion. Every year, on average, 20 to 25 percent of the country is submerged due to flooding; however, during extreme flooding, submerged areas can comprise up to 50–60 percent of the total landmass (Rentschler et al., 2022). Furthermore, northern parts of the country experience erratic rainfall patterns and drier climactic conditions leading to exacerbated droughts (Rahman et al., 2023). Temperature rise and change in rainfall due to climate change is expected to increase droughts in this region of Bangladesh, resulting in water stress and depletion leading to crop failure and drinking water crises. In the last 50 years, Bangladesh has experienced 20 droughts that caused severe reductions in agricultural production. Drought has become more frequent in recent years happening once in every 2.5 years (Rahman et al., 2023).

## 15.3 Climate-Related Risk Factors and Mental Health in Bangladesh

The complex relationship between mental health and climate change in Bangladesh is made evident by the country's frequent exposure to natural catastrophes and vulnerabilities associated with a changing climate. Numerous climate-related issues confront the nation, such as extended monsoons, sea level rise, floods, and cyclones. These stressors have profound impacts on the mental health and well-being of individuals, as well as the aggregate social well-being and stability of communities. According to the research, affected communities experience higher levels of stress, anxiety, sadness, depression, and post-traumatic stress disorder (PTSD) as a result of these dynamic climate-related events. These effects of such disasters on survival, physical health and injuries, property destruction, displacement, loss of livelihoods, and disruption of social networks exacerbate psychological suffering and have implications on long-term mental health and well-being. In this section, each unique climate-related risk factor for mental health in Bangladesh is presented and contextualized in a body of evidence that has been accumulating in the country.

### 15.3.1 Elevated Temperature and Humidity

In Bangladesh, the correlation between heat and mental health is particularly pronounced due to the country's geographic location and vulnerability to extreme temperatures (Eckstein, 2021). Recently conducted nationally representative research in Bangladesh (See Box 15.1 for details) has established that populations with exposure to elevated temperature and humidity are susceptible to a higher likelihood of anxiety and co-occurrence of depression and anxiety (Wahid et al., 2023). Heatwaves, which have become more frequent and intense in the region in recent years (Im et al., 2017), pose a significant threat to mental well-being. Prolonged exposure to high temperatures can amplify stress, anxiety, and irritability among the population (Rony & Alamgir, 2023). Moreover, heat-related physical health issues like heatstroke and dehydration contribute to discomfort and fatigue, which can exacerbate mental distress (Lõhmus, 2018; McMorris et al., 2006). Vulnerable groups, including the elderly, children, and individuals with pre-existing mental health conditions, are especially at risk of experiencing the detrimental effects of extreme heat on mental health in Bangladesh (Nahar et al., 2014; Wahid et al., 2023). The impact of heat on mental health is compounded by socioeconomic factors and limited access to resources. Many communities lack adequate infrastructure, such as reliable access to cooling systems or proper shelter (Shahid, 2012), exacerbating the challenges posed by extreme heat. Furthermore, the agricultural sector, a crucial part of Bangladesh's economy, faces risks from heat stress impacting crop yields (Miah et al., 2016), thereby affecting food security and livelihoods, which in turn contribute to mental health stressors among affected communities.

**Box 15.1: Featured research on the connection between heat, humidity, exposure to floods, and mental health outcomes in Bangladesh.**
A recently conducted study titled "Climate-related shocks and other stressors associated with depression and anxiety in Bangladesh: A nationally representative panel study" was one of the first research efforts in Bangladesh to examine the link between heat, humidity, and flood exposure, and depressive and anxiety disorders (Wahid, Raza, Mahmud, & Kohrt, 2023). The study represents an important contribution to the knowledge about mental health and climate change in Bangladesh, as it was one of the first research efforts on the topic designed to be nationally representative. The study utilized a two-staged stratified sampling design to achieve this goal. For data collection, several geographic units were constructed as primary sampling units based on the population size, with units comprising larger populations having a higher probability of inclusion into the study for data collection, in a probability proportional to size approach. Sampling units covered urban, rural and peri-urban areas of the country. Once these primary sampling units were determined, every household in these sampling units were screened for the presence of key vulnerable populations: women; children younger than 5 years; and elderly populations (age

≥66 years). Once the set of eligible households was created, a randomized approach was utilized to select households into the study for data collection. This approach was constructed to align with the population distribution of Bangladesh. There were two rounds of data collection from 3,606 individuals, at two time points: at the peak of summer and winter, to maximize temperature and weather variability. Taken together, these methodological considerations allowed the study to collect data that could be used to generate findings from a small sample and make inferences and draw conclusions about the whole country's population.

Several climate-related factors were included in the study as key stressors of mental health. These included (1) Ambient temperature, measured in degree Celsius; (2) Humidity, measured in grams of moisture per cubic meter (gm/m3); and (3) Exposure to severe flooding, including river overflow, surging sea water rise, flash floods, and excessive rise in ground water levels. Mental health outcomes included (1) Depression, as measured by the Patient Health Questionnaire-9 (PHQ-9), a scale consisting of nine questions inquiring about the presence and severity of depressive symptoms; (2) Generalized Anxiety Disorder-7 (GAD-7), an instrument that asks seven questions about the presence and severity of generalized anxiety disorder symptoms; and (3) Co-occurrence of both depression and anxiety, constructed from the GAD-7 & PHQ-9 scales.

The study found that for every 1-degree Celsius increase in ambient temperature, there was a statistically significant 21 percent higher odds of anxiety, and 24 percent higher odds of the co-occurrence of depression and anxiety. Temperature was not found to be associated with depression by itself. For humidity, for every 1 gm/m3 increase, there was six percent higher odds of co-occurring depression and anxiety, but no connection with depression and anxiety alone. Exposure to flooding was strongly associated with all three outcomes: 31 percent higher likelihood of depression; 69 percent higher odds of anxiety; and 87 percent higher likelihood of co-occurrence of both depression and anxiety.

### *15.3.2 Floods*

Research in Bangladesh consistently demonstrates the profound impact of floods on the mental health of affected communities. The loss of homes, livelihoods, and personal possessions during flooding episodes contributes significantly to emotional distress and trauma. Moreover, displacement and the subsequent challenges in resettlement amplify mental health burdens, particularly among vulnerable populations like women, children, and the elderly, who often experience heightened psychological vulnerabilities in the aftermath of floods. Recurrent and severe flooding events in the country have been linked to a range of adverse psychological outcomes. In the study profiled in Box 15.1, nationally representative research indicates exposure to flooding to be a major risk factor for poor mental health outcomes, with strong associations with depression, anxiety, and the co-occurrence of both conditions simultaneously (Wahid et al., 2023). Other studies highlight elevated levels of stress, anxiety, depression, and PTSD among individuals directly impacted by floods. One study (Mostafizur Rahman et al., 2023) conducted with female survivors of severe flash flooding in 2022 found that at least 65 percent of the sample of women recruited for the study screened for depression or anxiety, far higher than national prevalence rates of 6.7 and 4.5 percent for depression and anxiety, respectively (National Institute of Mental Health, 2019). Compounding these findings were reports that some women experience family violence during flooding events. Around 89 and 88 percent of those women reported severely worse depressive and anxiety outcomes, respectively. Specific flood-related risk factors associated with adverse mental health outcomes were experiencing the loss of family, injury or disease due to the flood, family violence, and property damage from flooding.

Exposure to floods also places those affected at higher risk of suicide. A study in Kurigram (Mamun et al., 2021), a climate vulnerable northern district of Bangladesh, found over 57 percent of flood survivors to have suicidality, with a subset of 5.7 percent actually making an active suicide plan, and 2 percent having made a suicide attempt. The study also illuminated connections between other forms of social and structural vulnerability to be associated with suicidality, such as co-morbid mental illness, lower education, and lower income. This underscores the idea that climate-related stressors do not work in a vacuum, but in conjunction with existing vulnerabilities, amplifying their impact on mental health and well-being. This idea was reinforced by findings from recent research in Sylhet (Gepp et al., 2022), where it was identified that flooding leads to a cascade of interconnected vulnerabilities to manifest. These included making households economically insecure leading to incurring high-interest debt, and leaving the most vulnerable households more food insecure. Around 45 percent of women in such food insecure households reported higher odds of depression, as measured almost two and a half years from initial flood exposure, providing empirical evidence that possibly points to persistent and long-term mental health impacts of index climate events such as floods.

### *15.3.3 Cyclones*

Research conducted in Bangladesh consistently underscores the profound impact of cyclones on mental health within affected populations. Cyclones, frequent in coastal regions, lead to devastating consequences that extend beyond physical damage. The loss of lives, homes, and livelihoods during these calamities contributes significantly to emotional trauma and mental health issues. Studies highlight heightened levels of psychological distress, including anxiety, depression, and PTSD, among individuals directly impacted by cyclones (Akhter et al., 2015; R. Kabir et al., 2016; Mullick et al., 2014; Tasdik Hasan et al., 2020). One recent study examined the impact of cyclone *Amphan* on the food security, livelihoods, and psychological outcomes of affected populations in Satkhira, one of the impacted coastal districts (Hossain et al., 2021). Around 55.7 percent of the sample population reported moderate or severe psychological symptoms, while an alarming 10.9 percent reported suicidal ideation. The cyclone left almost 40 percent of study participants with severe food insecurity, and among those, the psychological severity of symptoms was found to be even higher (66 percent). Other stressors tied to poor mental health were being of female biological sex and facing disruptions to jobs and other livelihoods.

Moreover, displacement and the disruption of social support networks worsen mental health problems, particularly among vulnerable groups such as women, children, and the elderly, who experience amplified psychological vulnerabilities following cyclones (Hayward & Ayeb-Karlsson, 2021; Tasdik Hasan et al., 2020). Research also emphasizes the enduring effects of cyclones on mental health in Bangladesh. Individuals and communities affected by these disasters often have to deal with prolonged psychological distress due to ongoing concerns about future cyclones and their consequences. The chronic stress resulting from the unpredictability and recurrence of cyclones perpetuates anxiety and mental health challenges. A qualitative study that examined perspectives of mental health in the context of cyclones in Khulna district found reports of the onset of panic and anxiety triggered by warning sirens, hydraulic horns, thunder, and other loud sources of noises, even after the threat of the disaster had subsided (Tasdik Hasan et al., 2020). Additionally, studies highlight the interplay between cyclones, economic hardships, food insecurity, and mental health, revealing how the loss of livelihoods and financial strain further compound psychological distress among cyclone-affected populations (Hossain et al., 2021). In Box 15.2, a case story detailing the devastating mental health implications of a cyclone is presented from the lived experience of a survivor. The case is provided courtesy of the SAJIDA Foundation, one of several non-governmental organizations that have been providing community-based mental health and psychosocial support for climate vulnerable communities in Bangladesh.

**Box 15.2: Case story of the mental health impacts of surviving a cyclone**

This case story was compiled from a focus group discussion conducted in 2021 for a research study by SAJIDA Foundation. The participant is a male in his 50s.

"Few days ago, we heard that a cyclone is heading towards us. So, we hurriedly prepared everything, along with our children, to move to the cyclone shelter. Then, they told that the cyclone moved away in another direction. We often need to be in this type of pressurized situation. Everyone face this pressure, except the children [who are too young to understand]. People didn't take cyclone warning seriously before the devasting cyclone Sidr back in

2007. When their own family members died in the cyclone, people started to take cyclone warnings seriously. Four members of my family died during that cyclone—My wife who was pregnant and my two sons. This is why people now have a fear when they hear about cyclone, and they try to go to the cyclone shelter hurriedly."

"In the 2007 cyclone, I lost two children. Since then, whenever I see bad weather I cannot sleep at night. The night passes by thinking about what to do, where to go, etc. My child was 4-year-old. He died in my arms. Water and wind were all over. The child was in one of my hands, and with other hand I was holding a tin. Due to the cold, my hand got a bit frozen and I couldn't feel it. Thus, the current swept my child away from my hand."

"After Sidr, whenever I see any bad weather, I become worried about what to do and where to go. I can't sleep, eat or concentrate to anything. I constantly think whether I will lose my children, or my house will be blown away again. I cannot build another house in my entire life with this little income. Suppose, I earned only 60 Taka today. Will I buy vegetables with it or rice? At that time, my brain does not work."

### *15.3.4 Drought*

Studies examining how Bangladesh's drought affects mental health reveal a range of complex and multifaceted issues that impacted populations have to deal with. While not as direct as cyclones or elevated temperatures, the extended periods of water shortage and agricultural hardship, including dynamic shifts in the agrarian economy that accompany a drought have substantial negative impact on mental health (Hayward & Ayeb-Karlsson, 2021). These include loss of livestock, loss of crops, forced migration, debt incurrence, etc., among other stressors. Research reveals elevated levels of stress, anxiety, and depression in people and communities dealing with the aftermath of drought. The reduction in water availability, crop loss, and ensuing food insecurity lead to increased psychological and emotional strain. For example, research conducted on the social and health impacts of drought among the *Santal*, an indigenous group in northwestern Bangladesh, revealed chronic water insecurity to cascade and trigger several interconnected social vulnerabilities (Ahmed et al., 2019). During the hotter season, the region dries up considerably pushing communities into water insecurity. As a result, women and children, who are often tasked with water collection responsibilities for their households, have to walk further and carry a higher number of water receptacles to collect potable water. Such experiences were found to take not only a physical toll but also trigger higher levels of mental distress among affected populations.

Studies highlight how the rural agrarian population mental health in the long term is profoundly impacted by recurrent drought in negative ways. Long-term psychological discomfort is experienced by communities that confront chronic water scarcity and ongoing agricultural disruptions as a result of drought and poverty (Hayward & Ayeb-Karlsson, 2021; Maîtrot et al., 2021; Miah et al., 2016). Moreover, the financial burden brought on by crop failures and decreased agricultural output aggravates mental health issues, especially for underprivileged communities whose primary source of income is agriculture. Anxiety and vulnerability related to mental health are exacerbated by the extended impact on livelihoods and food security, as well as the uncertainty around when the drought will end. In order to mitigate the immediate and long-lasting psychological effects of drought on individuals and communities, it is necessary to address the mental health implications of drought in Bangladesh through holistic interventions that integrate drought-resistant agricultural practices, livelihood diversification, and mental health support services.

### *15.3.5 Migration*

Throughout Bangladesh, migration brought on by the climate crisis unfolds primarily from rural to urban areas. Leaving behind familiar surroundings, losing homes, and facing uncertainty about the future have a profound psychological toll and create a complex web of difficulties that considerably increases the risk of adverse mental health outcomes for impacted communities. As elaborated upon in previous sections, due to the nation's vulnerability to cyclones, floods, drought, and rising sea levels, many people have been widely displaced or are forced to shift from disaster-prone or coastal/riverine areas to the country's urban centers. Migrants often find themselves settling in urban slums or informal settlements. The conditions of such settlements are often socially volatile and fraught with pronounced risk factors for mental illness, such as crime, infectious disease, injuries, overcrowded housing, insecure land tenure, among other stressors (Afsana & Wahid, 2013). Migration to cities does not necessarily translate to upward social mobility, and economic vulnerability for migrants can continue in the urban space for protracted periods of time (Ayeb-Karlsson et al., 2020) with urban slums functioning as concentration points of rampant urban poverty (Wahid, Sarker, Arafat, Apu, & Kohrt, 2021a, 2021b). As a result of the disruptions to social networks, the break from traditional livelihoods, and the uncertainty about the future caused by this forced relocation, research consistently finds migrants to report increased levels of stress, anxiety, and depression (Rashid, 2013; Wahid et al., 2021a, 2021b; Syed Shabab Wahid et al., 2021a, 2021b). The difficulties associated with relocation, subpar housing, and restricted access to essential services in cities all contribute to the worsening of mental health issues among these groups. Individuals who are displaced not only experience the loss of material assets but also undergo a deeper sense of disconnection, tied to a loss of place and a ruptured sense of belonging (Azad & Khan, 2015; Rashid, 2013). Furthermore, in metropolitan environments, migrants frequently report experiencing marginalization, loss of status, and prejudice (Ayeb-Karlsson et al., 2020; Sams, 2019), which can further exacerbate their susceptibility to mental health problems. Urban centers in Bangladesh often face unique climate threats as well which adversely impact mental health and well-being for urban residents but are especially exacerbated for the urban poor. "Heat island" effects in urban areas due to the lack of vegetation trap heat, making people susceptible to the pathways through which heat affects mental health, as described earlier. Urban areas, especially urban slums, often face flooding hazards as well, triggering similar vulnerabilities for mental health outcomes for poorer urbanites in Bangladesh as well. Among migratory groups, women, children, and the elderly are consistently found to be the most vulnerable (Hayward & Ayeb-Karlsson, 2021).

### *15.3.6 Gender*

Women in Bangladesh face particular vulnerabilities regarding mental health in the context of climate change. The disproportionate impact of environmental adversities amplifies stressors that uniquely affect women's mental well-being. With their gender roles often tied to caregiving, household responsibilities, and agricultural labor, women bear the harshest of climate-related challenges, including increased workloads due to water scarcity, crop failures, and resource shortages (Ferdous & Mallick, 2019). Displacement caused by floods or other climate-related disasters disrupts family structures, leading to heightened distress and psychological strain as women manage household and familial needs amidst the chaos of environmental upheavals (Akhter et al., 2015; Ferdous & Mallick, 2019; Mostafizur Rahman et al., 2023). The initiation of migration or displacement can be an especially vulnerable period for women, with an increased risk of experiencing sexual violence exacerbating trauma and mental distress—even temporary displacement to shelters in the face of a climate threat can exacerbate these risks for women (Hayward & Ayeb-Karlsson, 2021). Additionally, the cultural norms of Bangladesh often restrict women's mobility and access to resources, limiting their ability to cope with and adapt to the mental health implications of climate change (Ferdous & Mallick, 2019). Additionally, the intersectionality of gender and socioeconomic status amplifies the mental health vulnerabilities of women in Bangladesh (Hayward & Ayeb-Karlsson, 2021). Limited access to education and economic opportunities restricts their ability to cope with climate-related shocks and recovery pathways can be delayed due to low prioritization of women's needs, intensifying mental health burdens (Shahriar & Shepherd, 2019). Addressing the mental health challenges specific to women in the context of climate change in Bangladesh necessitates integrative approaches that work with communities to co-create interventions that seek to empower women, enhance resilience, and prioritize their access to mental health support services, within the framework of broader and equitable climate adaptation and disaster response strategies.

## 15.4 The Way Forward: The Need for Interventions, Policy, and Research

Efforts to address the mental health impacts of climate change in Bangladesh will require multifaceted approaches, and pathways toward progress in this critical area are evolving. There is a growing recognition of the need to integrate mental health considerations into climate adaptation and disaster response strategies. Initiatives focusing on community resilience-building, psychosocial support, and mental health awareness are emerging to mitigate the mental health impacts of climate-related adversities. Interventions need to focus on providing psychosocial support, mental health services, and community-based resilience-building programs for affected populations. Additionally, policies that integrate mental health considerations into migration management strategies and urban development plans are crucial to mitigate the mental health vulnerabilities stemming from climate-induced migration. Collaborative efforts involving government agencies, NGOs, and community stakeholders are underway to create sustainable solutions that prioritize the mental well-being of climate-affected populations in Bangladesh. Comprehensive solutions will require sustained investments in mental health infrastructure, capacity building, and policy frameworks that prioritize both environmental resilience and psychological well-being in the face of ongoing climate challenges in Bangladesh. In Box 15.3, a case story of a climate migrant receiving services from the SAJIDA Foundation's mental health program is presented. The case demonstrates the viability of community-based interventions in bringing about positive mental health and well-being outcomes, using community-based resources.

**Box 15.3: Case story of a climate migrant receiving mental health services in Mongla.**

This case story was collected by SAJIDA Foundation staff working in Mongla. The beneficiary received mental health intervention and related support from SAJIDA Foundation's Climate Change Programme.

Fatima Begum (name has been changed), a mother of two, lives in an urban slum in the climate vulnerable town of Mongla. A climate migrant, she moved to the port city of Mongla with her husband around 12 years ago. She got married at a very early age and moved to Mongla for a better life. Her husband used to work in Mongla port.

"We weren't rich, but life was not so bad. My husband was abusive. He would torture me both physically and mentally. I accepted it for sake of my children, but last year he just abandoned me and never returned home. With two children and no income I was in deep trouble. I was so anxious, so depressed and full of fear for the future. I didn't know how to survive. I couldn't eat, sleep or think straight. I couldn't share my ordeals with others as I was full of shame. I blamed myself for everything, even though it wasn't my fault."

"Last year, I got to know about SAJIDA Foundation in a courtyard meeting. In that meeting, I first heard the words "Mental health" and I connected with it instantly. It was like the apa (female community mobilizer) was telling my story. I realized what I was going through is a mental health problem, and that it could happen due to lots of reasons. Like our physical health, our mental health also needs to be taken care of. After discussing my situation with SAJIDA Foundation's community mobilizer, I decided to attend the mental health sessions, and took five sessions. At the sessions we discussed my problems and develop a plan to overcome the issues step by step. Based on the plan I become a member of SAJIDA's income generating activities and got support with poultry, vegetables for homestead vegetable cultivation, and treatment for physical health issues. Slowly I began to recover from my depression and start planning for my future. Now I have a small cloth business and some poultry. I grow most of my vegetables in my homestead. I got the right intervention at the right time. Now I am doing much better both mentally and financially."

There is also a pronounced need for further research into the psychosocial vulnerabilities of Bangladeshi populations due to climate change. Specifically, research needs to examine risk and vulnerability across the life course, to identify age-stratified risk profiles for mental illness, to inform tailored strategies for the young, middle-aged, and older populations. Similarly, utilizing a lens of equity to inform research is paramount so the compounding effects of climate change on the well-being of minority populations, those affected disproportionately by poverty, disability, gender status, religious affiliations, migrants, etc., can be elucidated. There is also a critical need to identify causal mechanisms of change that connect exposure to heat and humidity to mental health outcomes, e.g., emotional dysregulation, thermoregulation disruption, sleep disturbances, etc. From a climate change adaptation perspective, identifying such mechanisms can inform the development of specific strategies that can target the salient pathways via which risk of mental illness manifests due to exposure to such climate-related stressors. Such an approach, therefore, would hypothetically have a higher likelihood of leading to salutary outcomes if interventions were designed to address empirically verified pathways via which mental illnesses emerge or worsen. Additionally, there is a crucial need to examine the effects of climate change on the full spectrum of mental illness—while the majority of research in Bangladesh has examined common mental disorders such as PTSD, depression, anxiety, etc., there needs to be research that examines impacts on dementia, schizophrenia, bipolar disorder, suicidality, etc., to understand the full scope of vulnerability faced by Bangladesh's population due to climate change. Finally, interventions need to be carefully adapted to the local culture and context to make efforts acceptable, destigmatized, and accessible for communities.

## 15.5 Conclusion

Bangladesh faces unique threats to mental health and well-being due to the unfolding climate crisis. There are multifaceted stressors that combine with existing sociocultural and economic vulnerabilities, to exacerbate suffering and distress. A holistic approach, involving research, policy, and practice, is necessary to fully understand and respond to this dynamic threat and safeguard the well-being of millions of vulnerable Bangladeshis living on the frontlines of climate change.

## References


Afsana, K., & Wahid, S. S. (2013). Health care for poor people in the urban slums of Bangladesh. *Lancet, 382*(9910), 2049–2051. https://doi.org/10.1016/s0140-6736(13)62295-3

Aguilar-Gaxiola, S., Al-Hamzawi, A., Alonso, J., Benjet, C., Bruffaerts, R., Chatterji, S., … Ten Have, M. (2018). Socio-economic variations in the mental health treatment gap for people with anxiety, mood, and substance use disorders: results from the WHO World Mental Health (WMH) surveys. *Psychol Med, 48*(9), 1560-1571. https://doi.org/10.1017/S0033291717003336.

Ahmed, B., Kelman, I., Kamruzzaman, M., Mohiuddin, H., Rahman, M. M., Das, A., … Shamsudduha, M. (2019). Indigenous people's responses to drought in northwest Bangladesh. *Environmental Development, 29*, 55-66. https://doi.org/10.1016/j.envdev.2018.11.004

Akhter, S. R., Sarkar, R. K., Dutta, M., Khanom, R., Akter, N., Chowdhury, M. R., & Sultan, M. (2015). Issues with families and children in a disaster context: A qualitative perspective from rural Bangladesh. *International Journal of Disaster Risk Reduction, 13*, 313–323. https://doi.org/10.1016/j.ijdrr.2015.07.011

Ayeb-Karlsson, S., Kniveton, D., & Cannon, T. (2020). Trapped in the prison of the mind: Notions of climate-induced (im) mobility decision-making and wellbeing from an urban informal settlement in Bangladesh. *Palgrave Communications, 6*(1), 1–15.

Azad, M. A. K., & Khan, M. M. (2015). Post disasters social pathology in Bangladesh: A case study on AILA affected areas. *Sociology and Anthropology, 3*(2), 85–94.

Bathiany, S., Dakos, V., Scheffer, M., & Lenton, T. M. Climate models predict increasing temperature variability in poor countries. *Science Advances, 4*(5), eaar5809. https://doi.org/10.1126/sciadv.aar5809.

Charlson, F., Ali, S., Benmarhnia, T., Pearl, M., Massazza, A., Augustinavicius, J., & Scott, J. G. (2021). Climate change and mental health: A scoping review. *Int J Environ Res Public Health, 18*(9). https://doi.org/10.3390/ijerph18094486.

Chen, Y., Tao, M., & Liu, W. (2020). High temperature impairs cognitive performance during a moderate intensity activity. *Building and Environment, 186*, 107372. https://doi.org/10.1016/j.buildenv.2020.107372

Costello, A., Abbas, M., Allen, A., Ball, S., Bell, S., Bellamy, R., … Patterson, C. (2009). Managing the health effects of climate change: Lancet and University College London Institute for Global Health Commission. *Lancet, 373*(9676), 1693-1733. https://doi.org/10.1016/s0140-6736(09)60935-1.

Eckstein, D. K. V., & Schafer, L. (2021). *Global Climate Risk Index 2021*. Retrieved from https://www.germanwatch.org/en/cri.

Ferdous, J., & Mallick, D. (2019). Norms, practices, and gendered vulnerabilities in the lower Teesta basin, Bangladesh. *Environmental Development, 31*, 88–96. https://doi.org/10.1016/j.envdev.2018.10.003

Gepp, S., Waid, J. L., Brombierstäudl, D., Kader, A., Müller-Hauser, A. A., Wendt, A. S., … Gabrysch, S. (2022). Impact of unseasonable flooding on women's food security and mental health in rural Sylhet, Bangladesh: a longitudinal observational study. *The Lancet Planetary Health, 6*, S14. https://doi.org/10.1016/S2542-5196(22)00276-5.

Hayes, K., & Poland, B. (2018). Addressing mental health in a changing climate: Incorporating mental health indicators into climate change and health vulnerability and adaptation assessments. *Int J Environ Res Public Health, 15*(9). https://doi.org/10.3390/ijerph15091806.

Hayward, G., & Ayeb-Karlsson, S. (2021). 'Seeing with empty eyes': A systems approach to understand climate change and mental health in Bangladesh. *Climatic Change, 165*(1), 29. https://doi.org/10.1007/s10584-021-03053-9

Hossain, A., Ahmed, B., Rahman, T., Sammonds, P., Zaman, S., Benzadid, S., & Jakariya, M. (2021). Household food insecurity, income loss, and symptoms of psychological distress among adults following the Cyclone Amphan in coastal Bangladesh. *PLoS ONE, 16*(11), e0259098. https://doi.org/10.1371/journal.pone.0259098

Im, E.-S., Pal Jeremy, S., & Eltahir Elfatih, A. B. (2017). Deadly heat waves projected in the densely populated agricultural regions of South Asia. *Science Advances, 3*(8), e1603322. https://doi.org/10.1126/sciadv.1603322

IPCC. (2021). *Climate Change 2021: The Physical Science Basis*. Retrieved from https://www.ipcc.ch/report/ar6/wg1/downloads/factsheets/IPCC_AR6_WGI_Regional_Fact_Sheet_Asia.pdf.

Kabir, R., Khan, H. T. A., Ball, E., & Caldwell, K. (2016). Climate change impact: the experience of the coastal areas of Bangladesh affected by Cyclones Sidr and Aila. *Journal of Environmental and Public Health, 2016*, 9654753. https://doi.org/10.1155/2016/9654753

Kabir, S. M. S. (2018). Psychological health challenges of the hill-tracts region for climate change in Bangladesh. *Asian Journal of Psychiatry, 34*, 74–77. https://doi.org/10.1016/j.ajp.2018.04.001

King, A. D., & Harrington, L. J. (2018). The inequality of climate change from 1.5 to 2 °C of global warming. *Geophysical Research Letters, 45*(10), 5030–5033. https://doi.org/10.1029/2018GL078430.

Liu, J., Varghese, B. M., Hansen, A., Xiang, J., Zhang, Y., Dear, K., ... Bi, P. (2021). Is there an association between hot weather and poor mental health outcomes? A systematic review and meta-analysis. *Environment International, 153*, 106533. https://doi.org/10.1016/j.envint.2021.106533.

Lõhmus, M. (2018). Possible biological mechanisms linking mental health and heat-a contemplative review. *Int J Environ Res Public Health, 15*(7). https://doi.org/10.3390/ijerph15071515.

Mahendran, R., Xu, R., Li, S., & Guo, Y. (2021). Interpersonal violence associated with hot weather. *The Lancet Planetary Health, 5*(9), e571–e572. https://doi.org/10.1016/S2542-5196(21)00210-2

Maîtrot, M., Wood, G., & Devine, J. (2021). Understanding resilience: Lessons from lived experiences of extreme poverty in Bangladesh. *Development Policy Review, 39*(6), 894–910. https://doi.org/10.1111/dpr.12543

Mamun, M. A., Safiq, M. B., Hosen, I., & Al Mamun, F. (2021). Suicidal behavior and flood effects in Bangladesh: a two-site interview study. *Risk Manag Healthc Policy, 14*, 129–142. https://doi.org/10.2147/rmhp.S282965

McMorris, T., Swain, J., Smith, M., Corbett, J., Delves, S., Sale, C., ... Potter, J. (2006). Heat stress, plasma concentrations of adrenaline, noradrenaline, 5-hydroxytryptamine and cortisol, mood state and cognitive performance. *Int J Psychophysiol, 61*(2), 204-215. https://doi.org/10.1016/j.ijpsycho.2005.10.002.

Miah, M., Rahman, M., Rahman, M., & Saha, S. (2016). Impacts of climate variability on major food crops in selected agro-ecosystems of Bangladesh. *Annals of Bangladesh Agriculture, 20*, 61–74.

Mostafizur Rahman, M., Alam Shobuj, I., Tanvir Hossain, M., & Tasnim, F. (2023). Impact of disaster on mental health of women: A case study on 2022 flash flood in Bangladesh. *International Journal of Disaster Risk Reduction, 96*, 103935. https://doi.org/10.1016/j.ijdrr.2023.103935

Mullick, M. S., Nahar, J. S., Chowdhury, N. F., Rahman, W., Islam, M. M., Qusar, M. S., … Shahidullah, M. (2014). Psychiatric disorders among the children of 5 to 18 years old of'SIDR'affected areas. *Bangabandhu Sheikh Mujib Medical University Journal, 7*(1), 20-26.

Nahar, N., Blomstedt, Y., Wu, B., Kandarina, I., Trisnantoro, L., & Kinsman, J. (2014). Increasing the provision of mental health care for vulnerable, disaster-affected people in Bangladesh. *BMC Public Health, 14*(1), 708. https://doi.org/10.1186/1471-2458-14-708

National Institute of Mental Health. (2019). *National Mental Health Survey of Bangladesh 2018–19: Provisional Fact Sheet*. Retrieved from https://www.who.int/docs/default-source/searo/.

Rahman, M., Tumon, M. S. H., Islam, M. M., Chen, N., Pham, Q. B., Ullah, K., … Dewan, A. (2023). Could climate change exacerbate droughts in Bangladesh in the future? *Journal of Hydrology, 625*, 130096. https://doi.org/10.1016/j.jhydrol.2023.130096.

Rashid, M. M. (2013). Migration to big cities from coastal villages of Bangladesh: An empirical analysis. *Glob J Hum Soc Sci, 13*(5), 28–36.

Rentschler, J., Salhab, M., & Jafino, B. A. (2022). Flood exposure and poverty in 188 countries. *Nature Communications, 13*(1), 3527. https://doi.org/10.1038/s41467-022-30727-4

Romanello, M., Napoli, C. d., Green, C., Kennard, H., Lampard, P., Scamman, D., … Costello, A. The 2023 report of the <em>Lancet</em> Countdown on health and climate change: the imperative for a health-centred response in a world facing irreversible harms. *The Lancet*. https://doi.org/10.1016/S0140-6736(23)01859-7.

Rony, M. K. K., & Alamgir, H. M. (2023). High temperatures on mental health: Recognizing the association and the need for proactive strategies—A perspective. *Health Science Reports, 6*(12), e1729. https://doi.org/10.1002/hsr2.1729

Sams, I. (2019). Climate induced migration and social mobility among migrants: Evidence from the southwest coastal region of Bangladesh. *Social Sciences, 8*(4), 147–159.

Shahid, S. (2012). Vulnerability of the power sector of Bangladesh to climate change and extreme weather events. *Regional Environmental Change, 12*(3), 595–606. https://doi.org/10.1007/s10113-011-0276-z

Shahriar, A. Z. M., & Shepherd, D. A. (2019). Violence against women and new venture initiation with microcredit: Self-efficacy, fear of failure, and disaster experiences. *Journal of Business Venturing, 34*(6), 105945. https://doi.org/10.1016/j.jbusvent.2019.06.006

Tasdik Hasan, M., Adhikary, G., Mahmood, S., Papri, N., Shihab, H. M., Kasujja, R., … Nasreen, M. (2020). Exploring mental health needs and services among affected population in a cyclone affected area in costal Bangladesh: a qualitative case study. *International Journal of Mental Health Systems, 14*(1), 12. https://doi.org/10.1186/s13033-020-00351-0.

Wahid, S. S., Raza, W. A., Mahmud, I., & Kohrt, B. A. (2023). Climate-related shocks and other stressors associated with depression and anxiety in Bangladesh: A nationally representative panel study. *The Lancet Planetary Health, 7*(2), e137–e146. https://doi.org/10.1016/S2542-5196(22)00315-1

Wahid, S. S., Sandberg, J., Sarker, M., Arafat, A., Apu, A. R., Rabbani, A., … Kohrt, B. A. (2021). A distress-continuum, disorder-threshold model of depression: a mixed-methods, latent class analysis study of slum-dwelling young men in Bangladesh. *BMC Psychiatry, 21*(1), 291. https://doi.org/10.1186/s12888-021-03259-2.

Wahid, S. S., Sarker, M., Arafat, A. S. M. E., Apu, A. R., & Kohrt, B. A. (2021b). Tension and other idioms of distress among slum dwelling young men: A qualitative study of depression in urban Bangladesh. *Culture, Medicine, and Psychiatry*. https://doi.org/10.1007/s11013-021-09735-4

# Chapter 16
# Technology-Based Interventions for Mental Health Support in Bangladesh

**Faisal Muhammad and S. M. Yasir Arafat**

**Abstract** This chapter explores the potential presence and role of technology-based interventions in addressing mental health challenges in Bangladesh. The technology landscape in Bangladesh is examined, focusing on the growth of information and communication technology, mobile internet usage, and smartphone adoption. E-mental health initiatives, including tele-psychiatry and tele-counseling platforms, mobile apps, and virtual reality applications, are promising approaches to bridge gaps in mental health support. The importance of combating stigma and raising mental health awareness is discussed, focusing on the role of technology, online campaigns, and collaborations between tech companies and mental health institutions. Challenges and future directions for technology-based interventions are addressed, including digital divide concerns, cultural relevance, data privacy, and funding. It emphasizes the transformative potential of technology-based interventions and the need for collaboration, evidence-based practices, and awareness-building efforts to foster a supportive mental health ecosystem in Bangladesh.

**Keywords** Bangladesh · Mental health · Technology-based interventions · Stigma · Online support groups

F. Muhammad
Department of Public Health, Faculty of Allied Health Sciences, Daffodil International University (DIU), Dhaka, Bangladesh

Faculty of Medicine and Health Sciences, Department of Public and Community Health, Frontier University Garowe (FUG), Garowe, Somalia

Otu Institute of Research and Training (OIRT), London, UK

S. M. Y. Arafat (✉)
Department of Psychiatry, Bangladesh Specialized Hospital Limited, Dhaka, Bangladesh
e-mail: arafatdmc62@gmail.com



S. M. Y. Arafat (ed.), *Mental Health in Bangladesh*,
https://doi.org/10.1007/978-981-97-0610-5_16

## 16.1 Introduction

Mental health is critical to overall well-being, and its significance is increasingly recognized in Bangladesh. Despite progress in various sectors, the country faces significant challenges in addressing mental health issues and ensuring adequate support for individuals with mental health disorders.

### *16.1.1 Overview of Mental Health Challenges in Bangladesh*

Bangladesh is home to a vast population, and mental health challenges affect people from all walks of life. Common mental health disorders in the country include depression, anxiety, bipolar disorder, and post-traumatic stress disorder (PTSD). These conditions can severely impact individuals' lives, affecting their relationships, work performance, and overall quality of life (Ministry of Health & Family Welfare, 2021). Several factors, including poverty, unemployment, natural disasters, and exposure to violence, further exacerbate mental health challenges (Makwana, 2019; Thurston et al., 2021). In addition, the stigma surrounding mental health remains a significant barrier to seeking help and support. Many individuals with mental health issues hesitate to seek professional help due to fear of judgment and discrimination (Ministry of Health & Family Welfare, 2021).

### *16.1.2 Prevalence of Mental Health Disorders & Barriers to Accessing Mental Health Services*

The prevalence of mental health disorders in Bangladesh is substantial. According to a recent mental health survey, approximately 18.7% of the population suffers from mental disorders (Ministry of Health & Family Welfare, 2021). However, the numbers might be higher as mental health issues are often underreported. The survey also revealed that the mental health treatment gap was 91%. One of the primary barriers to accessing mental health services is the country's scarcity of mental health professionals. There is a significant shortage of psychiatrists, psychologists, and other mental health specialists, particularly in rural areas (Arafat et al., 2024). As a result, many individuals do not have easy access to mental health care. The stigma surrounding mental health also acts as a deterrent to seeking help. Negative attitudes and misconceptions about mental illnesses prevent people from openly discussing their mental health concerns and seeking appropriate treatment. This stigma can lead to social isolation and hinder the recovery process.

Moreover, insufficient awareness about available mental health services and resources contributes to low help-seeking behavior (Sanghvi & Mehrotra, 2020).

Many individuals and communities may not be aware of the options for mental health support and treatment.

## 16.2 Technology Landscape in Bangladesh

Technology has rapidly advanced in Bangladesh, contributing to various aspects of daily life, including healthcare and mental health support. In recent years, the country has witnessed significant progress in information technology, telecommunications, and digital infrastructure, paving the way for developing and implementing technology-based interventions for mental health.

### *16.2.1 Overview of Technological Advancements in Bangladesh*

Bangladesh has experienced remarkable technological advancements, particularly in information and communication technology (ICT) (Eusuf et al., 2022). The government and private sector have actively invested in developing the ICT sector, fostering innovation, and expanding digital services nationwide. The growth of the ICT sector has led to improved digital infrastructure, making high-speed internet connectivity more accessible to the population.

- ***Telecommunications and Internet Penetration:*** Bangladesh's telecommunications sector saw significant growth in the 2000s, with the introduction of mobile phones and the expansion of telecommunication networks (Aminuzzaman et al., 2003; Bayes et al., 1999). According to recent statistics, internet penetration has surged by about 38.9% of the population (Kemp, 2023), compared to less than 1% in the early 2000s (Internet Live Stats, 2016).
- ***E-Governance and Digital Services:*** In the current decade (2020s), Bangladesh has made substantial progress in e-governance and digital services (Al Mamun et al., 2021; Hossain, 2022). Initiatives like the National Portal (Bangladesh.gov.bd) offer various online government services, reducing bureaucratic hurdles. Adopting digital systems has contributed to increased efficiency, transparency, and citizen engagement.
- ***Fintech and Digital Payments:*** Fintech has emerged as a transformative force in the financial sector in the current decade (Noor, 2021). Mobile financial services and digital payment platforms have gained widespread acceptance. The percentage of adults with access to formal financial services has grown from around 10% in the early 2000s (Khalily, 2016; Mujeri, 2015) to over 50% in recent years (Mahmud, 2023; TBS Report, 2023).
- ***IT Industry and Outsourcing:*** In the early 2000s, the IT industry in Bangladesh was in its nascent stage, with limited recognition on the global stage (Centre for

Research and Information, 2017). However, in this decade (2020s) Bangladesh's IT industry has expanded significantly, especially in software development and outsourcing (Hossain et al., 2012). The country has become a notable player in the global IT outsourcing market, with an annual growth rate of around 30%. The sector's contribution to the GDP has risen from less than 1% to over 2% in the past two decades (Rahman, 2014; THOLONS, 2015; Ahmed, 2019).

### 16.2.2 Internet Connectivity & Accessibility and Penetration Rates (Internet and Mobile)

Internet connectivity and accessibility have significantly improved in Bangladesh (Azad & Islam, 2022). In collaboration with private sector entities, the government's efforts have led to expanding internet infrastructure, particularly in urban areas. As a result, a more significant portion of the population now has access to the Internet. Mobile internet usage has also witnessed tremendous growth, thanks to the widespread adoption of smartphones and affordable data plans. Mobile phones have become a primary means of internet access for many Bangladeshis, even in rural and remote regions (Saif, 2023).

The evolution of internet connectivity and accessibility in Bangladesh has driven the nation's technological progress and socio-economic development (Ashraf et al., 2017). In the early 2000s, internet connectivity in Bangladesh was limited and primarily available in urban areas (Islam & Rahman, 2006; Azad & Islam, 2004). Internet penetration was extremely low, with only a small fraction of the population accessing online resources. The digital divide between urban and rural regions was stark, hindering the widespread adoption of the internet (Hasan & Zaman, 2023). As of the current decade (2020s), Bangladesh has experienced a remarkable surge in internet penetration, driven by increased availability and affordability of smartphones, data plans, and improved infrastructure (GSMA, 2021). According to recent data, the internet penetration rate in Bangladesh has surpassed 50% of the population (Bangladesh Telecommunication Regulatory Commission, 2021), showcasing a significant increase from less than 1% in the early 2000s (Azam, 2007; Roknuzzaman, 2006).

The expansion of mobile networks, particularly 3G and 4G technologies, has been a major catalyst for enhancing internet accessibility across Bangladesh (Haque et al., 2021). Bangladesh's government's efforts to promote digitalization and connectivity have played a crucial role in bridging the digital divide and boosting internet accessibility. The "Digital Bangladesh" vision launched in 2009 aimed to transform the nation into a knowledge-based society, promoting information technology in all spheres of life (Islam & Grönlund, 2011).

### *16.2.3 Utilization of Smartphones and Digital Devices*

Smartphones and digital devices have become increasingly prevalent in Bangladesh (Hossain & Ahmed, 2016; Islam et al., 2021c; Ratan et al., 2022). The popularity of smartphones has opened up new opportunities for technology-based interventions, including mobile apps for mental health support, tele-psychiatry, and virtual reality applications. These devices enable individuals to access mental health resources and support conveniently, regardless of location (Thomee, 2018). The technology landscape in Bangladesh presents an optimistic outlook for implementing e-mental health initiatives (WHO, 2020). Leveraging the increasing internet connectivity, smartphone adoption, and digital literacy, technology-based interventions can bridge the gap in mental health support and reach more individuals in need of assistance.

The adoption and utilization of smartphones and digital devices have profoundly impacted Bangladesh's technological landscape, revolutionizing communication, information access, and service delivery (Hossain et al., 2023).

## 16.3 E-Mental Health Initiatives in Bangladesh

In response to the growing mental health challenges and the increasing potential of technology, Bangladesh has seen the emergence of various e-mental health initiatives. These interventions aim to leverage digital platforms and technology to provide accessible and effective mental health support to the population.

Several e-mental health programs have been established in Bangladesh to address the mental health needs of its citizens (WHO, 2020). These initiatives encompass a range of approaches, from online counseling platforms to mobile applications and tele-psychiatry services. Online counseling platforms offer virtual counseling sessions with mental health professionals. These platforms provide a safe and confidential space for individuals to discuss their mental health concerns and receive professional guidance. Mobile apps for mental health support have gained popularity in Bangladesh (Islam et al., 2021a). These apps offer a variety of features, including mood tracking, meditation, mindfulness exercises, and access to mental health resources. Tele-psychiatry services utilize telecommunications technology to connect mental health professionals with individuals seeking support (Chakrabarti, 2015). This approach is precious for remote or underserved individuals with limited access to in-person mental health services. Although still in the early stages, virtual reality applications have been explored as a potential tool for mental health interventions in Bangladesh (Koly et al., 2022a). Virtual reality can create immersive and interactive experiences that aid in therapeutic interventions.

Several non-governmental organizations (NGOs) have played vital roles in supporting mental health initiatives and addressing mental health challenges in Bangladesh (Hasan et al., 2021; Sen et al., 2023; UNICEF, 2021). These organizations have contributed significantly to raising awareness, counseling, and promoting mental well-being. While their roles may vary, their collective efforts have helped advance mental health services and reduce stigma.

- ***Mental Health and Psychosocial Support (MHPSS) Program:*** It is implemented by various organizations, including the United Nations Children's Fund (UNICEF) and Bangladesh Rehabilitation Assistance Committee (BRAC); this program aims to provide mental health and psychosocial support services to vulnerable populations, especially children and adolescents (Uddin et al., 2020).
- ***Moner Bondhu:*** An online platform that offers mental health counseling and support services through trained mental health professionals. It gives individuals a confidential space to discuss their mental health concerns.
- ***Somoy Foundation:*** It offers needy individuals online counseling services and mental health resources. They aim to reduce the stigma surrounding mental health and promote emotional well-being (https://www.facebook.com/handsforbetterment/).
- ***Anjuman Mufidul Islam:*** Anjuman Mufidul Islam operates several mental health clinics in Bangladesh, offering counseling and treatment services for individuals experiencing mental health issues (https://www.anjumanmibd.org/).

## 16.4 Tele-Psychiatry and Tele-Counseling Services

Tele-psychiatry involves conducting psychiatric consultations and assessments through video conferencing or telecommunication platforms. It allows individuals to access mental health services from the comfort of their homes, overcoming geographical barriers and reducing travel needs (Malhotra et al., 2022). In Bangladesh, where there is a shortage of mental health professionals (Arafat et al., 2024), especially in rural and remote regions, tele-psychiatry holds immense potential. It can help address the inequitable distribution of mental health services and extend the reach of psychiatrists to underserved communities. Additionally, tele-psychiatry can be instrumental in providing specialized care to individuals with complex mental health conditions who may not have easy access to specialized psychiatric facilities.

- ***International Centre for Diarrhoeal Disease Research, Bangladesh (ICDDR, B):*** ICDDR, B has been involved in tele-psychiatry projects that focus on providing mental health services to underserved and vulnerable populations in Bangladesh (Arafat et al., 2024)
- ***Tele-psychiatry Research and Innovation Network Ltd (TRIN):*** TRIN has been working in Bangladesh to promote, foster development, and assist the studies of the acquisition, dissemination, and application of knowledge and information concerning technology-aided health research in all its aspects, including mental health and psychosocial issues.

## 16.5 Mobile Technology and Mental Health in Bangladesh

Mobile technology has become a powerful tool for addressing Bangladesh's mental health challenges (Koly et al., 2022a). It enables the delivery of mental health information, support, and interventions directly to individuals, bridging gaps in access to traditional services. Several mobile apps have been developed to provide a spectrum of mental health support. Here are some potential apps in Bangladesh and their spectrum of use:

- ***Moner Bondhu:*** Moner Bondhu's mobile app extends its tele-counseling services to a digital platform. Users can access confidential mental health counseling, connect with trained professionals, and seek support for various mental health concerns.
- ***Daktarbhai:*** Healthcare Information System Ltd. presents "Daktarbhai," a one-stop digital health service solution for the people of Bangladesh. Daktarbhai is an initiative to facilitate the next generation of healthcare in Bangladesh by providing services in Psychiatry, family medicine, Internal medicine, dental, and many more.
- ***Zaynax Health***: This app provides access to proper healthcare wherever and whenever required to bridge the gap between healthcare service providers and service seekers across Bangladesh. Their services are in Psychiatry, Cardiology, General Medicine, Urology, etc. The app is owned by Zaynax Health, Bangladesh.
- ***MILVIK Health + :*** This app provides home-based remove doctor support and financial protection. This app is owned by MILVIK (Known globally as BIMA) Bangladesh Ltd., which uses mobile technology to deliver affordable insurance and health products. This app provides healthcare services, including mental health support.
- ***LifePlus Bangladesh:*** It is a one-stop digital healthcare service in Bangladesh. This app brings ease to the healthcare journey in various fields such as Psychiatry, Nutrition, Cardiology, Medicine, Dermatology, Neurology, etc..
- ***DocTime:*** It is an online Medical Service provider in Bangladesh created to become the first point of contact for health, well-being, and happiness. Their services include Psychiatry, Psychology, Internal Medicine, Dermatology, gastroenterology and many more.
- ***Maya—It's OK to ask for help:*** It was created to ensure daily wellness. This app gathered hundreds of doctors, psychiatrists, and beauticians. A Bangladesh-origin and Singapore-based digital Healthcare company owns the Maya app.

### *16.5.1 Role of Mobile Technology in Global Mental Health Initiatives*

Mobile technology has played a significant role in global mental health initiatives, particularly in low- and middle-income countries (LMICs) like Bangladesh (Farrington et al., 2014; Carter et al., 2022). Mobile apps and digital platforms have been developed to provide mental health information, self-help resources, and evidence-based therapeutic interventions. Mobile technology enables individuals to access mental health support discreetly and conveniently. With mobile apps, people can self-assess, track their moods and progress, practice mindfulness, and access resources related to various mental health conditions (Flanagan, 2016).

### *16.5.2 Review of Mobile Apps for Mental Health Support in Other Contexts*

Mobile apps for mental health support have been widely adopted worldwide (Lipschitz et al., 2019). These apps offer diverse features like guided meditation, cognitive behavioral therapy exercises, stress management tools, and mental health assessments. Some apps use artificial intelligence and machine learning algorithms to personalize interventions and track users' progress (Gotzl et al., 2022). They also provide interactive and engaging content to keep users motivated and committed to their mental well-being.

### *16.5.3 Potential Benefits and Challenges of Using Mobile Apps in Bangladesh*

In the context of Bangladesh, mobile apps for mental health support offer several potential benefits:

i. Increased Accessibility: Mobile apps can reach individuals in urban and rural areas, expanding access to mental health support nationwide.
ii. Cost-Effectiveness: Mobile apps can be cost-effective compared to traditional in-person interventions, making mental health resources more affordable and scalable.
iii. Anonymity and Privacy: Mobile apps allow individuals to engage in self-help and therapy anonymously, which can reduce the stigma associated with seeking mental health support.

Despite these benefits, challenges exist in the implementation of mobile apps for mental health support in Bangladesh:

i. Digital Literacy: Some segments of the population may face challenges in using mobile apps due to limited digital literacy.
ii. Language Barriers: Ensuring that the content and resources in mobile apps are available in local languages is essential for widespread adoption.
iii. Cultural Relevance: Tailoring the content and interventions to be culturally relevant and sensitive is crucial for user engagement and effectiveness.

## 16.6 Virtual Reality (VR) and Augmented Reality (AR) Applications

Virtual Reality (VR) and Augmented Reality (AR) are innovative technologies that have shown promise in various fields, including mental health interventions. These immersive technologies offer unique opportunities to create impactful and engaging experiences that can be utilized to support mental health in Bangladesh.

### *16.6.1 VR and AR in Mental Health Interventions*

VR involves creating a computer-generated, three-dimensional environment that users can interact with using special headsets and controllers (Baker & Fairclough, 2022). AR, on the other hand, overlays digital content in the real-world environment, often viewed through smartphones or AR glasses.

In mental health interventions, VR and AR can be used in various ways:

- o Exposure Therapy: VR can create virtual environments to facilitate exposure therapy for individuals with anxiety disorders or phobias. This allows them to confront their fears in a controlled and safe setting (Boeldt et al., 2019; Rothbaum & Hodges, 1999).
- o Mindfulness and Relaxation: VR and AR applications can offer immersive mindfulness and relaxation experiences, helping individuals reduce stress and anxiety (Ma et al., 2023).
- o Coping Skills Training: These technologies can teach coping strategies and problem-solving skills by simulating challenging situations and guiding users through the process (Core et al., 2006).
- o Distraction during Medical Procedures: VR and AR can be utilized as distraction techniques during medical procedures, reducing anxiety and pain perception (Aminabadi et al., 2012; Koticha et al., 2019).

### *16.6.2 Overview of VR and AR in Bangladesh*

Certainly, while VR (Virtual Reality) and AR (Augmented Reality) applications are still in the early stages of development in Bangladesh, their potential for mental health support is promising. As technology infrastructure continues to improve and digital accessibility expands, these immersive technologies could significantly address mental health challenges.

a. **Existing VR and AR Applications**

- ***MindCalm VR:*** This VR application provides guided meditation and relaxation experiences using immersive virtual environments. Users can engage in calming scenarios that help reduce stress and anxiety.

- ***Virtually Better Bangladesh:*** Virtual reality exposure therapy could be adapted for various mental health conditions, helping individuals confront and manage their fears or triggers in a controlled, immersive environment.
- ***Therachat AR:*** An augmented reality app that encourages users to engage in positive mental health practices through interactive activities and reminders.

b. **Potential VR and AR Applications**

- ***Virtual Therapy Sessions:*** VR could create simulated therapy environments, allowing individuals to engage in counseling sessions or exposure therapy in a virtual setting, enhancing accessibility and comfort.
- ***Mindfulness and Relaxation:*** AR applications could offer interactive mindfulness exercises, helping users practice deep breathing, meditation, and relaxation techniques in their real-world surroundings.
- ***Virtual Support Groups:*** VR environments could simulate group therapy sessions, connecting individuals with similar challenges to share experiences, receive peer support, and engage in therapeutic discussions.
- ***Skills Training:*** VR and AR could be used to develop interactive modules for teaching coping skills, stress management techniques, and emotional regulation strategies.
- ***Cultural Sensitivity and Customization:*** VR and AR apps could be tailored to reflect Bangladesh's cultural context, making mental health support more relatable and relevant for users.
- ***Positive Visualization:*** AR could provide users with tools to create and interact with positive visualizations, helping them shift their focus to more uplifting perspectives.

### *16.6.3 Challenges and Prospects of VR and AR in Bangladesh*

The integration of VR and AR in mental health interventions in Bangladesh may face several challenges:

i. ***Technical Infrastructure:*** VR and AR technologies require robust technological infrastructure, including high-speed internet and advanced computing capabilities. Ensuring widespread access to such infrastructure may be challenging, especially in rural areas.
ii. ***Cost:*** VR and AR technologies can be expensive, including the equipment and software required. Cost considerations must be considered while developing and implementing VR and AR applications for mental health support.
iii. ***Training and Expertise:*** Mental health professionals need training to use VR and AR technologies effectively in therapeutic settings. Providing training and support for professionals may require additional resources.

Despite these challenges, the prospects of VR and AR in mental health interventions in Bangladesh are promising. As technology advances and becomes more affordable, VR and AR applications can become increasingly accessible and effective in addressing mental health challenges in the country.

## 16.7 Online Support Groups and Peer-To-Peer Platforms

Online support groups and peer-to-peer platforms have become valuable resources for individuals seeking mental health support and connection. These virtual communities provide a safe and supportive environment for individuals to share their experiences, seek advice, and offer mutual encouragement, fostering a sense of belonging and reducing feelings of isolation. Social support promotes mental health and well-being (Harandi et al., 2017). Connecting with others with similar experiences can reduce loneliness and help individuals cope with challenges more effectively. Supportive relationships can provide validation, empathy, and practical advice, leading to improved mental health outcomes. Online support groups and peer-to-peer platforms have gained traction in Bangladesh as effective means of providing mental health support, connecting individuals with similar experiences, and reducing feelings of isolation (Mantracare, 2023).

In Bangladesh the LGBTQ + organizations have support groups and peer-to-peer platforms like *Bandhu Social Welfare Society* and *Boys of Bangladesh (BoB).* These organizations play a crucial role in providing support, fostering a sense of community, and reducing isolation for LGBTQ + individuals in Bangladesh.

i. ***Bandhu Social Welfare Society:*** Bandhu is a prominent organization in Bangladesh that offers mental health and psychosocial support to sexual minority groups, including transgender individuals and men who have sex with men (MSM) (https://www.bandhu-bd.org/).
ii. ***Boys of Bangladesh (BoB):*** While Boys of Bangladesh (BoB) primarily focuses on creating a sense of community and providing social support for gay men in Bangladesh, they often serve as a platform for members to share their mental health concerns and seek peer support (http://www.boysofbangladesh.org/).

## 16.8 Combating Stigma and Raising Mental Health Awareness

### *16.8.1 The Role of Technology in Reducing Mental Health Stigma in Bangladesh*

Technology provides a practical and far-reaching platform to challenge misconceptions and stigma surrounding mental health (Rodriguez-Rivas et al., 2022). By disseminating accurate information, personal stories, and positive narratives about mental health, technology can destigmatize mental illnesses and promote open conversations. Digital platforms offer opportunities to educate the public, health professionals, and policymakers about mental health conditions, treatment options, and the importance of seeking support. Online resources can help dispel myths and provide evidence-based information, leading to a better-informed society that is more understanding and supportive of individuals with mental health challenges.

### 16.8.2 Online Campaigns and Social Media for Awareness-Raising

Online campaigns and social media have proven to be powerful tools for mental health awareness-raising globally (Latha et al., 2020). In Bangladesh, social media platforms such as Facebook, Twitter, and Instagram have a significant user base, making them ideal for disseminating mental health information and resources (Islam et al., 2021b; Koly et al., 2022b; Nandy et al., 2022). Mental health organizations, NGOs, and government agencies can launch online campaigns that promote mental health literacy, challenge stereotypes, and encourage help-seeking behavior. Engaging visuals, personal stories, and user-generated content can create a community and encourage mental health discussion. Social media influencers and celebrities can also play a positive role by using their platforms to raise awareness, share personal experiences, and advocate for mental health support. Online campaigns and social media initiatives have become powerful tools for raising awareness about mental health issues, combating stigma, and promoting open discussions in Bangladesh (Latha et al., 2020). Here are some specific names of campaigns and initiatives:

- #LetsTalkBD: Organized by the World Health Organization (WHO) Bangladesh. The campaign aims to encourage open conversations about mental health and raise awareness.
- #MentalHealthMatters: This hashtag is used to share information, stories, and resources related to mental health awareness and support in Bangladesh.

### 16.8.3 Overview of Collaborations Between Tech Companies and Mental Health Institutions

Collaborations between tech companies and mental health institutions can lead to innovative solutions that promote mental health awareness and support. Tech companies can provide resources, technical expertise, and digital platforms, while mental health institutions contribute clinical knowledge and evidence-based practices. These collaborations may result in the development of mental health apps, online screening tools, and digital resources that are user-friendly, culturally relevant, and accessible to a broad audience. Additionally, partnerships can help ensure the ethical use of technology and safeguard user data and privacy. By working together, tech companies and mental health institutions can leverage each other's strengths to create impactful initiatives that foster a supportive and inclusive environment for mental health in Bangladesh. In Bangladesh, the information regarding this type of collaboration is limited or unavailable.

## 16.9 Coping with Challenges

As technology-based interventions for mental health support continue to evolve in Bangladesh, it is essential to address various challenges and plan for future directions to ensure their effectiveness and sustainability.

### *16.9.1 Addressing Barriers to Technology-Based Mental Health Interventions*

To fully realize the potential of technology-based mental health interventions, several barriers must be addressed:

a. Digital Divide: Bridging the digital divide is crucial to ensure that technology-based interventions are accessible to all population segments, including those in rural and underserved areas (Chang et al., 2004; Vassilakopoulou & Hustad, 2023).
b. Internet Connectivity: Improving internet connectivity in remote regions is necessary to enable individuals to access online mental health resources and services (Too et al., 2020).
c. Affordability: Ensuring that technology and data plans are affordable for all individuals is essential to prevent further disparities in accessing mental health support (Teachman et al., 2022).
d. Technical Literacy: Promoting digital literacy among the population will empower individuals to use technology-based mental health tools effectively (Altaf et al., 2023).

### *16.9.2 Overcoming Digital Literacy and Language Challenges*

Digital literacy can pose a significant challenge in adopting technology-based mental health interventions (Li, 2023). Providing user-friendly interfaces and clear instructions can help individuals navigate these platforms more effectively. Additionally, offering resources in local languages will make interventions more inclusive and culturally relevant.

### 16.9.3 Integrating Technology with Traditional Mental Health Services

Integrating technology-based interventions with traditional mental health services is crucial in creating a comprehensive mental health support system (Graham et al., 2021; Feijt et al., 2022). Collaboration between mental health professionals, technology experts, and policymakers is essential to ensure seamless integration and data sharing while maintaining client confidentiality and ethical considerations. Hybrid models that combine in-person counseling with technology-based follow-up or support can be particularly effective in ensuring continuity of care and optimizing treatment outcomes (Wentzel et al., 2016).

### 16.9.4 Ensuring Data Privacy and Security

As technology plays a significant role in mental health support, safeguarding user data and privacy becomes paramount (Bondre et al., 2021). Organizations and developers must adhere to strict data protection guidelines to maintain trust and confidence among users. Implementing secure and encrypted communication channels can protect sensitive information and prevent data breaches (Arora et al., 2014).

### 16.9.5 Strengthening Evidence-Based Practices

Certainly, evidence-based practices are crucial for ensuring the effectiveness and impact of technology-based mental health interventions. In Bangladesh, as technology is increasingly integrated into mental health services, rigorous research and evaluation play a vital role in shaping these interventions. Here's an example of evidence-based practices in the Bangladeshi context:

**Example:** Mental Health and Psychosocial Support (MHPSS) Programs by BRAC and UNICEF.

BRAC, a prominent non-governmental organization in Bangladesh, and UNICEF have collaborated on Mental Health and Psychosocial Support (MHPSS) programs. These programs aim to provide evidence-based mental health interventions to vulnerable populations, particularly children and adolescents, who may have experienced trauma, conflict, or other psychosocial challenges. The MHPSS programs incorporate technology as a part of their interventions, utilizing evidence-based practices to deliver mental health support. Here's how the evidence-based approach is implemented:

- Assessment: The programs begin with thorough assessments to identify mental health needs within specific communities and populations.

- Culturally Appropriate Interventions: Interventions are culturally tailored and grounded in Bangladesh to ensure relevance and effectiveness.
- Use of Technology: Technology, including mobile phones and online platforms, is used to reach a larger audience and provide timely support.
- Training and Capacity Building: Mental health professionals and community workers are trained in evidence-based practices to deliver interventions effectively.
- Ongoing Monitoring and Evaluation: Rigorous monitoring and evaluation are conducted to measure the impact of interventions, gather feedback, and make necessary improvements.
- Research and Adaptation: Insights from the evaluation process are used to adapt and refine interventions over time, ensuring they remain evidence-based and effective.

By incorporating technology into evidence-based MHPSS programs, organizations like BRAC and UNICEF can provide scalable and accessible mental health support to a wider population. Integrating technology allows for innovative approaches while maintaining the rigor of evidence-based practices.

### *16.9.6 Capacity Building and Training*

Building mental health professionals' capacity to utilize technology-based interventions effectively is essential. Providing training on using tele-psychiatry platforms, mobile apps, and virtual reality applications will enable mental health professionals to integrate technology into their practice confidently.

### *16.9.7 Collaboration and Public–private Partnerships*

Collaboration among government agencies, mental health institutions, tech companies, NGOs, and community organizations is critical to foster a multi-dimensional approach to mental health support. Public–private partnerships can lead to innovative solutions, more significant resource mobilization, and broader reach.

### *16.9.8 Sustainable Funding and Resource Allocation*

Sustainable funding and resource allocation are essential for developing, implementing, and maintaining technology-based mental health interventions (Graham et al., 2020). Government support, international aid, and corporate social responsibility initiatives can play a vital role in ensuring the continuity and scalability of these programs.

## 16.10 Conclusion

Bangladesh's mental health support field is undergoing significant transformations, driven by advancements in technology and a growing recognition of the importance of mental well-being. Technology-based interventions have emerged as promising tools to address the mental health challenges in the country, providing innovative and accessible solutions to support individuals in need. E-mental health initiatives, such as online counseling platforms, mobile apps, tele-psychiatry, virtual reality, and peer-to-peer platforms, offer opportunities to reach a broader population and provide support regardless of geographical location. To fully harness the potential of technology-based mental health interventions, addressing challenges such as the digital divide, digital literacy disparities, data privacy concerns, and the need for culturally relevant content is crucial. Collaboration among mental health professionals, technology experts, government agencies, NGOs, and community organizations is essential to develop and implement comprehensive and evidence-based solutions. Technology can be pivotal in challenging misconceptions, disseminating accurate information, and fostering open conversations about mental health. As technology advances and becomes more accessible, investing in research and evaluation is essential to ensure the effectiveness and ethical use of technology-based interventions. Rigorous evaluation of these interventions will contribute to evidence-based practices and inform future developments in the field. The future of mental health support in Bangladesh lies in a balanced approach integrating technology with traditional mental health services. Bangladesh can foster a healthier and more resilient society by creating a supportive ecosystem that embraces technology, addresses challenges, and prioritizes mental health.

## References


Ahmed, A. (2019). How outsourcing jobs are booming in Bangladesh?. Retrieved September 15, 2023, from https://medium.com/@akibahmed/how-outsourcing-jobs-are-booming-in-bangladesh-2019-f6eebb31972c.

Al Mamun, A., Islam, S., Arifuzzaman, M., & Suhaimi, M. A. B. (2021). E-Government services for sustainable development: The challenges and strategies of implementing E-Government in Bangladesh. *International Journal of Computer Science and Information Technology Research, 9*(1), 65–74.

Altaf Dar, M., Maqbool, M., Ara, I., & Zehravi, M. (2023). The intersection of technology and mental health: Enhancing access and care. *International Journal of Adolescent Medicine and Health, 35*(5), 423–428. https://doi.org/10.1515/ijamh-2023-0113

Aminabadi, N. A., Erfanparast, L., Sohrabi, A., Oskouei, S. G., & Naghili, A. (2012). The impact of virtual reality distraction on pain and anxiety during dental treatment in 4–6 year-old children: A randomized controlled clinical trial. *Journal of Dental Research, Dental Clinics, Dental Prospects, 6*(4), 117.

Aminuzzaman, S., Baldersheim, H., & Jamil, I. (2003). Talking back! Empowerment and mobile phones in rural Bangladesh: A study of the village phone scheme of Grameen Bank. *Contemporary South Asia, 12*(3), 327–348.

Arafat, S. M. Y, Giasuddin, N. A., & Mazumder, A. H. (2024). Access to mental health care in Bangladesh – Current status, potential challenges, and ways out. In S. M. Y. Arafat & S. K. Kar (Eds.), *Access to mental health care in South Asia – Current status, potential challenges, and ways out*. Singapore: Springer Nature. https://doi.org/10.1007/978-981-99-9153-2_3

Arora, S., Yttri, J., & Nilsen, W. (2014). Privacy and security in mobile health (mHealth) research. *Alcohol Research: Current Reviews, 36*(1), 143–151. https://www.ncbi.nlm.nih.gov/pmc/articles/PMC4432854/

Ashraf, M., Grunfeld, H., Hoque, M. R., & Alam, K. (2017). An extended conceptual framework to understand information and communication technology-enabled socio-economic development at community level in Bangladesh. *Information Technology & People, 30*(4), 736–752.

Azad, K. A, & Islam, N. (2022). Overview of internet access in Bangladesh: Impact, barriers, and solutions. Retrieved July 30, 2023, from https://web.archive.org/web/20160103124803/https://www.isoc.org/inet97/proceedings/E3/E3_1.HTM.

Azam, S. (2007). Internet adoption and usage in Bangladesh. *Japanese Journal of Administrative Science, 20*(1), 43–54.

Baker, C., & Fairclough, S. H. (2022). Adaptive virtual reality. *Current Research in Neuroadaptive Technology*, pp. 159–176. https://doi.org/10.1016/B978-0-12-821413-8.00014-2.

Bangladesh Telecommunication Regulatory Commission. (2021). Internet Subscribers in Bangladesh. Retrieved September 15, 2023, from http://www.btrc.gov.bd/content/internet-subscribers-bangladesh-march-2021.

Bayes, A., Von Braun, J., & Akhter, R. (1999). *Village pay phones and poverty reduction: Insights from a Grameen Bank initiative in Bangladesh* (No. 8). ZEF Discussion Papers On Development Policy.

Boeldt, D., McMahon, E., McFaul, M., & Greenleaf, W. (2019). Using virtual reality exposure therapy to enhance treatment of anxiety disorders: Identifying areas of clinical adoption and potential obstacles. *Frontiers in Psychiatry, 10*, 773. https://doi.org/10.3389/fpsyt.2019.00773

Bondre, A., Pathare, S., & Naslund, J. A. (2021). Protecting mental health data privacy in India: the case of data linkage with Aadhaar. *Global Health: Science and Practice, 9*(3), 467–480. https://doi.org/10.9745/GHSP-D-20-00346

Carter, H., Araya, R., Anjur, K., Deng, D., & Naslund, J. A. (2021). The emergence of digital mental health in low-income and middle-income countries: A review of recent advances and implications for the treatment and prevention of mental disorders. *Journal of Psychiatric Research, 133*, 223. https://doi.org/10.1016/j.jpsychires.2020.12.016

Chakrabarti, S. (2015). Usefulness of telepsychiatry: A critical evaluation of videoconferencing-based approaches. *World Journal of Psychiatry, 5*(3), 286–304. https://doi.org/10.5498/wjp.v5.i3.286

Chang, B. L., Bakken, S., Brown, S. S., Houston, T. K., Kreps, G. L., Kukafka, R., ... & Stavri, P. Z. (2004). Bridging the digital divide: reaching vulnerable populations. *Journal of the American Medical Informatics Association, 11*(6), 448-457.

Core, M., Traum, D., Lane, H. C., Swartout, W., Gratch, J., & Marsella, S. (2006). Teaching negotiation skills through practice and reflection with virtual humans. *SIMULATION*. https://doi.org/10.1177/0037549706075542

CRI. (2017). Bangladesh's digital revolution. Retrieved July 30, 2023, from https://cri.org.bd/publication/digital-revolution/Bangladesh's%20Digital%20Revolution.pdf.

Eusuf, M. A., Ahmed, N., & Khan, M. M. Z. (2022). Stepping up ICT growth engine. UNDP Bangladesh. Retrieved July 8, 2023, from https://www.undp.org/bangladesh/news/stepping-ict-growth-engine.

Farrington, C., Aristidou, A., & Ruggeri, K. (2014). MHealth and global mental health: Still waiting for the mH2 wedding? *Globalization and Health, 10*(1), 1–8.

Feijt, M., Westerink, J., Bierbooms, J., Bongers, I., & IJsselsteijn, W. (2022). Integrating technology in mental healthcare practice: A repeated cross-sectional survey study on professionals' adoption of Digital Mental Health before and during COVID-19. *Frontiers in Psychiatry, 13*. https://doi.org/10.3389/fpsyt.2022.1040023.

Flanagan, T. (2016). With mobile health Apps, Smartphones, and Mental Health Collide. HealthCare Recruiters International. Retrieved July 30, 2023, from https://hcrnetwork.com/mobile-health-apps-smartphones-mental-health-collide/.

Götzl, C., Hiller, S., Rauschenberg, C., Schick, A., Fechtelpeter, J., Abaigar, U. F., Koppe, G., Durstewitz, D., Reininghaus, U., & Krumm, S. (2022). Artificial intelligence-informed mobile mental health apps for young people: A mixed-methods approach on users' and stakeholders' perspectives. *Child and Adolescent Psychiatry and Mental Health, 16*,. https://doi.org/10.1186/s13034-022-00522-6

Graham, A. K., Lattie, E. G., Powell, B. J., Lyon, A. R., Smith, J. D., Schueller, S. M., Stadnick, N. A., Brown, C. H., & Mohr, D. C. (2020). Implementation strategies for digital mental health interventions in health care settings. *The American Psychologist, 75*(8), 1080. https://doi.org/10.1037/amp0000686

GSMA. (2021). Achieving mobile-enabled digital inclusion in Bangladesh. Retrieved September 15, 2023, from https://www.gsma.com/mobilefordevelopment/wp-content/uploads/2021/03/Achieving-mobile-enabled-digital-inclusion-in-Bangladesh.pdf.

Haque, A., Islam, N., Samrat, N. H., Dey, S., & Ray, B. (2021). Smart farming through responsible leadership in Bangladesh: Possibilities, opportunities, and beyond. *Sustainability, 13*(8), 4511.

Harandi, T. F., Taghinasab, M. M., & Nayeri, T. D. (2017). The correlation of social support with mental health: A meta-analysis. *Electronic Physician, 9*(9), 5212–5222. https://doi.org/10.19082/5212.

Hasan, M., & Zaman, M. A. (2023). Digital divide points to disparity in rural-urban internet access. The Daily Star. Retrieved September 15, 2023, from https://www.thedailystar.net/business/economy/news/digital-divide-points-disparity-rural-urban-internet-access-3345526.

Hasan, M. T., Anwar, T., Christopher, E., Hossain, S., Hossain, M. M., Koly, K. N., Saif-Ur-Rahman, K. M., Ahmed, H. U., Arman, N., & Hossain, S. W. (2021). The current state of mental healthcare in Bangladesh: Part 1 – an updated country profile. *Bjpsych International, 18*(4), 78–82. https://doi.org/10.1192/bji.2021.41

Hassan, A., Ali, M. D., Ahammed, R., Bourouis, S., & Khan, M. M. (2021). Development of NLP-integrated intelligent web system for E-mental health. *Computational and mathematical methods in medicine, 2021*.

Hossain, M. (2022). Digital Bangladesh vision and the current state of digitalization. In *Digital Transformation and Economic Development in Bangladesh: Rethinking Digitalization Strategies for Leapfrogging* (pp. 29–56). Singapore: Springer Nature Singapore.

Hossain, M. B., Dewan, N., Senin, A. A., & Illes, C. B. (2023). Evaluating the utilization of technological factors to promote e-commerce adoption in small and medium enterprises. *Electronic Commerce Research*, pp. 1–20.

Hossain, M. E., & Ahmed, S. Z. (2016). Academic use of smartphones by university students: A developing country perspective. *The Electronic Library, 34*(4), 651–665.

Hossain, M. E., Dechun, H., & Tran, Q. (2012). The rise of offshore IT outsourcing industry: An attempt to assess Bangladesh's competitive advantages. *Available at SSRN 3941323*.

Internet Live Stats. (2016). Bangladesh Internet Users. Retrieved July 15, 2023, from https://www.internetlivestats.com/internet-users/bangladesh/.

Islam, A., & Rahman, A. (2006). Growth and development of information and communication technologies in Bangladesh. *The Electronic Library, 24*(2), 135–146.

Islam, M. N., Khan, S. R., Islam, N. N., Rezwan-A-Rownok, M., Zaman, S. R., & Zaman, S. R. (2021a). A mobile application for mental health care during covid-19 pandemic: Development and usability evaluation with system usability scale. In *Computational Intelligence in Information Systems: Proceedings of the Computational Intelligence in Information Systems Conference (CIIS 2020)* (pp. 33–42). Springer International Publishing.

Islam, M. R., Jannath, S., Moona, A. A., Akter, S., Hossain, M. J., & Islam, S. M. (2021b). Association between the use of social networking sites and mental health of young generation in Bangladesh: A cross-sectional study. *Journal of Community Psychology, 49*(7), 2276–2297. https://doi.org/10.1002/jcop.22675

Islam, M. S., Sujan, M. S., Tasnim, R., Mohona, R. A., Ferdous, M. Z., Kamruzzaman, S., Toma, T. Y., Sakib, M. N., Pinky, K. N., Islam, M. R., Siddique, M. A., Anter, F. S., Hossain, A., Hossen, I., Sikder, M. T., & Pontes, H. M. (2021c). Problematic smartphone and social media use among bangladeshi college and university students amid COVID-19: The role of psychological well-being and pandemic related factors. *Frontiers in Psychiatry, 12*, 647386. https://doi.org/10.3389/fpsyt.2021.647386

Kemp, S. (2023). Digital 2023: Bangladesh. Retrieved July 8, 2023, from https://datareportal.com/reports/digital-2023-bangladesh.

Khalily, M. A. (2016). Financial inclusion, financial regulation, and education in Bangladesh. ADBI Working Paper 621. Tokyo: Asian Development Bank Institute. Retrieved from https://www.adb.org/publications/financial-inclusion-financial-regulation-and-educationbangladesh.

Koly, K. N., Saba, J., Muzaffar, R., Modasser, R. B., Colon-Cabrera, D., & Warren, N. (2022a). Exploring the potential of delivering mental health care services using digital technologies in Bangladesh: A qualitative analysis. *Internet Interventions, 29*, 100544. https://doi.org/10.1016/j.invent.2022.100544

Koly, K. N., Tasnim, Z., Ahmed, S., Saba, J., Mahmood, R., Farin, F. T., & Reidpath, D. D. (2022b). Mental healthcare-seeking behavior of women in Bangladesh: Content analysis of a social media platform. *BMC Psychiatry, 22*(1), 1–12. https://doi.org/10.1186/s12888-022-04414-z

Koticha, P., Katge, F., Shetty, S., & Patil, D. P. (2019). Effectiveness of virtual reality eyeglasses as a distraction aid to reduce anxiety among 6–10-year-old children undergoing dental extraction procedure. *International Journal of Clinical Pediatric Dentistry, 12*(4), 297. https://doi.org/10.5005/jp-journals-10005-1640

Latha, K., Meena, K. S., Pravitha, M. R., Dasgupta, M., & Chaturvedi, S. K. (2020). Effective use of social media platforms for the promotion of mental health awareness. Journal of Education and Health Promotion, p. 9. https://doi.org/10.4103/jehp.jehp_90_20.

Li, J. (2023). Digital technologies for mental health improvements in the COVID-19 pandemic: A scoping review. *BMC Public Health, 23*(1), 1–10. https://doi.org/10.1186/s12889-023-15302-w

Lipschitz, J., Miller, C. J., Hogan, T. P., Burdick, K. E., Lippin-Foster, R., Simon, S. R., & Burgess, J. (2019). Adoption of mobile apps for depression and anxiety: Cross-sectional survey study on patient interest and barriers to engagement. *JMIR Mental Health, 6*(1). https://doi.org/10.2196/11334.

Ma, J., Zhao, D., Xu, N., & Yang, J. (2023). The effectiveness of immersive virtual reality (VR) based mindfulness training on improvement mental-health in adults: A narrative systematic review. *Explore, 19*(3), 310–318.

Mahmud, M. (2023). Financial inclusion in Bangladesh: Scope and Progress. Retrieved August 24, 2023, from https://bigd.bracu.ac.bd/financial-inclusion-in-bangladesh-scope-and-progress/.

Makwana, N. (2019). Disaster and its impact on mental health: A narrative review. *Journal of Family Medicine and Primary Care, 8*(10), 3090–3095. https://doi.org/10.4103/jfmpc.jfmpc_893_19

Malhotra, S., Chand, P., Chatterjee, K., & Brahma, A. (2022). Practice of telepsychiatry and its current legal status. *Indian Journal of Psychiatry, 64*(Suppl 1), S176. https://doi.org/10.4103/indianjpsychiatry.indianjpsychiatry_716_21

Mantracare. (2023). Online therapy in Bangladesh. Retrieved August 22, 2023, from https://mantracare.org/bangladesh/online-therapy/.

Ministry of Health & Family Welfare. (2021). National Mental Health Survey 2019. Retrieved March 10, 2023, from http://nimh.gov.bd/wp-content/uploads/2021/11/Mental-Health-Survey-Report.pdf.

Mujeri, M. K. (2015). Improving access of the poor to financial services. Retrieved July 30, 2023, from https://gedkp.gov.bd/wp-content/uploads/2021/02/1_Improving-Access-of-the-Poor-to-Financial-Services.pdf?post_id=744.

Nandy, A., Biswas, M., & Das, J. (2022). Social media & mental health: A narrative study on Bangladesh during the Lockdown time of COVID-19 Pandemic. *International Journal of Research and Innovation in Social Science (IJRISS). VI*, 680–689.

Noor, W. (2021). What's next for Bangladesh's fintech innovation?. Visa Economic Empowerment Institute. Retrieved August 24, 2023, from https://usa.visa.com/content/dam/VCOM/global/ms/documents/veei-whats-next-for-bangladesh.pdf.

Rahman, A. (2014). *Bangladesh–An emerging Market for IT/ITeS Outsourcing: An analysis of why Limelight Networks Inc. should outsource to Bangladesh* (Doctoral dissertation, INDEPENDENT UNIVERSITY, BANGLADESH).

Ratan, Z. A., Parrish, M., Alotaibi, M. S., & Hosseinzadeh, H. (2022). Prevalence of smartphone addiction and its association with sociodemographic, physical and mental well-being: A cross-sectional study among the young adults of Bangladesh. *International Journal of Environmental Research and Public Health, 19*(24). https://doi.org/10.3390/ijerph192416583.

Rodríguez-Rivas, M. E., Cangas, A. J., Cariola, L. A., Varela, J. J., & Valdebenito, S. (2022). Innovative technology–based interventions to reduce stigma toward people with mental illness: Systematic review and meta-analysis. *JMIR Serious Games, 10*(2). https://doi.org/10.2196/35099.

Roknuzzaman, M. (2006). A survey of Internet access in a large public university in Bangladesh. *International Journal of Education and Development using ICT, 2*(3).

Rothbaum, B. O., & Hodges, L. F. (1999). The use of virtual reality exposure in the treatment of anxiety disorders. *Behavior Modification, 23*(4), 507–525.

Saif, S. (2023). Internet connection in Bangladeshi households soars almost eightfold in a decade. THE BUSINESS STANDARD. Retrieved September 15, 2023, from https://www.tbsnews.net/bangladesh/telecom/internet-connection-bangladeshi-households-soars-almost-eightfold-decade-662658.

Sanghvi, P. B., & Mehrotra, S. (2021). Help-seeking for mental health concerns: A review of Indian research and emergent insights. *Journal of Health Research, 36*(3), 428–441.

Sen, K. K., Nilima, S., Zahura, F. T., & Bari, W. (2023). Do education and living standards matter in breaking barriers to healthcare access among women in Bangladesh? *BMC Public Health, 23*(1), 1431.

TBS Report. (2023). Growth in financial account ownership has slowed down in Bangladesh: findings. THE BUSINESS STANDARD. Retrieved August 24, 2023, from https://www.tbsnews.net/economy/growth-financial-account-ownership-has-slowed-down-bangladesh-findings-569290.

Teachman, B. A., Silverman, A. L., & Werntz, A. (2022). Digital mental health services: Moving from promise to results. *Cognitive and Behavioral Practice, 29*(1), 97–104.

THOLONGS 2015. Bangladesh IT/ITeS Industry Development Strategy: Global Demand Assessment Competitive Landscape and Industry Statistics. Retrieved September 15, 2023, from https://bcc.portal.gov.bd/sites/default/files/files/bcc.portal.gov.bd/notices/57e936e0_dd8c_4eea_a0b1_3c3195adb36e/Draft%20Report%20Global%20Demand%20Assessment,%20Competitive%20Landscape,%20and%20Industry%20Statistics.pdf.

Thomée, S. (2018). Mobile phone use and mental health. A review of the research that takes a psychological perspective on exposure. *International Journal of Environmental Research and Public Health*, 15(12). https://doi.org/10.3390/ijerph15122692.

Thurston, A. M., Stöckl, H., & Ranganathan, M. (2021). Natural hazards, disasters and violence against women and girls: A global mixed-methods systematic review. *BMJ Global Health, 6*(4). https://doi.org/10.1136/bmjgh-2020-004377.

Too, L. S., Leach, L., & Butterworth, P. (2020). Mental health problems and internet access: Results from an Australian national household survey. *JMIR Mental Health, 7*(5). https://doi.org/10.2196/14825.

Uddin, M. J., Alam, M. T., Ahmed, H. U., Khan, N. M., & Talukder, S. K. (2020). Mental health and psychosocial support (MHPSS) in COVID-19 outbreak. *Bangladesh Journal of Infectious Diseases, 7*, S45.

UNICEF. (2021). Empowerment and independence: In pursuit of adolescent-friendly mental health. Retrieved August 22, 2023, from https://www.unicef.org/stories/pursuit-of-adolescent-friendly-mental-health-bangladesh.

Vassilakopoulou, P., & Hustad, E. (2023). Bridging digital divides: A literature review and research agenda for information systems research. *Information Systems Frontiers, 25*(3), 955–969. https://doi.org/10.1007/s10796-020-10096-3

Wentzel, J., & Bohlmeijer, E. T. (2016). Mixing online and face-to-face therapy: How to benefit from blended care in mental health care. *JMIR Mental Health, 3*(1). https://doi.org/10.2196/mental.4534.

World Health Organization. (2020). Bangladesh WHO special initiative for mental health situational assessment. *World Health Organization.*

# Chapter 17
# Mental Health of Vulnerable Populations in Bangladesh

**Madhurima Saha Hia and Muhammad Kamruzzaman Mozumder**

**Abstract** Being in a vulnerable community in a resource-constrained setting is a double burden. With the limited availability of psychosocial support services in Bangladesh, people from vulnerable communities are often left without any support for their mental health conditions. This chapter presents the current state, and mental health concerns along with challenges and recommendations for providing psychosocial services to four vulnerable communities living in Bangladesh, namely, stranded Pakistanis, forcibly displaced Myanmar nationals, sexually diverse communities and climate change victims. Apart from providing clarity on mental health and associated features of these four communities, this chapter may help researchers look forward towards strategies for the improvement of services.

**Keywords** FDMN · Rohingya · Bihari · Psychosocial support · Challenges · Vulnerable community

## 17.1 Introduction

Vulnerability is a relative term and its interpretation is dependent on the type of impact being considered. It generally indicates future prospects or the possibility of a single or multiple negative outcome(s). Poverty, lack of education, adverse exposure and precarious living conditions are the most common vulnerabilities that are linked with multiple negative outcomes including mental illness and psychosocial dysfunctions. Generally, people with such vulnerabilities are systematically oppressed, and become victims of violations of economic, civil, political, social and cultural rights, discrimination and social exclusion (Taket et al., 2009). They have limited or no access to health care and social welfare services, and thus are vulnerable or susceptible to physical and psychosocial harm or risk. Thus, the existing vulnerability of a person can lead to additional vulnerabilities including long-term unemployment,

M. S. Hia · M. K. Mozumder (✉)
Department of Clinical Psychology, University of Dhaka, Dhaka, Bangladesh
e-mail: mozumder@du.ac.bd



S. M. Y. Arafat (ed.), *Mental Health in Bangladesh*,
https://doi.org/10.1007/978-981-97-0610-5_17

low income, limited access to education and health care or exclusion from social policies (Taket et al., 2009).

## 17.2 Vulnerable Communities in Bangladesh

One simple way of describing a vulnerable community is the portion of society to whom inequality and disorganization have become a normative reality (Pearlin, 1999). Bangladesh is a low-resource country with a huge population of 160 million, and almost all people are faced with different kinds of vulnerabilities. However, there are groups of populations who are faced with multiple vulnerabilities. These vulnerable groups often face the most devastating impact in terms of mental health concerns. This chapter will briefly discuss four of such vulnerable populations, namely, the stranded Pakistani; the Forcibly Displaced Myanmar Nationals (FDMN) community; lesbian, gay, bisexual and transgender (LGBT) communities; and the climate change victims. However, it should be noted that the complete list of vulnerable communities in Bangladesh would be much bigger and may take an entire book to discuss.

The stranded Pakistanis who are also known as the Bihari community have been living in camp-like settlements in different parts of Bangladesh since 1971. The FDMN, i.e. the Rohingya communities from Myanmar have been seeking refuge and living in camps in Bangladesh since the 1970s which has peaked with a recent large influx in 2017. Sexually diverse communities, namely, the lesbian, gay, bisexual and transgender people are generally hidden populations due to their sexual practices and behaviours which are unacceptable in the mainstream societal perception of Bangladesh. Finally, the rural communities affected by the climate changes in disaster-prone Bangladesh suffer from loss of livelihood, displacement and loss of social empowerment.

### *17.2.1 Stranded Pakistanis in Bangladesh*

Stranded Pakistanis or ‘Biharis’ are an Urdu-speaking Muslim community, originally from Indian provinces (e.g. Bihar, Uttar Pradesh, Madhya Pradesh) who, due to the partition during the independence of Indian subcontinent in 1947, moved to the then East Pakistan, i.e. present-day Bangladesh (Mantoo, 2013). They left their ancestral home in India to escape persecution in a Hindu-majority country, where communal conflicts between the two religions are claimed to have taken an estimated 30,000 lives of this Urdu-speaking Bihari community in 1946 (Mantoo, 2013). The huge distance of 2200 km between the two parts of Pakistan separated by India in the middle made the country difficult to survive and inherently unstable. When war broke out between the two parts, with Indian support, East Pakistan gained independence and became Bangladesh. During the 9 months of the war, the Bihari community, due to their cultural difference with the Bangladeshi community and identification with the Pakistani community, took a position against the independence of Bangladesh and supported the Pakistani army. Unfortunately for them, when Pakistan lost the war, they became the enemy of the newly formed state of Bangladesh. Predictably, after the war, they faced immense hostility and aggression from the Bangali community (Mantoo, 2013) and a large number of Bihari Muslims were consequently killed as retribution for their active engagement in the genocidal operations against the pro-liberation Bangali community during the war (Haider, 2016; Mantoo, 2013). Soon afterwards the Bihari communities across the country were placed into camp settlements under the Geneva Convention. They became stranded in the camp because (i) they perceived themselves as Pakistanis, not as Bangladeshi; (ii) they were originally from India and (iii) Pakistan did not want to take them as they were not from Pakistan.

An estimated 3,00,000 stranded Pakistanis are living under impoverished conditions where large families have to live in small households with limited privacy, poor sanitation systems and little supportive structures in 116 camps across Bangladesh (Akter et al., 2022; Haider, 2016). These people are still being discriminated against in the education and employment sectors. A recent survey of members of the Bihari community reported that most of the Urdu-speaking children do not have access to school, and the rest had to hide their identity as Bihari to avoid stigmatization (Haider, 2016). The Bihari community mostly rely on low-paid menial jobs as day labourers or rickshaw pullers, while some of them operate small tea stalls or grocery shops. As a result of limited access to education and decent employment opportunities, their income level remains relatively much lower than others in the surrounding mainstream society (Haider, 2016).

To summarize, even after 50 years of independence, the Bihari community is living in extreme poverty in abysmal conditions, devoid of basic rights. In recent times, many individuals from the community, especially from the younger generations, expressed their interest in being recognized as Bangladeshi rather than being labelled as 'Stranded Pakistani' (Begum, 2023). A survey with the Bangali and Bihari populations indicated that Bangali participants do not see cultural integration and economic rehabilitation of the Bihari community as a security threat for the country which shows hope for the possibility of integration of these communities (Haider, 2016). The Bihari participants of the survey, on the other hand, reported that they did not have any intention to migrate to Pakistan, as the younger generation was born in Bangladesh (Haider, 2016). All participants from the Bihari community expressed their wish to have a normal life like any Bangladeshi citizen, where they no longer had to stay in camps, and are warmly welcomed in the education and employment sector of the country (Haider, 2016).

### 17.2.2 Forcibly Displaced Myanmar Nationals

The Forcibly Displaced Myanmar Nationals (FDMC) are members of the Rohingya community, a Muslim minority living in the Rakhine State of Myanmar, who have been forced to flee their homeland to Bangladesh, due longstanding to systematic discrimination and targeted persecution by the government in their own country. They have never been recognized as citizens by the Government of Myanmar and hence were perceived as not entitled to basic rights including access to health and education (Riley et al., 2020). State policies in Myanmar restricted their freedom of movement, getting married, having children or building permanent households (Riley et al., 2020). As early as the 1970s, this community started to flee to neighbouring Bangladesh to avoid illegal arrests, harassment and violence by Myanmar's armed forces. Due to escalated military atrocities, a major influx of Rohingya people to Bangladesh took place in 1978, 1992 and 2012 while the largest influx of 700,000 Rohingya individuals happened in 2017 (Hossain, 2023). Since then, they have been living in overcrowded camp settlements in the Cox's Bazar area of Bangladesh. Currently, approximately 945,953 Rohingya people are living in 33 extremely congested camps in Ukhiya and Teknaf Upazilas of Cox's Bazar, and are entirely dependent on humanitarian aid from national and international agencies for food and living (Ahmad et al., 2020; Inter-Sector Coordination Group, 2023). Despite consistent efforts by international humanitarian organizations and regional associations, the Myanmar government refused to repatriate the Rohingya.

Despite constant support from aid agencies along with government, non-government and UN organizations, the Rohingya communities are still facing numerous challenges including limited scope of education, safety at camps, food insecurity and vulnerability to natural disasters. Almost half of the Rohingya population is children who do not have enough opportunities for nutrition, education recreation and development. Currently, there are 5735 learning centres for approximately 400,000 learners. Despite relentless efforts from humanitarian organizations, around 100,000 children still cannot go to school most of whom are female (Inter-Sector Coordination Group, 2023). The accommodations at the camps lack the durability to withstand natural calamities, such as storm, heavy rainfall, fire outbreak or landslides and 95% of households has been reported to be vulnerable to moderate-to-high level of natural disaster (Inter-Sector Coordination Group, 2023). The people from camps are not allowed to move freely or work, they have to accept the amount of food they are provided with even when it is perceived as inadequate (Ahmad et al., 2020). In the Multi-sectoral Need Assessment Programme, the displaced Rohingya people reported their needs for access to food and education, protection, opportunities for learning skills, shelter and cooking materials (Inter-Sector Coordination Group, 2023).

There are frequent reports of multiple forms of sexual- and gender-based violence against women and girls, including rape, child marriage and domestic violence (Inter-Sector Coordination Group, 2023). A recent survey suggested that there is a tendency to normalize violence against women in this context, by addressing 'domestic violence' as a 'family affair' by the camp dwellers (Guglielmi et al., 2020). Moreover, because of the social stigma associated with gender-based violence, many survivors hesitate to report such crimes. Estimation suggests that at least 2.6% of women in the camps die due to sexual violence and lack of proper post-assault medical care (Médecins Sans Frontières, 2018).

In the post-migration context, the relationship between the host and displaced population is very crucial for resilience development. Initially, the local people of Bangladesh were very supportive and sympathetic towards the Rohingya migrants and were willing to help them (Sohel & Siddiqui, 2019). However, gradually the Rohingya refugee community outnumbered the host community population in Ukhiya Upazila and took shelter in their productive agricultural lands (Inter-Sector Coordination Group, 2023). At the beginning of this Rohingya crisis, a number of local people were recruited as relief workers; however, as time progressed they started to lose jobs because the humanitarian organizations started to hire more from the Rohingya community (Sohel & Siddiqui, 2019). These resulted in the developing negative attitudes towards the Rohingya community among the hosts. Survey of the host community indicated mixed attitudes towards the Rohingya people (Jerin & Mozumder, 2019). Reports of antisocial or criminal activities by the Rohingya community have also exacerbated the dispute between them and the local people (Zafar, 2020).

Recently, the Government of Bangladesh took an initiative to decongest camps and relocate the Rohingya community to Bhasan Char, an island in the coastal region of the country. Despite some resistance from the Rohingya community, 30,000 of the initially planned 100,000 Rohingya people have been moved to Bhasan Char since 2022 (Inter-Sector Coordination Group, 2023). From the overall description of the current scenario in Rohingya camps, it can be said that, despite, genuine efforts from government and aid agencies, the Rohingya migrants are living in a poor condition where their basic rights and dignity are not protected. Moreover, with the increasing need around the ongoing crisis in Afghanistan and Ukraine, international assistance for the Rohingya issue is gradually declining creating a serious concern for this aid-dependent community of a million people (Zahed, 2023).

### *17.2.3 Sexually Diverse Communities*

The sexually diverse community generally referred to as lesbian, gay, bisexual or transgender (LGBT) are sexual minorities across the world. Although the exact size of the LBGT population has not been established in Bangladesh, the estimate suggests the approximate size of male homosexuals to be between 21,833 and 110,581 and transgenders to be between 4504 and 8882 (icddrb & Government of Bangladesh, 2012). Perception towards the sexually diverse community in mainstream society is generally negative. Bangladesh is a Muslim-majority country where homosexuality contradicts Islamic values (Jahangir & Abdul-Latif, 2016). The legal system prohibits homosexual intercourse where it connoted as 'against the order of nature' (The Penal Code-1860, 1860). There have been several attacks and murders of LGBT activists which resulted in widespread terror and a deep sense of insecurity among the sexually diverse communities in Bangladesh (Shovon, 2019). Therefore, the LGBT becomes a hidden community in Bangladesh and they rarely seek support due to the fear of disclosure and subsequent humiliation and discrimination.

Across the world, sexually diverse communities face a number of challenges including stigma and discrimination, financial hardships, physical, emotional, and sexual abuse and legal problems (Emlet, 2016), which is much more common in Bangladesh considering legal, religious and moral codes and values in Bangladesh against the behaviour and practices of the LGBT community. Male homosexuals in Bangladesh have been reported to face discrimination including exclusion from family, and humiliation from society (Mozumder et al., 2016). Study findings also reported extreme social exclusion; humiliation and verbal, physical and sexual abuse towards the Hijra community in Bangladesh (Khan et al., 2009). Wong and Noriega (2013) through an in-depth qualitative exploration reported commonplace experiences of blackmailing, sexual as well as physical assault, deprivation and humiliation among the sexually diverse communities in Bangladesh. The stigma and discrimination faced by the LGBT communities in Bangladesh limits their participation in society and threatens their existence taking a heavy toll on their health and well-being.

The government of Bangladesh recognizes the sexually diverse community as a vulnerable group and acknowledges the gap in knowledge about this community as reflected in the following excerpt from the National Mental Health Strategic Plan 2020–2030,

> A particularly vulnerable and understudied group is the "lesbian, gay, bisexual, transgender and queer" group. Although Bangladesh recognizes a third gender, little has been done to study their psychological and social well-being within the larger community (p-11, Government of Bangladesh, 2022).

### *17.2.4 Climate Change Victims*

The geographic location made Bangladesh a climatic disaster-prone country. It has been hit by numerous cyclones, flooding, riverbank erosion and droughts throughout the century. The recent and rapid changes in climatic conditions are making these much more common nowadays. Global warming and associated climate change threaten the increase of sea level causing the drowning of low-lying coastal lands and increasing salinity in the upstream. Both cause significant concern for housing and food insecurity. Climate change is likely to result in the death of thousands of people, creating threats to shelter and essential infrastructures, and declining supply and quality of food, water and energy (Nelson et al., 2018). This is also one of the primary reasons for increased displacement all over the world (Schwerdtle et al., 2018). Bangladesh is considered the most vulnerable South Asian country for internal migration. Riverbank erosions alone are believed to internally displace 13.3 million people in Bangladesh by 2050 (The World Bank Group, 2022).

People affected by cyclones, flooding and riverbank erosion in Bangladesh often lose everything in a matter of days or a few hours. This is especially devastating as there is no or little social protection for the families affected by these from the government of the local communities. While floods in Bangladesh are generally associated with the most economic damage, cyclones are responsible for the most casualties (see The World Bank Group, 2022). Communities at different localities are faced with different climatic challenges. While the cyclone is a major concern for the coastal region in the southwest, the landslide is a concern in the southeastern hilly region and drought is a major challenge in the northwest of the country. All these increased the risk of poverty which is a core vulnerability for many negative outcomes.

Bangladesh was ranked as the world's seventh most vulnerable country to climate change (Ahmed, 2006). Climate change and its consequences have caused human suffering across the globe in recent times. However, the sufferings and impacts vary based on a number of factors including financial capacity, existing infrastructure, quality of housing and demographics of the person affected by the changes (Eaton et al., 2022; Hallegatte & Rozenberg, 2017). Developing preparedness and resilience to natural disasters is one of the major agenda for the Government of Bangladesh. Initiatives have been taken to develop community resilience and agricultural adaptation to reduce harm caused by disasters and climate change (Ahmed, 2006; The World Bank Group, 2022). The Ministry of Environment, Forest and Climate Change in coordination with other relevant ministries including energy, agriculture and disaster management has developed a robust policy framework focussing on climate change adaptation (Ahmed, 2006; The World Bank Group, 2022).

## 17.3 Mental Health Concerns Among the Vulnerable Communities

There has been very limited data on the mental health aspects of the stranded Pakistani community. However, it is evident from the historical overview that this Urdu-speaking Bihari Muslim community has been subjected to violence, stigma and discrimination, social exclusion, poverty and rights violations since 1946 because of their religious and cultural identity and political position, behaviour and opinion. The mental health impact of communal violence can be drastic, including persistent insecurity, anxiety, trauma symptoms, helplessness and hopelessness (Farooqui & Ahmad, 2021). Evidence suggests that trauma response can be transmitted across generations through learning, parenting and family environment (Lehrner & Yehuda, 2018) In addition, the newer generations are still facing discrimination and social exclusions. Stigma and discrimination are the major impediments to one's search for value as a human being. Perceived discriminatory experiences and social exclusion have significant negative effects on the psychosocial well-being of people (Precupetu et al., 2019).

Literature labelled stranded Pakistanis as 'de facto stateless people' (Haider, 2016), and studies showed that statelessness or ineffective citizenship is associated with poor mental health consequences (Herberholz, 2022). The community has been living in poverty for decades. Reviews of the literature suggested that poverty is one of the important contributing factors to mental disorders (Saraceno & Barbui,

1997). It is also argued that if poverty arises from systemic social inequality and power imbalance, the impact on mental health could be even more drastic (Burns, 2015). In light of all this evidence, it can be hypothesized that stranded Pakistanis or Bihari Muslims are vulnerable to developing psychological disorders. However, being a left-over community, no one seems to care much about mental health, not even the researchers. Some social activists are working on enhancing the livelihood, education and health of the community but a thorough assessment or intensive intervention towards the improvement of mental health of this vulnerable community is yet to be carried out.

Compared to the stranded Pakistani community, the mental health state and needs of the Rohingya community are well researched and documented (see Ager et al., 2019). Targeted persecution, systematic human rights violations, traumatic migrations and stressful camp settlements take a heavy toll on the mental health and well-being of the Rohingya community (Riley et al., 2020). Research suggested that the interaction between trauma exposure and daily-life stressors at camps in the context of limited access to health care, education and work opportunities is contributing to negative mental health consequences among the Rohingya community (see Ritsema & Armstrong-Hough, 2023). A systematic review of this community revealed that the prolonged deprivation made them vulnerable to developing a range of mental health problems, such as posttraumatic stress disorder, anxiety, depression and suicidal ideation (Tay et al., 2019). A secondary cross-sectional survey indicated that 4.9% of the Rohingya were suffering from PTSD while 30% were suffering from depression (Ritsema & Armstrong-Hough, 2023).

Depression was found to be mostly linked with daily stressors, whereas trauma symptoms were directly correlated with traumatic experiences mediated by present life stress (Riley et al., 2017). A screening survey conducted with the camp children showed that 52% of the children had emotional problems and 25% had relationship problems with peers (Khan et al., 2019). Around 4.8% of children below the age of 2 years and 7.3% of children between the age of 2 and 16 years were screened positively for neurodevelopmental disorders (Khan et al., 2019). Incidents of sexual- and gender-based violence induce anxiety and depression in Rohingya women (Tay et al., 2019).

The LGBT communities go through a number of stressors in their lives, including rejection, humiliation and neglect from family and maltreatment in wider society. A considerable proportion of them also experience childhood sexual abuse by homosexual and heterosexual perpetrators (Mozumder & Ahmed, 2016). They have to deal with negative social perception, public humiliation, discrimination in employment and limited access to legal support due to their non-normative sexual orientation (Mozumder & Ahmed, 2016). Heterosexual normativity and expectations, combined with stigma and discrimination against people with homosexual orientation, has been known to contribute towards distress and mental health consequences in the form of minority stress (Kelleher, 2009). A number of studies suggest that individuals from the LGBT community are more vulnerable to developing mental health and psychological problems than the general population. High prevalence of depression, anxiety, suicidal ideation and substance abuse among sexually diverse communities are widely reported. A survey finding showed that around 30% of male homosexuals have attempted suicide and around 40% expressed suicidal ideation and self-harm behaviour (Mozumder et al., 2023). A significant proportion of them have experiences of being victims of sexual abuse in childhood and adulthood (Mozumder et al., 2016). A comprehensive mixed-method study of the LGBT population across Bangladesh reported significantly higher levels of hopelessness, depression, perceived stress and somatic symptoms among the sexually diverse communities compared to the general population (Mozumder & Ahmed, 2016). They found a severe level of hopelessness among 11.8% lesbian, 8.2% gay, 4.6% bisexual and 7.7% transgender participants while for the general population, it was only 1.2% (Mozumder & Ahmed, 2016). Lesbians are more prone to engage in self-harm and suicidal thoughts while gays reported a higher rate of attempted suicide (Mozumder & Ahmed, 2016).

The consequences of climate change have a huge impact on people's health and well-being. A pilot study conducted by the SAJIDA Foundation reported that 37.3% of climate change victims have mental health needs (Diaz & Rahaman, 2022). Analysing possibilities of variations in temperature, rainfall, humidity, drying out safe water resources and salinity intrusion, Rahman et al. (2019) presented projected impacts of climate change in Bangladesh. They predicted increase in vector-borne diseases (e.g. malaria, dengue), increased water-borne diseases (e.g. diarrhoea, dysentery), heightened risks of cardiovascular diseases and pre-eclampsia in pregnant women (see Rahman et al., 2019). These changes in the environment also have negative impacts on people's mental health and well-being. In a recent nationwide survey in Bangladesh, it was found that stressors related to climate change are strongly correlated with the prevalence of depression and anxiety (Wahid et al., 2023). They found a strong connection between increase in temperature and exposure to flood (within 12 months) with anxiety and depression providing very strong evidence of increased mental health risk associated with climate change (Wahid et al., 2023). It is important to mention that the influence of climate change on people's physical and mental health is mediated by several social and demographic factors. Climate-related shocks and natural calamities have a disproportionate impact on certain groups of people. In Bangladesh, marginalized rural women and girls, who are restricted by social norms, dependent on others for livelihood and have limited access to information and support suffer the most from climate change impacts (Rahman et al., 2019).

## 17.4 Key Players in Mental Health Service Delivery for the Vulnerable Communities

The vulnerable communities are generally minorities in society, hence there is a general lack of concern for their betterment and well-being in the wider community. Generic mental health services are available from the government at the district level. With some exceptions, the mental health services at the government hospitals are generally open for all and not catered for a specific vulnerable group. While government organizations are focussed on enhancing mental health services in a generic manner, non-government organizations are more focussed on addressing the specific mental health needs of vulnerable communities. Due to fund dependency, these NGOs often lack the capacity to go beyond the scope of specific projects aiming at specific target groups. This allows them to stay focussed and this serves the specific vulnerable community. Fund dependency often results in the lack of continuity of the service and sometimes oversaturation of service when increased fund is available.

### *17.4.1 Government Organization*

Mental health has been placed on the list of the top 10 priority health conditions in Bangladesh. The country has already updated and drafted the necessary legal frameworks to support mental health activities. The legal framework includes a complete set consisting of the National Mental Health Strategic Plan 2020–2030, National Mental Health Policy (2019) and National Mental Health Act 2018. Despite these affirmative attitudes and actions, a comprehensive and universal mental health service is still far from reality. With 0.16 psychiatrists, 0.34 professionally trained psychologists and 0.4 psychiatric nurses per 1,00,000 individuals, the scope of access to mental health services is pretty slim for the people in Bangladesh (World Health Organization, 2020). The staggering 92.3% treatment gap for mental health therefore is not surprising at all (World Health Organization, 2020). In the context of limited availability of service for the mainstream society, ensuring adequate service for all the vulnerable groups would be a far-fetched expectation. While the 2020–2030 Strategic Plan discussed the mental health needs and strategies for some of the vulnerable groups, it failed even to mention some other groups with multiple vulnerabilities, for example, the stranded Pakistani community and the climate change victims.

The mental health impact of climate change is recognized by the government and is well documented as an area of work in numerous technical and policy documents. However, service development to support mental health initiatives for climate change victims is yet to be implemented. The existing mental health facilities can be utilized and mobilized in case of crisis; however, it should be noted that the existing services are already overloaded with work.

The Reginal Trauma Counselling Centres (RTCC) has been established by the Ministry of Women and Children Affairs to address the psychosocial needs of the vulnerable communities affected by trauma. They have in-person service in eight district headquarters through government hospitals along with telephone counselling through hotline numbers. The RTCC also has developed infrastructure and resources to provide mental health and psychosocial support services for the FDMN community living in the camps in Cox's Bazar District of Bangladesh.

### 17.4.2 Non-government Organization

Among the four vulnerable groups discussed above, mental health and psychosocial services for the FDMN community have been the most organized and accessible to the beneficiary group. Due to international attention and the availability of funds, numerous local and international NGOs started to work on addressing the mental health and psychosocial needs of the FDMN community. Among the numerous organizations providing mental health services to the FDMN community, Brac, Caritas, Gono Swastha, Action against Hunger, FIVDB, Humanity and Inclusion, and Save the Children are only a few to name.

Only a handful of organizations work with the secretive LGBT community in Bangladesh. For over two decades, the Bandhu Social Welfare Society (BSWS) has been providing psychosocial counselling (through in-house psychosocial counsellors) and advanced psychological support (through referral) for this community. Due to the increased risk of sexually transmitted infections (including HIV), several other organizations have also been working with the LGBT community with partial psychosocial support with a primary focus on preventing STIs and HIV.

Although many NGOs work with climate change victims to provide health and livelihood support, only a few consider mental health aspects in their service delivery. SAJIDA Foundation has been providing mental health services to climate change victims through its comprehensive programme. Initially, they started with well-being sessions and counselling support as mental health components for their beneficiaries with needs. Overtime they have upgraded their mental health service delivery to a three-tier model involving (i) the community mobilizer for initial support and screening, (ii) the para-counsellor for basic psychological support (4–6 sessions structured work for anxiety and depression) and (iii) the clinical psychologist for advanced support through referral from para-counsellors. A recent startup named Moner Bondhu has also initiated work on mental health services for climate change victims.

### 17.4.3 United Nations Entities

United Nations works with the government to support the national development priorities of Bangladesh. A total of 17 UN entities with different focuses and priorities are contributing to Bangladesh. The UN in Bangladesh, through its partnership, provides humanitarian assistance to the Rohingya refugees that include education, food, shelter, sanitation, physical health and mental health. Among all the UN agencies, the United Nations High Commissioner for Refugees (UNHCR) and the International Organization for Migration (IOM) are the most closely linked with the psychosocial support services for the Rohingya community at Cox's Bazar. The World Health Organization (WHO) in collaboration with the government and the NGOs is also extending their work in supporting mental health service improvement through mhGap training which is expected to increase access to treatment for mental health conditions.

The UN System is also collaborating and aiding the government of Bangladesh in its effort towards strengthening risk reduction, preparedness and humanitarian initiatives around disaster management for the people affected by natural calamities and climate change. The WHO has developed a policy brief on mental health and climate change which can be used as the leading document for supporting mental health programmes and activities around climate change (World Health Organization, 2022). The United Nations Development Programme (UNDP) also has an interest in incorporating mental health support in their Local Government Initiatives on Climate Change (LoGIC) project.

## 17.5 Challenges and Recommendations for Psychosocial Service to Vulnerable Communities

Based on the nature of the vulnerability, the specific communities often present with or develop unique features of having considerable differences from the mainstream society. Understanding the vulnerable communities and the putative challenges is necessary for ensuring quality mental health support for them. This section will discuss a few of these challenges considering the Bangladesh context.

### *17.5.1 Linguistic and Cultural Differences*

Cultural and linguistic aspects of any community influence the way they express their symptoms and help-seeking behaviour (Helman, 2007). Therefore, understanding or minimizing these differences between mental health service providers is crucial. This is especially true for the Rohingya and Bihari communities (see Islam & Mozumder, 2021); however, it would be inaccurate to automatically assume that the linguistic and cultural differences will not be an issue for the sexual minority communities and climate change victims. Developing resources and professionals from within the vulnerable communities through training can be a useful approach to addressing the challenges of linguistic and cultural differences. This approach has already been tested with positive results in providing psychosocial support for the LGBT community in Bangladesh.

### 17.5.2 Limited Understanding of the Vulnerable Communities

Research-based data on the vulnerable community are generally lacking in Bangladesh. However, effective mental health service development and delivery requires a deeper understanding of the beneficiary group. Evidence-informed policymaking therefore mandates generating data before the development and deployment of any service. Among the four vulnerable communities discussed in this chapter, only the Rohingya community has been well researched; however, further data may be required depending on the nature of the service and its deployment. Considerable resources and efforts need to be allocated to research to understand these communities.

### 17.5.3 The Top-Down Approach of Policymaking

Policymakers as well as service developers, with their extended experience and confidence in their expertise, often heavily rely on the top-down process of service development. The limited availability of data on vulnerable communities further strengthens this reliance on the top-down approach. In this process, the service providers lose connection with the recipients which results in underutilization and inappropriateness of the service. It is therefore necessary to consult with the representatives of the vulnerable communities in designing, implementing and monitoring services for them.

### 17.5.4 Resource Limitation

As mentioned earlier in Sect. 3.1, mental health service professionals are scarce in Bangladesh. Growing qualified mental health professionals is a time- and resource-intensive process. Additionally, the vulnerable communities lack the necessary resources (information, finance, transportation, support or courage) to access the limited available mental health services. Accessing the service may become additionally difficult with specific features of the vulnerable community, for example, the Rohingya committees living in the camp are not allowed to go outside the fencing, the climate change victims may have migrated to a new and unfamiliar place and the LGBT community may fear disclosure. The NGO approach of moving into the vulnerable community may be a better approach to help them access the service.

### 17.5.5 Perception of the Wider Community

Vulnerable communities, being minorities, are generally looked at negatively by the mainstream society. They are often poor and require support from mainstream society which is commonly perceived as the draining of resources. This can be especially frustrating to mainstream society where the vulnerable community takes necessary support from the same pool of limited reservoir of resources. This can initiate or escalate conflicts between the two communities. Psychosocial care for vulnerable communities should therefore have a community awareness and integration component to avoid conflict.

### 17.5.6 Geological and Regional Priorities

In the context of the global village, no country or issue can stay separate from the remaining world. Economic recession in America will trigger a financial crisis in the remaining world. Priorities shift over time and with influences from recent incidents. The escalation of conflict in Ukraine and Afghanistan has led to the shrinkage of funding for the Rohingya community in Bangladesh. Current geopolitical contexts are supportive of the mental health aspects of climate change activities; however, no one can be certain that this will remain the same after 5 years.

## 17.6 Conclusion

With a focussed discussion on four vulnerable communities, their context and their mental health state, this chapter attempted to orient the readers on the scenario of mental health services for specific population groups in Bangladesh. The discussion indicates variations in available services for each of the communities and raises concerns regarding the lack of services for some of the communities. The challenges and recommendations can be useful for designing effective interventions for these communities.

## References

Ager, W., Horn, R., Mozumder, M., Riley, A., & Ventevogel, P. (2019). From the editors: Introducing Intervention's special issue on the mental health and psychosocial wellbeing of Rohingya refugees [Editorial]. *Intervention, 17*(2), 117–121. https://doi.org/10.4103/intv.intv_54_19

Ahmad, A. A., Ramlan, A. Z., Ladiqi, S., & Noor, N. (2020). Importance of food security: Rohingya refugee in Cox's Bazar camp. *International Journal of Psychosocial Rehabilitations, 24*(1), 5153.

Ahmed, A. U. (2006). *Bangladesh climate change impacts and vulnerability: A synthesis*. Climate Change Cell, Department of Environment.

Akter, F., Afroz, T., & Mahbub, M. (2022). *Challenges & Prospects of Bihari Camp Residents in Bangladesh: A Report on a Pilot Survey Project in Center Community Relief (CCR) Camp and Mohammadpur Market Camp in Bangladesh*. O. H. Inc.

Begum, T. (2023). 'We have a right to live in dignity': Biharis in Bangladesh fight for equality—and jobs. *The Guardian*. https://www.theguardian.com/global-development/2023/may/09/we-have-a-right-to-live-in-dignity-biharis-in-bangladesh-fight-for-equality-and-jobs.

Burns, J. K. (2015). Poverty, inequality and a political economy of mental health. *Epidemiology and Psychiatric Sciences, 24*(2), 107–113. https://doi.org/10.1017/S2045796015000086

Diaz, M. L., & Rahaman, M. M. (2022). Deep scars of climate change: The need for addressing mental health issues in Bangladesh. *The Business Standard*. https://www.tbsnews.net/thoughts/deep-scars-climate-change-need-addressing-mental-health-issues-bangladesh-557982.

Eaton, J., Nwefoh, E., Duncan, J., Sangare, O., Weekes, Y., & Adams, B. (2022). Addressing mental health and wellbeing in the context of climate change: Examples of interventions to inform future practice. *Intervention Journal of Mental Health and Psychosocial Support in Conflict Affected Areas, 20*(1), 107–113. https://doi.org/10.4103/intv.intv_35_21

Emlet, C. A. (2016). Social, economic, and health disparities among LGBT older adults. *Generations, 40*(2), 16–22.

Farooqui, N., & Ahmad, A. (2021). Communal violence, mental health and their correlates: A cross-sectional study in two Riot affected districts of Uttar Pradesh in India. *Journal of Muslim Minority Affairs, 41*(3), 510–521. https://doi.org/10.1080/13602004.2021.1999139

Government of Bangladesh. (2022). *National Mental Health Strategic Plan 2020–2030*. Dhaka.

Guglielmi, S., Jones, N., Muz, J., Baird, S., Mitu, K., & Ala Uddin, M. (2020). Age-and gender-based violence risks facing Rohingya and Bangladeshi adolescents in Cox's Bazar. *Policy Brief. London: Gender and Adolescence: Global Evidence.*

Haider, Z. (2016). Rejected people in Bangladesh: If the biharis were counted. *Journal of Muslim Minority Affairs, 36*(3), 427–443. https://doi.org/10.1080/13602004.2016.1212496

Hallegatte, S., & Rozenberg, J. (2017). Climate change through a poverty lens. *Nature Climate Change, 7*(4), 250–256. https://doi.org/10.1038/nclimate3253

Helman, C. (2007). *Culture, health and illness* (7th ed.). Hodder Arnold.

Herberholz, C. (2022). 'We are inferior, we have no rights': Statelessness and mental health among ethnic minorities in Northern Thailand. *SSM - Population Health, 19*, 101138. https://doi.org/10.1016/j.ssmph.2022.101138.

Hossain, A. N. M. Z. (2023). Educational crisis of Rohingya refugee children in Bangladesh: Access, obstacles, and prospects to formal and non-formal education. *Heliyon, 9*(7), e18346. https://doi.org/10.1016/j.heliyon.2023.e18346.

icddrb, & Government of Bangladesh. (2012). *Counting the numbers of males who have sex with males, males sex workers and Hijra in Bangladesh to provide HIV prevention services*. N. A. S. Programme. http://www.slideshare.net/ntuhin/participatory-situation-assessment-for-msm-msw-hijra-in-bangladesh-by-icddrb.

Inter-Sector Coordination Group. (2023). *2023 Joint Response Plan: Rohingya Humanitarian Crisis*. https://reliefweb.int/attachments/f421e91f-6a0e-4bf6-8514-d8ad24e28c96/bangladesh_2023_jrp_rhc_appeal_en.pdf.

Islam, S., & Mozumder, M. K. (2021). Challenges to providing quality mental health services for forcibly displaced populations: The case of Rohingya refugees in Bangladesh. *Asian American Journal of Psychology, 12*(3), 234–240. https://doi.org/10.1037/aap0000195

Jerin, M., & Mozumder, M. (2019). Exploring host community attitudes towards Rohingya refugees in Bangladesh [Article]. *Intervention, 17*(2), 169–173. https://doi.org/10.4103/intv.intv_27_19

Kelleher, C. (2009). Minority stress and health: Implications for lesbian, gay, bisexual, transgender, and questioning (LGBTQ) young people. *Counselling Psychology Quarterly, 22*(4), 373–379. https://doi.org/10.1080/09515070903334995

Khan, S. I., Hussain, M. I., Parveen, S., Bhuiyan, M. I., Gourab, G., Sarker, G. F., … Sikder, J. (2009). Living on the extreme margin: Social exclusion of the transgender population (hijra) in Bangladesh. *Journal of Health, Population and Nutrition, 27*(4), 441–451. http://www.jstor.org/stable/23499634.

Khan, N. Z., Shilpi, A. B., Sultana, R., Sarker, S., Razia, S., Roy, B., . . . McConachie, H. (2019). Displaced Rohingya children at high risk for mental health problems: Findings from refugee camps within Bangladesh. *Child: Care, Health and Development, 45*(1), 28–35. https://doi.org/10.1111/cch.12623.

Lehrner, A., & Yehuda, R. (2018). Trauma across generations and paths to adaptation and resilience. *Psychological Trauma: Theory, Research, Practice, and Policy, 10*(1), 22–29. https://doi.org/10.1037/tra0000302

Mantoo, S. A. (2013). Bihari refugees stranded in bangladesh since 1971. *Journal of South Asian Studies, 1*(2), 123–129.

Médecins Sans Frontières. (2018). *No one was left: death and violence against the Rohingya in Rakhine state, Myanmar*. http://archive.nyu.edu/handle/2451/42262.

Mozumder, M. K., & Ahmed, S. (2016). *Exploration of Mental Health Needs and Support Systems among LGBT Population in Bangladesh*. Bandhu Social Welfare Society.

Mozumder, M. K., Haque, M. A., Jasmine, U. H., Royal, R. I., & Sharmin, R. (2016). Behavior and experience of male homosexuals in Bangladesh. *Bangladesh Journal of Psychiatry, 30*(22), 41–44. https://doi.org/10.3329/bjpsy.v30i2.45364

Mozumder, M. K., Jasmine, U. H., Haque, M. A., & Haque, S. (2023). Mental health and suicide risk among homosexual males in Bangladesh. *PLoS ONE, 18*(8), e0289597. https://doi.org/10.1371/journal.pone.0289597

Nelson, G., Bogard, J., Lividini, K., Arsenault, J., Riley, M., Sulser, T. B., … Rosegrant, M. (2018). Income growth and climate change effects on global nutrition security to mid-century. *Nature Sustainability, 1*(12), 773-781. https://doi.org/10.1038/s41893-018-0192-z.

Pearlin, L. I. (1999). The Stress Process Revisited. In C. S. Aneshensel & J. C. Phelan (Eds.), *Handbook of the Sociology of Mental Health* (pp. 395–415). Springer US. https://doi.org/10.1007/0-387-36223-1_19.

Precupetu, I., Aartsen, M., & Vasile, M. (2019). Social exclusion and mental wellbeing in older Romanians. *Social Inclusion, 7*(3), 4–16. https://doi.org/10.17645/si.v7i3.2008.

Rahman, M. M., Ahmad, S., Mahmud, A. S., Hassan-uz-Zaman, M., Nahian, M. A., Ahmed, A., … Streatfield, P. K. (2019). Health consequences of climate change in Bangladesh: An overview of the evidence, knowledge gaps and challenges. *WIREs Climate Change, 10*(5), e601. https://doi.org/10.1002/wcc.601.

Riley, A., Akther, Y., Noor, M., Ali, R., & Welton-Mitchell, C. (2020). Systematic human rights violations, traumatic events, daily stressors and mental health of Rohingya refugees in Bangladesh. *Conflict and Health, 14*(1), 60. https://doi.org/10.1186/s13031-020-00306-9

Riley, A., Varner, A., Ventevogel, P., Taimur Hasan, M. M., & Welton-Mitchell, C. (2017). Daily stressors, trauma exposure, and mental health among stateless Rohingya refugees in Bangladesh. *Transcultural Psychiatry, 54*(3), 304–331. https://doi.org/10.1177/1363461517705571

Ritsema, H., & Armstrong-Hough, M. (2023). Associations among past trauma, post-displacement stressors, and mental health outcomes in Rohingya refugees in Bangladesh: A secondary cross-sectional analysis [Original Research]. *Frontiers in Public Health, 10*. https://doi.org/10.3389/fpubh.2022.1048649

Saraceno, B., & Barbui, C. (1997). Poverty and mental illness. *The Canadian Journal of Psychiatry, 42*(3), 285–290. https://doi.org/10.1177/070674379704200306

Schwerdtle, P., Bowen, K., & McMichael, C. (2018). The health impacts of climate-related migration. *BMC Medicine, 16*(1), 1. https://doi.org/10.1186/s12916-017-0981-7

Shovon, F. (2019). কমেন আছনে বাংলাদেশের সমোমীরা [State of the homosexuals in Bangladesh] *DW News*. https://p.dw.com/p/3J2TR.

Sohel, I. M., & Siddiqui, P. (2019). Tensions and potential conflict between host communities and Rohingya refugees. *the.independent*. https://www.academia.edu/download/60483985/

Tensions_and_potential_conflict_between_host_communities_and_Rohingya_refugees_20190904-98795-rsd236.pdf.

Taket, A., Crisp, B. R., Nevill, A., Lamaro, G., Graham, M., & Barter-Godfrey, S. (2009). *Theorising social exclusion*. Routledge.

Tay, A. K., Riley, A., Islam, R., Welton-Mitchell, C., Duchesne, B., Waters, V., & Ventevogel, P. (2019). The culture, mental health and psychosocial wellbeing of Rohingya refugees: A systematic review. *Epidemiol Psychiatr Sci, 28*(5), 489–494. https://doi.org/10.1017/s2045796019000192

The Laws of Bangladesh, ACT NO. XLV Of 1860. (1860). http://bdlaws.minlaw.gov.bd/act-11/section-3233.html?hl=1.

The World Bank Group. (2022). *Bangladesh Country Climate and Development Report*. T. W. Bank. http://hdl.handle.net/10986/38181.

Wahid, S. S., Raza, W. A., Mahmud, I., & Kohrt, B. A. (2023). Climate-related shocks and other stressors associated with depression and anxiety in Bangladesh: A nationally representative panel study. *The Lancet Planetary Health, 7*(2), e137–e146. https://doi.org/10.1016/S2542-5196(22)00315-1

Wong, C., & Noriega, S. (2013). *Exploring gender-based violence among men who have sex with men, male sex worker and transgender communities in Bangladesh and Papua New Guinea.*

World Health Organization. (2020). *Bangladesh: WHO special initiative for mental health, Situational assessment*. W. H. Organization. https://www.who.int/docs/default-source/mental-health/special-initiative/who-special-initiative-country-report---bangladesh---2020.pdf?sfvrsn=c2122a0e_2.

World Health Organization. (2022). *Mental health and climate change: policy brief*. (9240045120). World Health Organization Retrieved from https://iris.who.int/bitstream/handle/10665/354104/9789240045125-eng.pdf.

Zafar, A. (2020). The rohingya refugees: A review of security threats for ban. *GSJ*, *8*(9).

Zahed, I. U. M. (2023). Impact of the geopolitical status quo vis-à-vis the Rohingya crisis on the social, economic, and political aspects of Bangladesh. *Asian Politics & Policy*, *15*(4), 643–667. https://doi.org/10.1111/aspp.12716.

# Chapter 18
# Geriatric Psychiatry in Bangladesh

**S. M. Yasir Arafat, Atiqul Haq Mazumder, and Mohammad Muntasir Maruf**

**Abstract** Being a densely populated country, Bangladesh contains about 15.7 million populations aged above 60 years making up about 9.3% of the population with an increased proportion over the decades. Mental disorders are prevalent among elderly adults in Bangladesh, particularly among those in rural and marginalized communities. Geriatric psychiatric disorders are frequently under-diagnosed due to a lack of awareness and a focus on physical health problems. In this chapter, we discuss the current status of the geriatric population, their proportion, and demography in Bangladesh. We discuss the available evidence determining the prevalence and burden of psychiatric disorders in old age in the country. We highlighted the available specialized services for geriatric psychiatry in the country. The unmet need in geriatric psychiatry is mounting. However, there is a dearth of research and holistic services for geriatric psychiatry. As an entity geriatric psychiatry is in a rudimentary state in Bangladesh with similar challenges of psychiatry and other branches of psychiatry in Bangladesh that warrant policy-level attention and implications.

**Keywords** Geriatric psychiatry · Old-age psychiatry · Bangladesh psychiatry · Mental health · Psychiatric services

S. M. Y. Arafat (✉)
Department of Psychiatry, Bangladesh Specialized Hospital Limited, Dhaka, Bangladesh
e-mail: arafatdmc62@gmail.com

A. H. Mazumder
Ministry of Health and Family Welfare, Government of Bangladesh, Dhaka, Bangladesh

M. M. Maruf
Department of Addiction Psychiatry, National Institute of Mental Health, 1207 Dhaka, Bangladesh



S. M. Y. Arafat (ed.), *Mental Health in Bangladesh*,
https://doi.org/10.1007/978-981-97-0610-5_18

## 18.1 Introduction

Approximately 14% of adults aged 60 and above are living with a mental disorder, according to the Global Health Estimates (GHE) 2019. These conditions represent 10.6% of the total disability (measured in disability-adjusted life years, DALYs) among this age group. Depression and anxiety are the most prevalent mental health issues for older individuals. The GHE 2019 data also reveals that nearly a quarter (27.2%) of global suicide deaths occur among those aged 60 or above (WHO, 2023).

Bangladesh is a hugely populated country in South Asia with an area of 147,570 $km^2$ and about 170 million populations (Bangladesh Bureau of Statistics, 2023; adjust population). Of this population about 30% live in urban and the rest about 70% live in rural areas of the country. After its independence, Bangladesh made tremendous progress in several aspects of public health, especially in reducing maternal and child mortality (GBD, 2019 Bangladesh Burden of Disease Collaborators, 2023). Life expectancy has been improved significantly in the country. It was below 50 years in the 1970s; below 60 years in the 1980s; and in 2023, it reached above 73 years (Macrotrends, 2023; Statista, 2023). According to the latest *Population & Housing Census* 2022, among the total population, more than 9% (9.3%) were geriatric population making a count of 15.7 million (Bangladesh Bureau of Statistics, 2023). The proportion of geriatric (age above 60 years) populations has been increasing day by day. It was 5.7% in 1974, 6.4% in 2001, 7.5% in 2011, and 9.3% in 2022 (Bangladesh Bureau of Statistics, 2023; Barikdar et al., 2016).

The distribution of physical diseases and mental disorders is different from adulthood. There is a continuation of non-communicable diseases that started in mid-life and there are newer illnesses started in this period. Due to the changes happening in the body, family dynamics, societal roles, and friends, old people have different needs. Mental health care is an inevitable part of geriatric health care. There isn't a specific age at which individuals may start seeing a geriatrician, a doctor who focuses on the health care of elderly individuals (Somme et al., 2011). In literature from the 1950 and 1960s, the age of 55 years was often noted as the cut-off point at which one is categorized as geriatric. The age of 65 years is often cited as the cut-off for being classified as geriatric (Fisher et al., 2013). Other cut-offs, like 60 years (Ates et al., 2018) and 75 years (Somme et al., 2011), have also been used.

Though Bangladesh made remarkable progress in the health sector, still there are challenges especially in mental health (Arafat, 2024; Arafat et al., 2024). Various domains of mental health services are neglected due to high stigma, low literacy, inadequate research, and budget (Arafat, 2024; Arafat et al., 2024). Geriatric psychiatric services is one of the neglected domains of mental health services in the country. In this chapter, we discuss the current status of the geriatric population, their mental illness burden, and current specialized services for geriatric psychiatry in Bangladesh.

## 18.2 Epidemiology and Burden of Mental Disorders Among Elderly People in Bangladesh

Assessment of psychiatric disorders among older population is an under-studied area in Bangladesh. Whatever evidence we have, the majority of the studies assessed depression and anxiety (Table 18.1) with little attention to neurocognitive disorders.

### *18.2.1 Findings from Empirical Studies*

A cross-sectional study conducted in the rural Mirzapur sub-district involved 130 healthy individuals aged 40 and above, with no history of hypertension, cardiovascular diseases, hepatic or renal dysfunction, or diabetes (Das et al., 2014). Depression was measured by using the *Geriatric Depression Scale* (GDS-30). The study found 42% of participants had mild depression, while 17% were severely depressed. Depression was 2.8 times more common among females than males, and individuals aged 60 and above were 2.8 times more likely to have depression than those aged 40–59. Those on a vegetable-based diet, with low income, or a poor wealth index were at a higher risk of depression. These findings remained consistent even after controlling for factors like vitamin $B_{12}$, folic acid, liver function, and blood hemoglobin levels. The study underscores the prevalence of depression among healthy elders and highlights the impact of gender, age, diet, and socioeconomic status on depression risk.

Another cross-sectional study was conducted on 471 individuals over 60 years old in a rural area of Bangladesh (Palmer et al., 2014). This study included a physical examination to diagnose bodily disorders, an organized interview to investigate sociodemographic and social elements, and blood tests to evaluate nutritional and clinical factors. Dementia prevalence was determined on the basis of age and sex, and its links with clinical, social, and nutritional factors were investigated using logistic regression. Dementia was assessed by using the *Diagnostic and Statistical Manual of Mental Disorders* (DSM-IV) standards. The study found the prevalence were 11.5% and 3.6% for questionable dementia and definite dementia, respectively. The prevalence of dementia rose with age and fell with higher education levels. Malnutrition amplified the risk of dementia nearly six times (adjusted OR: 5.9; 95% CI = 1.3–26.3), while regular involvement in social activities decreased the risk. A significant link was discovered between malnutrition and dementia, emphasizing the importance of further research in this field within low-income countries.

Another cross-sectional study aimed to assess the risk of dementia development, including *mild cognitive impairment* (MCI) and Alzheimer's disease, among older age group (Uddin et al., 2019). The study included 390 adults aged between 60 and 70 years. The *Takeda Three Colors Combination* (TTCC) test was utilized to identify MCI and mild dementia, while the Clinical Dementia Rating determined the level of dementia. Results showed that among 60–65 year olds, MCI was found in

154 respondents, mild dementia was found in 76 persons, moderate dementia was found in 1, severe dementia was found in 4, and no dementia was identified in 29 respondents. Among 66–70 year olds, MCI was noted in 75, mild dementia in 36, severe dementia in 2, and no dementia in 13 respondents. The TTCC test had a sensitivity of 75% for mild dementia and 58% for MCI, with a specificity of 52%.

The same study assessed the prevalence of depressive symptoms using Self-Reporting Questionnaire (SRQ 20, n = 625), and investigated potential social network and economic associations (Wahlin et al., 2015). The presence of depression and suicidal ideation was assessed in a subsample (n = 471). Analyses were conducted on items corresponding to DSM-IV criteria resulting in a dichotomous manner. The prevalence of depressive symptoms was 45%, with the highest rate seen in the oldest females (70%). Suicidal ideation was found among 23% of the respondents. Female gender, low education (illiterate), and living without partners were the risk factors for depression and suicidal ideation. These relationships were not explained by social network and economic factors. Living with children and having good social were noted as resilient factors for both of the conditions.

In 2017, a study was conducted to evaluate the Quality of Life (QOL) and investigate its relationship with factors like depression among older adults in Bangladesh (Uddin et al., 2017). The study used a cross-sectional design and included participants aged between 60 and 75 years old who speak Bangla, cognitively sound, and willing to participate. Those with severe chronic diseases like heart, respiratory or renal failure, and those requiring assisted living were excluded. The sample comprised 280 participants from 10 villages in the southern districts of Bangladesh—Lakshmipur and Noakhali. The study aimed to provide insights into the association between depression and QOL in the aging population of Bangladesh. 84.6% participants perceived moderate level and 13.9% perceived low level of QOL in psychological domain. Findings indicated that there was a significant and moderate negative correlation between QOL and individuals experiencing depression.

In 2019, a cross-sectional study was conducted among 168 participants (100 females and 68 males) from Patuakhali City and its surrounding villages to assess geriatric depression using the GDS-15 (Disu et al., 2019). The geriatric depression prevalence rate was 36.9% among the participants. 71–80-year age group and 60–65-year age group had more depression (41.4 and 38.5%, respectively) compared to 66–70-year age group (31.3%). Exclusion of elderly people with current illness or sickness might be related to the lower prevalence rate of depression.

A cross-sectional study utilized multi-level cluster random sampling to select 2425 adults, including 1249 women, aged between 18 and 90 years from the Narail upazilla to detect psychological stress (Islam, 2019). The Kessler 10 item questionnaire was employed to evaluate psychological distress. Among the participants 1278 were adults (18–59 years of age) and 1147 older adults (60–90 years of age). The geriatric population (60–90 years) had significantly higher rate of moderate and severe psychological distress when compared to the younger adults (18–59 years). Severe psychological distress was more prevalent in women than men, and this disparity widened with age.

Another study cross-sectionally assessed the risk factors linked to depressive symptoms among 400 individuals aged 65 or older (Rahman et al., 2020a, 2020b). The prevalence of depressive symptoms was found to be 55.5%, with 23% exhibiting mild, 19% moderate, and 13.5% severe depression. Factors such as advanced age, gender, living situation, nuptiality, presence of other medical conditions, visual problem, past falls, feelings of loneliness, and a fear of falling were all significant contributors to developing depression.

A cross-sectional study was conducted in 2020 among 1032 geriatric persons (≥60 years) via telephone interviews using the 15-item GDS-15 (Mistri et al., 2021). Depressive symptoms were observed in 40.1% of the participants. This prevalence was significantly greater in the oldest age group (52.7%), women (48.9%), those who were widowed (51.6%), illiterate (43.9%), those in the lowest family income bracket (62.1%), individuals living alone (68.4%), and those who received COVID-19 pandemic-related information (62.5%).

A community-based cross-sectional study with a total of 400 participants was designed to ascertain the rate and severity of depressive symptoms and malnutrition among geriatric population and to examine the relationship between the two (Alam et al., 2021). The mean age of the participants in the study was 72.1 ± 7.0 years, with an equal number of males and females. Elderly individuals residing in institutions such as hospitals, nursing homes, or old-age homes, as well as those with terminal illnesses or mental retardation, were not included in the study. Nutritional status was determined using the Mini Nutritional Assessment (MNA), while the GDS was utilized to evaluate depression. Roughly 84% of participants exhibited various symptoms of depression. The occurrence of malnutrition and depression was higher among males. Those who were malnourished and those at risk of malnutrition had a significantly greater likelihood of experiencing depression. Good physical health, a healthy lifestyle, and a supportive family environment can help alleviate depression in the elderly population.

A cross-sectional comparative research was done among 600 elderly (aged ≥ 60 years) participants in three rural communities in 2019 (Islam et al., 2021). The study involved two groups of respondents: 300 depressed (cases) and 300 non-depressed (comparison group), matched for age and living area. Data was collected using a semi-structured questionnaire, and depression was determined using the GDS-15. The MNA-Short Form was used to assess nutritional status. There was no significant gender difference between depressed (44.0% male, 56.0% female) and non-depressed (46.0% male, 54.0% female) older adults. However, malnutrition was significantly higher in cases (56.0%) than in comparison group (18.0%) ($p < 0.01$). Malnourished participants were around three times more likely to experience depression than well-nourished counterparts. Depression was more prevalent among unemployed older adults, those from lower and middle classes, those with a "poor diet", single older adults, and tobacco users.

A 2019 cross-sectional study of 2795 individuals, aged 60 and above, in Bangladesh found that the prevalence of dementia was 8.0% (Naheed et al., 2023). The study used the *Mini Mental State Examination* (MMSE) to measure dementia, defined as an MMSE score of less than 24 out of 30. Factors such as age, sex, educational attainment, nuptiality, and occupation influenced dementia prevalence, but urban/rural location or socioeconomic status did not. After adjusting for certain factors, the study found that women were twice as likely as men to have dementia, those aged 90 and above were nine times more likely than those aged 60–69 to have dementia, and individuals with no education were three times more likely than those with primary school education to have dementia.

Another cross-sectional survey targeted 200 geriatric people (age 60–80 years), living in old homes at Dhaka and collected data via face-to-face interviews (Akter et al., 2023). The MMSE and GDS were used to assess cognitive function and depression levels, respectively. The study revealed moderate cognitive impairment in 43%, mild cognitive impairment in 36%, and normal cognition in 19.5%. Severe depression was found in 56% of the participants.

A cross-sectional study was carried out in an urban setting, involving in-person interviews using the GDS-15 to assess depression (Tabassum et al., 2023). This study included 230 elderly outpatients, aged between 60 and 80, who were visiting a hospital for medical purposes in Dhaka City. The prevalence of depression was 81.7%, with mild, moderate, and severe depression seen in 52.6, 25.2, and 3.9% of the subjects (scoring 5–8, 9–11, and 12–15 on the GDS, respectively). This rate of depression prevalence was generally higher compared to other studies conducted elsewhere, which could be attributed to the use of the GDS-15 scale and the particular environment in which the study was conducted. Depression was more common in individuals who were divorced, separated, never married, or widowed, as well as those who were retired or jobless. Additionally, individuals with an education level below primary and those who were socially isolated were more susceptible to depression. Those who regularly drank coffee were less likely to have depressive symptoms. This could be linked to the possibility that coffee consumption is often associated with a higher socioeconomic status.

Another community-based, cross-sectional study was conducted among elderly Forcibly Displaced Myanmar Nationals (FDMN) in Kutupalong Refugee Camp, Cox's Bazar, Bangladesh, from November 2021 to March 2022 (Alam et al., 2023). The study, which involved 430 participants aged $\geq 60$ years, used the MNA-Short Form and GDS-Short Form to determine malnutrition and geriatric depression (GD), respectively. Malnutrition was prevalent in 25.3% of subjects, with an additional 29.1% at risk. GD was found in 57.9% of participants, with 17.5% also experiencing malnutrition. Depression was significantly higher among malnourished geriatric people. The study concludes that agencies in Cox's Bazar should prioritize addressing geriatric malnutrition and GD among elderly FDMN.

### *18.2.2 The First National Mental Health Survey on in Bangladesh (2003–2005)*

The first national survey conducted in Bangladesh from 2003 to 2005 underscores the significant influence of mental disorders on the country (NIMH, B and WHO, 2007). This nationwide survey was conducted in both rural and urban settings among 13,080 participants with age of 18 and above. The prevalence rate of mental disorder was 16.1%. The most common disorder was neurotic disorders (8.4%). Females suffered more than males. Older age was associated with higher prevalence.

### *18.2.3 National Mental Health Survey 2019*

This nationwide cross-sectional survey was conducted both rural and urban settings, among 7270 study population with the age $\geq$ 18–99 years (Ministry of Health & Family Welfare, 2021). Overall prevalence of mental disorder was 18.7%. The highest prevalence of mental disorders was observed in people aged 60 and above (28.1%), followed by those aged 50 to 59 (22.1%), 30 to 39 (20.0%), 40 to 49 (17.2%), and 18 to 29 (14.6%). The rise in mental disorders among older age groups could be due to the prevalence of physical comorbidities within these groups. Additionally, the emergence of new disorders as people age can contribute to the increased prevalence of mental disorders in older individuals.

## 18.3 Available Services in Geriatric Psychiatry in Bangladesh

Bangladesh has inadequate resources dedicated to geriatric care overall, let alone geriatric mental health care. There is no geriatric health and/or geriatric psychiatrist in the country. Human resources, funding, social protection, and publicly available data are specially limited in the country (Barikdar et al., 2016). There is a Masters course in Gerontology in Dhaka University and a 100-mark course on geriatric nursing in the graduation program in nursing at the nursing colleges and institutes (Nayak, 2018). No recognition of geriatric psychiatry as established specialty as well as a lack of suitable planning or strategic interventions for rendering holistic care confers significant barrier to health care for old-age population. However, various qualified and semi-qualified healthcare providers from allopathy and alternative care background provide healthcare services to the people irrespective of age, both in government and non-government sectors in Bangladesh. Besides, unqualified, traditional, and informal carers also have major impact in providing health care in the country (Ministry of Health and Family Welfare, 2021).

## *18.3.1 Government Services*

### 18.3.1.1 Primary and Secondary Health Care

In the government healthcare settings at union, upazilla, and district levels, there is no facility of specialized mental health care, let alone services for geriatric mental health. However, many primary and secondary care physicians and nurses have been trained on mental health conditions with the mhGAP initiatives of the World Health Organization, implemented by Directorate General of Health Services of Bangladesh and National Institute of Mental Health (NIMH).

### 18.3.1.2 Tertiary Health Care

National Institute of Mental Health, Dhaka

There is a department in NIMH dedicated to the geriatric population in addition to the disorders due to general medical conditions. This *Department of Geriatric and Organic Psychiatry* has been providing its services from 2001. It has inpatient services, outpatient services, specialized clinic, and academic activities. There are currently 24 inpatient beds for geriatric male and 20 beds for female, 70% of which are non-paying. There is a separate outpatient consultation room specially dedicated for the geriatric population. Moreover, there was a specialized clinic for older age persons with mental health conditions every week in Tuesday, run by the psychiatrists, the activities of which has been suspended since the emergence of COVID-19.

Other Tertiary Care Centers

Mental Hospital Pabna, the oldest mental healthcare facility in Bangladesh, is a 500-bed hospital having no inpatient bed for geriatric population, though any person irrespective of age can get outpatient consultation. There is no dedicated inpatient bed or outpatient clinic only for geriatric population in medical colleges and not even in *Bangabandhu Sheikh Mujib Medical University* (BSMMU). However, older age patient with psychiatric disorders can get inpatient treatment, if indicated, in BSMMU and medical colleges having psychiatric inpatient beds. Dhaka Medical College Hospital has a 28-bed geriatric inpatient unit, which is the only one of such kind in government facilities running from 2014, but this unit has no specific allocation for psychiatric patients (Nayak, 2018). National Institute of Neuroscience in Dhaka runs a dementia clinic every Thursday where older patients from all corners of the country can have outdoor consultation for dementia.

#### 18.3.1.3 Other Government Services for Older Population

Elders Rehabilitation Centre (Boyoshko Punorbashon Kendro), registered under the Department of Social Service, was established in 1987. It is a center in Gazipur, near the capital city Dhaka, having free accommodation for about 1200 old persons as well as food, clothing, and health care, though no psychiatrist provides mental health services there (Nayak, 2018).

### *18.3.2 Non-Government Organization (NGO) Services*

Psychiatrists and psychologists provide outpatient services for the geriatric population with mental health conditions in their regular private chambers. Some NGOs operate specific healthcare and rehabilitation programs for geriatric population, of them *Bangladesh Association for the Aged and Institute of Geriatric Medicine (BAAIGM)* is of special mention. Starting from 1960, BAAIGM, popularly known as *Probin Hitoishi Sangha (PHS)*, provides a holistic care including accommodation and healthcare services for geriatric population. There it runs a 50-bed hospital and a 50-bed residential facility for geriatric peoples (Kabir et al., 2016). *Subarta Trust* operates a residential complex with healthcare services but being paid services, these may be unaffordable to many. *Sir William Beveridge Foundation* provides domiciliary services for geriatric population since 2007 with the opportunity to access to trained geriatric health professionals (Kabir et al., 2016). Senior Citizen Hospital (SCH) in Dhaka is a specialized private hospital dedicated to elderly people (SCH, 2023). But all of these facilities lack dedicated mental healthcare services. *Parents lounge* in Chattogram is a model of keeping sound mental health through the arrangement of recreational activities as well as free healthcare services (Nayak, 2018). *Retired officers Welfare Association* and *Retired Police Officers Welfare Association* in Dhaka, *Rehabilitation Center for Aged and Child, Service Center for Elderly People* in Rajshahi, *Elderly Development Initiative* in Manikganj, etc. are also providing such services toward the elderly (Alam et al., 2018). In our culture, support of the family members play a vital role in mental well-being of geriatric age group (Rahman et al., 2020a, 2020b). Sometimes a distant relative or any other person from village-home of the concerned affluent family in town is brought to act as an informal carer of the elderly person in the family.

## 18.4 Conclusion

Among the psychiatric disorders, anxiety, depression, stress, and dementia have been studied in Bangladesh. Mental health services for old-age population are underdeveloped and service demand for psychiatric problems in old age has been mounting in Bangladesh. However, specialist services for geriatric psychiatry are in a rudimentary state in the country. Likewise, the other branches of psychiatry have similar challenges that need policy-level changes and field-level implications of the policy in the country.

## References


Akter, N., Banu, B., Chowdhury, S. H., Islam, K. R., Tabassum, T. T., & Hossain, S. M. (2023). Astute exploration of collective mental health events among the residents of elderly care homes. *Heliyon, 9*(7), e18117. https://doi.org/10.1016/j.heliyon.2023.e18117

Alam, M., Hossain, I., Islam, N., & Mamun, M. (2018). Service requirements for the aged in Bangladesh. *SSRN Electronic Journal*. https://doi.org/10.2139/ssrn.3117272

Alam, M. M., Das, R., Clara, A. A., Mohsin, F. M., Rumi, M. A. H., Wahab, A., Hasan, M. A., & Hawlader, M. D. H. (2023). The assessment of geriatric malnutrition, geriatric depression and associated co-morbidities among forcibly displaced Myanmar nationals in Bangladesh. *Public Health Nutrition, 26*(10), 2048–2055. https://doi.org/10.1017/S1368980023001556

Alam, M. R., Karmokar, S., Reza, S., Kabir, M. R., Ghosh, S., & Mamun, M. A. A. (2021). Geriatric malnutrition and depression: Evidence from elderly home care population in Bangladesh. *Preventive Medicine Reports, 23*, 101478. https://doi.org/10.1016/j.pmedr.2021.101478

Arafat, S.M.Y, Giasuddin, N.A., Mazumder, A.H. (2024). Access to Mental Health Care in Bangladesh – Current Status, Potential Challenges, and Ways Out. Arafat SMY, Kar SK, eds. Access to Mental Health Care in South Asia - Current Status, Potential Challenges, and Ways Out. Springer Nature Singapore. https://doi.org/10.1007/978-981-99-9153-2_3

Arafat, S.M.Y., (2024). Mental Health Services in Bangladesh. Arafat SMY, ed. Mental Health in Bangladesh: From Bench to Community. Springer Nature Singapore. https://doi.org/10.1007/978-981-97-0610-5_3

Ates Bulut, E., Soysal, P., & Isik, A. T. (2018). Frequency and coincidence of geriatric syndromes according to age groups: Single-center experience in Turkey between 2013 and 2017. *Clinical Interventions in Aging, 13*, 1899–1905. https://doi.org/10.2147/CIA.S180281

Bangladesh Bureau of Statistics, (2023). Population & Housing Census 2022. https://bbs.gov.bd/site/page/47856ad0-7e1c-4aab-bd78-892733bc06eb/Population-&-Housing (accessed on 12 December 2023).

Barikdar, A., Ahmed, T., & Lasker, S. P. (2016). The Situation of the Elderly in Bangladesh. *Bangladesh Journal of Bioethics, 7*(1), 27–36. https://doi.org/10.3329/bioethics.v7i1.29303

Das, J., Farzana, FD, Ferdous, F., Ahmed S, Sarah Tegenfeldt, et al. (2014). Factors Associated with Elderly Depression among Rural Bangladeshi Individuals. *American Journal of Psychiatry and Neuroscience, 2*(1), 1–7. https://doi.org/10.11648/j.ajpn.20140201.11

Disu, T. R., Anne, N. J., Griffiths, M. D., & Mamun, M. A. (2019). Risk factors of geriatric depression among elderly Bangladeshi people: A pilot interview study. *Asian Journal of Psychiatry, 44*, 163–169. https://doi.org/10.1016/j.ajp.2019.07.050

Fischer, C. E., Ismail, Z., & Rapoport, M. J. (2013). Geriatric Psychiatry or Psychogeriatrics? Partnership at the CAGP/CCSMH 2012 Scientific Meeting. *Canadian Geriatrics Journal : CGJ, 16*(1), 3–5. https://doi.org/10.5770/cgj.16.66

GBD 2019 Bangladesh Burden of Disease Collaborators. (2023). The burden of diseases and risk factors in Bangladesh, 1990–2019: A systematic analysis for the Global Burden of Disease Study 2019. *The Lancet. Global Health, 11*(12), e1931–e1942. https://doi.org/10.1016/S2214-109X(23)00432-1

Islam, F. M. A. (2019). Psychological distress and its association with socio-demographic factors in a rural district in Bangladesh: A cross-sectional study. *PLoS ONE, 14*(3), e0212765. https://doi.org/10.1371/journal.pone.0212765

Islam, M. Z., Disu, T. R., Farjana, S., & Rahman, M. M. (2021). Malnutrition and other risk factors of geriatric depression: A community-based comparative cross-sectional study in older adults in rural Bangladesh. *BMC Geriatrics, 21*(1), 572. https://doi.org/10.1186/s12877-021-02535-w

Kabir, R., Kabir, M., Uddin, M. S. G., Ferdous, N., & Chowdhury, M. R. K. (2016). Elderly population growth in Bangladesh: Preparedness in public and private sectors. *IOSR Journal of Humanities and Social Science, 21*, 58–73. https://doi.org/10.9790/0837-2108025873

macrotrends, 2023. Bangladesh Life Expectancy 1950–2023. https://www.macrotrends.net/countries/BGD/bangladesh/life-expectancy#:~:text=The%20life%20expectancy%20for%20Bangladesh,a%200.39%25%20increase%20from%202019 (accessed on 12 December, 2023).

Ministry of Health & Family Welfare, 2021. National Mental Health Survey 2019. http://nimh.gov.bd/wp-content/uploads/2021/11/Mental-Health-Survey-Report.pdf (accessed 29 March, 2023).

Mistry, S. K., Ali, A. R. M. M., Hossain, M. B., Yadav, U. N., Ghimire, S., Rahman, M. A., Irfan, N. M., & Huque, R. (2021). Exploring depressive symptoms and its associates among Bangladeshi older adults amid COVID-19 pandemic: Findings from a cross-sectional study. *Social Psychiatry and Psychiatric Epidemiology, 56*(8), 1487–1497. https://doi.org/10.1007/s00127-021-02052-6

Naheed, A., Hakim, M., Islam, M. S., Islam, M. B., Tang, E. Y. H., Prodhan, A. A., Amin, M. R., Stephan, B. C. M., & Mohammad, Q. D. (2023). Prevalence of dementia among older age people and variation across different sociodemographic characteristics: A cross-sectional study in Bangladesh. *The Lancet Regional Health. Southeast Asia, 17*, 100257. https://doi.org/10.1016/j.lansea.2023.100257

National Institute of Mental Health & Hospital (Bangladesh). (2007). WHO Bangladesh: Prevalence, Medical Care, Awareness and Attitude Towards Mental Illness in Bangladesh. In M. E. Karim & M. M. Zaman (Eds.), pp. 1–27. Retrieved from http://books.google.com.bd/books/about/Prevalence_Medical_Care_Awareness_and_At.html?id=cixINwAACAAJ&redir_esc=y.

Nayak, H. S. (2018). The felt need of home-based geriatric care in Bangladesh. *Journal of Nursing and Health Studies, 3*(2), 7. https://doi.org/10.21767/2574-2825.1000036

Palmer, K., Kabir, Z. N., Ahmed, T., Hamadani, J. D., Cornelius, C., Kivipelto, M., & Wahlin, Å. (2014). Prevalence of dementia and factors associated with dementia in rural Bangladesh: Data from a cross-sectional, population-based study. *International Psychogeriatrics, 26*(11), 1905–1915. https://doi.org/10.1017/S1041610214001392

Senior citizen hospital (2023). https://seniorcitizenhospital.com/. Accessed on 14.12.2023

Rahman, M. S., Rahman, M. A., Afroze, L., & Islam, S. M. S. (2020a). Unmet needs for mental care services for older people in Bangladesh during the COVID-19 pandemic. *General Psychiatry, 33*(6), e100294. https://doi.org/10.1136/gpsych-2020-100294

Rahman, M. S., Rahman, M. A., Ali, M., Rahman, M. S., Maniruzzaman, M., Yeasmin, M. A., Ahmed, N. A. M. F., Abedin, M. M., & Islam, S. M. S. (2020b). Determinants of depressive symptoms among older people in Bangladesh. *Journal of Affective Disorders, 264*, 157–162. https://doi.org/10.1016/j.jad.2019.12.025

Somme, D., Lazarovici, C., Dramé, M., Blanc, P., Lang, P. O., Gauvain, J. B., Voisin, T., Gonthier, R., De Wazières, B., Jeandel, C., Couturier, P., Blanchard, F., & Saint-Jean, O. (2011). The geriatric patient: Use of acute geriatrics units in the emergency care of elderly patients in France. *Archives of Gerontology and Geriatrics, 52*(1), 40–45. https://doi.org/10.1016/j.archger.2010.01.018

Statista, 2023. Life expectancy (from birth) in Bangladesh from 1865 to 2020*. https://www.statista.com/statistics/1071009/life-expectancy-bangladesh-historical/ (accessed on 12 December, 2023).

Tabassum, T., Suzuki, T., Iwata, Y., & Ishiguro, H. (2023). Depression and Associated Factors Among the Elderly Population in an Urban Tertiary Geriatric Hospital in Bangladesh. *Gerontology & Geriatric Medicine, 9*, 23337214231178144. https://doi.org/10.1177/23337214231178145

Uddin, M. A., Soivong, P., Lasuka, D., & Juntasopeepun, P. (2017). Factors related to quality of life among older adults in Bangladesh: A cross sectional survey. *Nursing & Health Sciences, 19*(4), 518–524. https://doi.org/10.1111/nhs.12385

Uddin, M. S., Mamun, A. A., Takeda, S., Sarwar, M. S., & Begum, M. M. (2019). Analyzing the chance of developing dementia among geriatric people: A cross-sectional pilot study in Bangladesh. *Psychogeriatrics : The Official Journal of the Japanese Psychogeriatric Society, 19*(2), 87–94. https://doi.org/10.1111/psyg.12368

Wahlin, Å., Palmer, K., Sternäng, O., Hamadani, J. D., & Kabir, Z. N. (2015). Prevalence of depressive symptoms and suicidal thoughts among elderly persons in rural Bangladesh. *International Psychogeriatrics, 27*(12), 1999–2008. https://doi.org/10.1017/S104161021500109X

World Health Organization (2023, October 20). Mental health of older adults. Retrieved December 19, 2023, from https://www.who.int/news-room/fact-sheets/detail/mental-health-of-older-adults

# Chapter 19
# NGOs Working on Mental Health in Bangladesh

**Rubina Jahan, Md. Ashiquir Rahaman, and Arun Das**

**Abstract** The presence and active engagement of non-governmental organizations (NGOs) in the mental health sector have been instrumental in popularizing and shaping the narrative around mental health in Bangladesh. Through their dedicated efforts, these NGOs have played a pivotal role in raising awareness, reducing stigma, and expanding the accessibility of mental health services, contributing significantly to the sector's increased recognition and acceptance within the broader societal discourse. Given the context, this chapter meticulously examines the multifaceted involvement of NGOs in the mental health sector, unraveling a narrative that spans historical contexts, describes roles, explores service approaches, presents work around vulnerable communities, highlights innovations through case studies, addresses challenges faced, and casts a perceptive gaze into the future. Each section within this comprehensive exploration contributes to a nuanced understanding of the collective efforts that NGOs have undertaken to address the complex challenges of mental health in Bangladesh over the years.

**Keywords** Mental health · NGO · Historical context · Localized innovations · Challenges · Approach · Bangladesh

R. Jahan (✉)
Head of Programme, Mental Health, SAJIDA Foundation, Dhaka, Bangladesh
e-mail: rumirj@gmail.com

Md. A. Rahaman
Department of Clinical Psychology, University of Dhaka, Dhaka, Bangladesh

A. Das
Helpline Operations, Kaan Pete Roi Emotional Support & Suicide Prevention Helpline, Dhaka, Bangladesh



S. M. Y. Arafat (ed.), *Mental Health in Bangladesh*,
https://doi.org/10.1007/978-981-97-0610-5_19

## 19.1 Historical Context: NGOs Work in Mental Health Sector in Bangladesh

In the historical context of Bangladesh, the social development scene has been significantly shaped by the extensive involvement of non-governmental organizations (NGOs). This influence extends prominently to the development and enhancement of mental health services as well in the country. The inception of NGOs' engagement with mental health can be traced back to the post-liberation phase (December 16, 1971) when these organizations, originally focused on post-war rehabilitation and aiding communities in distress, began to recognize the pressing need for addressing psychosocial challenges.

### *19.1.1 The Early Years: 1970 to 1980s*

In the early 1970s to the 1980s, a significant phase of NGO involvement in mental health development unfolded in Bangladesh. Organizations such as *Bangladesh Rural Advancement Committee* (BRAC) and *Gonosasthaya Kendra* (G.K.) emerged during this period. BRAC, for instance, initially began its activities by providing crucial relief and rehabilitation assistance to the community of fishermen in the north-east, who had faced displacement due to the atrocities during 1971 (MacMillan, 2022). In tandem with their rehabilitation efforts, these organizations recognized the essential need for psychosocial support to empower the affected communities. Similarity, G.K. had its origins in a mobile medical unit that provided crucial support to the freedom fighters in 1971 (Islam, 2016). In response to the pressing needs of the time, G. K. also partially stepped into addressing psychosocial support, recognizing the importance of holistic care. During this period, many such NGOs emerged such as *Rangpur Dinajpur Rural Service* (RDRS), *Bangladesh Rural Development Academy* (BARD), *Caritas Bangladesh, Ain O Salish Kendra* (ASK), etc. backed by local, national, and international funding who played a crucial role in shaping the field gradually.

Importantly, during this period, the formal development of the mental health field had yet to materialize. The historical trajectory reveals a progressive shift from immediate post-war relief initiatives to a more nuanced and comprehensive approach, laying the groundwork for the development and enhancement of mental health services in Bangladesh later on.

### *19.1.2 1980 to 1990s*

One of the other earliest concerns addressed by mental health NGOs in Bangladesh was working with substance dependence. This issue arose due to the historical use of substances like opium and cannabis, and the subsequent smuggling of drugs like heroin into the country in the 1980s (Ambekar et al., 2005). This led to a surge in heroin consumption and a growing demand for rehabilitation programs for those dependent on heroin. In response to this need, the *Bangladesh Rehabilitation and Assistance Center for Addicts* (BARACA) was established by the *Holy Cross Brothers* in Bangladesh in 1988. *BARACA* became the first drug treatment and rehabilitation center in Bangladesh, providing services for the treatment and rehabilitation of drug-dependent individuals, both male and female. It also offered awareness programs on drug use, harm and risk reduction, as well as voluntary counseling and testing (VCT) for those with substance dependencies. CREA, *Ashokti Punorbashon Kendra* (APON), and *Addiction Management and Integrated Care* (AMIC) are few of the major institutions formed and worked in the field during this period.

During the 1990s and early 2000s, the issue of drug addiction gained prominence through extensive media campaigns. These campaigns not only increased public awareness but also emphasized the urgent need for rehabilitation services for individuals struggling with substance dependence. Numerous mental health NGOs have conscientiously directed their endeavors toward addressing this pivotal aspect of mental health care. They not only played a significant role in raising awareness at the community level but also established facilities and contributed in developing inclusive, culturally sensitive, and cost-effective evidence-based treatment programs that enhanced the chances of successful recovery while reducing the risk of relapse in response to this need. Presently, the landscape boasts an extensive network of over 364 (Department of Narcotics Control, 2023) licensed rehabilitation facilities spread across the country, each functioning at varying capacities determined by their revenue-generating models. However, the accessibility to these facilities is not uniform, creating a nuanced scenario where individuals' financial affordability becomes a critical determinant.

### *19.1.3 The Transition 2000s to Present*

In the early 2000s, there has been a growing recognition of the importance of mental health in Bangladesh. The increasing involvement of NGOs in this field has been instrumental in not only elevating awareness but also in formalizing the mental health sector, demonstrating a concentrated commitment to addressing the diverse mental health needs of the population.

Another prominent sphere within the domain of mental health that has accumulated significant attention from NGOs is children's mental health, particularly within the realm of intellectual disabilities and autism spectrum disorder (ASD). The *Shuchona Foundation*, a prominent entity in the country known for its significant contributions to reforming legislation, policy, and quality services within the government health system, has earned accolades internationally for its expertise in neurodevelopmental disorder (NDD).

Many NGOs started working primarily in the specialized education and service provision for children with NDD; employed specialized teaching methods, including Verbal Prompt, Treatment and Education of Autistic and related Communication-handicapped Children (TEACCH), Picture Exchange Communication System (PECS), and the Applied Behavior Analysis (ABA) therapy, to provide individualized support for each. Organizations like *Beautiful Mind*, *Proyash* and *Inner Circle* pioneered catering services to the unique needs of children with a range of symptoms and broadened the scope of child mental health services to include conditions of varying severity, such as attention-deficit hyperactivity disorder (ADHD). These NGOs are offering outpatient and school-based services tailored to children experiencing a wide spectrum of neurodevelopmental disorders, ranging from mild to severe in nature.

Concurrently, there has been a rising emphasis on community-based mental health care, with NGOs assuming a pivotal role in both the development and execution of programs at the grassroots level. In recent years, NGOs like BRAC, *SAJIDA Foundation*, and *Innovation for Wellbeing Foundation* (IWF) are few of the many organizations concentrated more in community mental health to ensure increased access to mental healthcare support. These community-based interventions expanded through diverse and hard-to-reach areas such as rural and urban marginalized settings, humanitarian settings, climate change and disaster vulnerable regions, etc.

Apart from that, the country has also witnessed a handful of organizations making substantial investments in mental health research, advocacy, and policy reformation, contributing significantly to the evolving landscape of mental health in the country. The various roles of NGOs and its impact in the national landscape will be further elaborated in the later sections of this chapter. It is needless to say, as a whole, NGOs are filling gaps in service provision, raising awareness about mental health issues, and advocating for policy changes to improve mental healthcare accessibility and quality in Bangladesh.

## 19.2 Role of NGOs in Mental Health

In the context of being a densely populated and resource-limited country, Bangladesh faces numerous challenges in its healthcare infrastructure. One significant hurdle is the scarcity of health professionals, particularly in the field of mental health. To address this critical gap in mental health service provision, NGOs play a pivotal role through various activities encompassing education, enhancing service accessibility, fostering collaboration, developing resources, and advocating for policy changes. The following provides an illustrative overview of the roles undertaken by NGOs in the realm of mental health in Bangladesh.

### 19.2.1 Raising Awareness and Reducing Stigma

Addressing the global challenge of mental health stigma, particularly pronounced in low- and middle-income countries (LMICs) like Bangladesh, is crucial. As highlighted in the national mental health survey 2019 (Ministry of Health & Welfare, 2021), stigma significantly impedes treatment-seeking behavior due to the fear of negative labeling, such as being deemed "mad". NGOs in Bangladesh are actively involved in multifaceted efforts to raise awareness and mitigate stigma. They employ diverse strategies, including campaigns, workshops, training, seminars, and informational materials, to disseminate knowledge about mental health and stress the importance of seeking mental health services. Although progress may be gradual, these initiatives by NGOs such as *Kaan Pete Roi Emotional Support and Suicide Prevention Helpline* (KPR), *Society for Voluntary Association* (SOVA), *Moshal Foundation, Achol Foundation, HEAL Bangladesh,* IWF, BRAC, and *SAJIDA Foundation* contribute to reducing stigma and cultivating a more accessible mental health infrastructure in Bangladesh, where resources are often limited.

### 19.2.2 Advocating for Policy Changes

NGOs have been playing a crucial role in advocating for policy changes to strengthen the mental health service structure and promote mental well-being. In 2018, Bangladesh achieved a significant milestone in its mental health landscape by introducing the National Mental Health Act, thereby replacing the age-old Lunacy Act of 1912 (Mental Health Act, 2018). One of the key contributors to this achievement includes the dedicated efforts of the *Shuchona Foundation* who played a pivotal role in advocating for and drafting the progressive legislation. *Bangladesh Mental Health Network* (BMHN) also played a significant role to enable the process. The enactment of the National Mental Health Act marks a crucial step forward for Bangladesh's mental health fraternity, signaling a commitment to modernizing and prioritizing mental health care in the country (Karim & Shaikh, 2021).

Notably, NGOs have been focusing on drawing the government's attention to address barriers to mental health, such as inadequate services, suboptimal care quality in psychiatric facilities, paternalistic and gender-insensitive service approaches, human rights violations, and the stigma attached to individuals with mental disorders. NGOs have been actively working to establish mental health as an inherent human right, ensuring access to the necessary care and support for maintaining good mental health. Additionally, NGOs have been advocating for individuals facing discrimination, abuse, or other injustices, emphasizing successful implementation of diverse mental health service programs. Their efforts extend to pushing for increased funding for mental health services and the seamless integration of mental health into primary health care, addressing critical gaps in mental health provision.

### 19.2.3 Expanding Access to Mental Health Services

NGOs have played a crucial role in broadening access to mental health services across Bangladesh. One primary avenue through which NGOs contribute to enhanced mental health access is by establishing and managing mental health clinics, hospitals, and psychosocial support centers. According to a nationwide mental health service mapping, *Gonoshasthaya Samaj Vittik Medical College and Hospital*, *Psychological Health and Wellness Clinic* (PHWC), *Dorpon Service*, *Monojogot Center*, *Center for Mental Health and Care, Bangladesh* (CMHC, B), and *Healing Heart* among many other entities providing facility-based mental health services (ADD International Bangladesh, 2021). These facilities serve as vital hubs for diagnosis, treatment, and support for individuals grappling with mental health conditions. NGOs have also undertaken initiatives to bolster the number of trained mental health professionals in the country. According to a 2015 mental health situation analysis article, 46% of mental health professionals, including psychiatrists, are employed by NGOs, for-profit mental health facilities, or in private practice (Islam & Biswas, 2015). In addition to physical infrastructure, NGOs leverage technological advancements such as telemedicine and tele-counseling services to overcome barriers to access. Through these technological means, mental health professionals from NGOs offer consultations and even remote monitoring, extending their services beyond traditional healthcare facilities. *Tele-Psychiatry Research and Innovation Network* (TRIN) and *SAJIDA Foundation* are few of the major players reaching hard-to-reach communities and offering mental health services utilizing tele-mental health platforms. Moreover, NGOs have expanded their scope to provide mental health services to vulnerable populations, including refugees, disaster survivors, and individuals who identify as gender and sexually diverse.

## 19.3 Approaches of NGOs

Bangladeshi NGOs employ various methodologies to offer mental health services, often aligning with three distinct approaches such as the fund-based approach, the revenue-generating approach, and the integration of mental health as a value-added service.

### 19.3.1 Fund-Based Approach

Most NGOs rely primarily on grants, donations, and financial aid from government bodies, philanthropists, corporations, and fundraising campaigns to sustain their mental health initiatives. These funds serve as the lifeblood, enabling NGOs to execute mental health programs and support services. Many medium- and small-sized mental health NGOs like IWF, KPR, and TRIN heavily rely on external fundings. Apart from that, prominent organizations such as BRAC and SAJIDA Foundation, many of their mental health initiatives are fund based. Leveraging these resources, NGOs conduct outreach programs and awareness campaigns, organize community interventions, and establish counseling centers or helplines to offer immediate assistance to those in need. This approach often allows them to offer free or subsidized mental health services, making it accessible to low-income as well as underserved and marginalized communities. NGOs, through this approach, aim to bridge the gaps in mental healthcare accessibility, ensuring that financial constraints do not hinder individuals from seeking essential support.

However, relying solely on funding can make these programs vulnerable to financial instability, impacting the continuity of services. NGOs employing this approach face constant pressure to secure resources and may struggle to maintain programmatic stability in the long run. This is applicable for NGOs in general and not limited to mental health NGOs only. For example, until May 21, 2021, donations and foreign grants to NGOs working in Bangladesh decreased by 14%. This reduction in funding is creating a serious crisis for many small- and medium-sized NGOs, putting their existence at risk. Even one of the most prominent NGOs, BRAC, in June 2021, faced a significant setback when the U.K. decided to cut aid worth 450 million British Pounds annually. The reasoning behind the cut was that the funds would be redirected to African countries facing more severe poverty challenges than Bangladesh. Unfortunately, this withdrawal of funds had a direct impact on women's and girls' education, as well as those in extreme poverty in Bangladesh, creating difficulties for ongoing initiatives and support programs in these areas (Baser & Abu Hasnath, 2023).

### *19.3.2 Revenue-Generating Approach*

Contrary to the fund-based model, some NGOs implement revenue-generating activities to sustain their mental health initiatives. These organizations create sustainable income streams through various channels, such as running social enterprises, selling mental health-related products or services, charging fees for specific interventions, or partnering with corporations. For example, outpatient clinics such as PHWC, *Monobikash Foundation,* and CMHC, B, providing psychotherapy and psychiatric consultations; drug addiction recovery centers such as *Promises BD, APON, and Prottoy*; and neurodevelopment support centers for children in Bangladesh such as *Inner Circle* and *Beautiful Mind* mostly employed revenue-generating financial models. By generating revenue, these NGOs create a self-sustaining ecosystem that ensures the continuity and quality of mental healthcare provisions.

While this approach offers NGOs financial independence and operational stability, it creates a potential risk of excluding individuals who cannot afford these services, potentially leaving behind vulnerable populations with limited resources, which could undermine the non-profit mission of the NGOs. However, NGOs often reinvest the surplus revenues to improve and expand their mental health programs or provide subsidized services for individuals who cannot afford the full cost, thereby maintaining a balance between financial viability and social impact.

### *19.3.3 Mental Health as a Value-Added Service*

In an evolving landscape, many NGOs and businesses have recognized mental health as a fundamental component of overall well-being. Integrating mental health services as part of their core offerings, these organizations consider it a value-added service. For instance, NGOs focusing on education, community development, or health care incorporate mental health components into their existing programs. Examples of such NGOs are *Hashimukh Somaj Kallayan Songstha, Care Bangladesh,* ASK, *Acid Survivors Foundation* (ASF), *Bangladesh Legal Aid and Services Trust* (BLAST), *Bandhu Social Welfare Society* (Bandhu) and *Praggroshor,* etc. By embedding mental health awareness, counseling, or support mechanisms into different initiatives, these organizations promote a comprehensive approach to the well-being of the communities they serve. Also, companies may provide employee assistance programs or wellness initiatives that encompass mental health support as an integral component.

This approach helps normalizing mental health discussions, promotes early identification of problems, reduces stigma, and encourages individuals to seek help by making these services more accessible in everyday settings. Integrating mental health as part of a comprehensive package empowers individuals to address mental health concerns while benefiting from other essential services, thus amplifying the overall impact. This approach leverages existing infrastructure and resources, reaching a wider population and highlighting the interconnectedness of mental health with other social issues. However, while it enhances awareness and accessibility, the depth and specialization of services might be limited compared to dedicated mental health-focused NGOs. Also, this approach may require additional staff training and careful planning to ensure effective implementation.

Each approach has its advantages and challenges. The fund-based approach ensures access to care for marginalized communities but faces financial uncertainties. The revenue-generating approach offers sustainability and quality but risks excluding individuals who cannot afford the fees. The value-added approach promotes holistic well-being and accessibility but might not provide the necessary depth of support for individuals with complex mental health needs. While choosing the appropriate approach depends on the organization's mission, resources, and target population, combining different approaches and adopting innovative strategies could potentially yield the most comprehensive impact.

## 19.4 NGOs Working with Vulnerable Communities

Vulnerable communities are groups facing a higher risk of discrimination, exploitation, and disparities in social, economic, political, and health outcomes compared to the general population (Rukmana, 2014). Factors contributing to vulnerability include age, socioeconomic status, disability, health, gender identity, sexual orientation, location, cultural background, and exposure to specific challenges. These communities, prone to negative health outcomes, especially in mental health due to discrimination and unequal opportunities, need special attention. In Bangladesh, NGOs play a crucial role in addressing the diverse needs of vulnerable communities, focusing on Forcibly Displaced Myanmar Nationals (Rohingya); survivors of climate change; indigenous populations; and lesbian, gay, bi-sexual, transgender and queer (LGBTQ) communities (Table 19.1).

### *19.4.1 Forcibly Displaced Myanmar National (Rohingya)*

Historically, the Rohingya, an ethnic, linguistic, and religious minority from Myanmar's northern Rakhine state, have faced political oppression and have been subjected to forced displacement in Bangladesh, occurring notably in 1978, 1992, 2012, and 2016. However, the most significant forced displacement took place in August 2017. According to UNHCR, as of August 2023, over 960,000 Rohingya refugees reside in Bangladesh, situated in 33 highly congested refugee camps primarily located in Ukhiya and Teknaf Upazilas of the Cox's Bazar District, as well as on the island of Bhasan Char (UNHCR, 2023). Moreover, the majority of the Rohingya refugees are children, with 51 percent composed of women and girls (UNHCR, 2021). The prolonged exposure to conflict compounded by adverse conditions of displacement and deprivation may have heightened the refugee's vulnerability to a wide spectrum of mental health disorders, including post-traumatic stress disorder, anxiety, panic disorder, depression, and suicidal ideation (Tay et al., 2019). Moreover, high rates of sexual- and gender-based violence prevail among this population, contributing to negative mental health outcomes and hindering help-seeking behavior. Therefore, the Rohingya influx and their multifaceted needs have prompted NGOs to address the humanitarian crisis. According to JRP, 2022, a total 74 NGOs are working as the implementing partners in the Rohingya camps in Bangladesh under the coordination of Government of Bangladesh (GoB) (JRP, 2022). In the beginning, the majority of NGOs used the task-shifting approach within border health initiatives to address the community's primary needs for mental health and psychosocial services (MHPSS). However, a small number of organizations created creative models to mainstream the population's mental health needs. A case study of such a successful innovation has been presented in Sect. 19.5 of this chapter.

### 19.4.2 Survivors of Climate Change

Climate change presents a multifaceted threat to vulnerable populations, extending its impacts beyond the physical realm to encompass profound psychological consequences, including anxiety, depression, and post-traumatic stress disorder (PTSD) (Wahid et al., 2023). In Bangladesh, where climate impacts are severe, a 2023 World Bank-funded study in Lancet Planetary Health linked higher temperatures, humidity, and floods to increased anxiety and depression (Wahid et al., 2023). SAJIDA Foundation's pilot study in Gabura and Mongla echoed these concerns, with 88% acknowledging disasters as a major cause of mental health issues (Diaz & Rahaman, 2022).

While climate change and mental health is a relatively new field with limited empirical research, NGOs like *SAJIDA Foundation*, BRAC, and *Friendship* are addressing the mental health challenges faced by climate-vulnerable communities. These organizations use a community-based approach, deploying trained volunteers to provide essential healthcare services, including mental health support. Fortunately, technology is now playing a crucial role in providing mental health services in remote areas, including climate-vulnerable populations. However, despite NGOs' increased focus in providing support to local communities, these efforts are often transient and may not be adequate to meet the sustained needs of the affected people.

### 19.4.3 Indigenous Community

As of the 2022 census report, Bangladesh is home to approximately 1,650,159 indigenous individuals, constituting about 1% of the total population (Bangladesh Bureau of Statistics, 2023). There are around 51 indigenous communities in Bangladesh, primarily residing in the Chittagong Hill Tracts, as well as other regions like Sylhet, Naogaon, Dinajpur, and Mymensingh (Bangladesh Bureau of Statistics, 2023). The indigenous people in Bangladesh face a range of challenges, including illiteracy, poverty, high conflict rates, human rights violations, limited employment opportunities, restricted healthcare access, lack of clean water and sanitation, and poor infrastructure development. These multifaceted challenges, coupled with their minority status, significantly impact the mental health of indigenous communities. Research indicates higher rates of anxiety and depression among these populations compared to the general population in Bangladesh (Faruk et al., 2021). Despite these challenges, culturally sensitive mental health services for this sizable population are nearly nonexistent. Only a handful of NGOs are currently working in these intersections, prioritizing the human rights, health, and livelihood aspect of indigenous people in Bangladesh. *Supporting People and Rebuilding Communities* (SPaRC), for example, focuses on gender equality, sustainable development, justice, peace, and both mental and physical health. Similarly, the *Manusher Jonno Foundation* (MJF) collaborates with local organizations to improve the well-being of poor and marginalized communities, including those belonging to indigenous communities in the Chittagong Hill Tracts. However, their efforts are presently confined to enhancing nutrition services, fostering community mobilization, promoting climate-resilient agriculture, and providing social safety-net services. Therefore, there is a pressing need for targeted, culturally sensitive mental health interventions to address the long-neglected mental health and well-being of historically marginalized indigenous populations in Bangladesh.

### *19.4.4 LGBTQ Community*

The LGBTQ community in Bangladesh frequently encounters distinctive challenges arising from societal stigma and discrimination, given that the concepts of gender diversity and sexual orientation are intricate and often considered taboo in the conservative, predominantly Muslim society of the country. Consequently, living in an invalidating and discriminatory society can significantly impact the mental health and well-being of LGBTQ individuals, compared to the general population (Wei et al., 2020). In response to this critical issue, few organizations are working to promote health and well-being, offer support, and advocate for the rights of LGBTQ individuals. One such organization is the *Bandhu Social Welfare Society* (Bandhu), focusing on improving access to legal support, reducing stigma and discrimination, mitigating gender-based violence (GBV), and addressing human rights violations. Additionally, they work to enhance access to healthcare services, covering sexual and reproductive health and rights (SRHR), HIV prevention, mental health support, non-communicable diseases (NCDs), and general health care. Additionally, ICDDR, B, although primarily a research-based organization, engages with sexual and gender diverse communities through a program named the Programme for HIV and AIDS. While initially centered on HIV prevention and STIs, their recent expansion includes services related to SRHR, mental health, psychosocial counseling, and addressing GBV.

Despite the significant presence of a large LGBTQ community in Bangladesh and their evident need for mental health support, organizations working with this community often face legal challenges that compel them to operate informally. Limiting their ability to openly advocate for LGBTQ rights and provide formalized mental health support to the community.

## 19.5 Mental Health Innovations—Case Studies

In this chapter, we delve into three unique initiatives, such as Kaan Pete Roi suicide prevention helpline, BRAC humanitarian play lab, and Shojon tele-mental health, each contributing unique and pioneering approaches to address mental health challenges in Bangladesh.

### 19.5.1 Kaan Pete Roi (KPR) Emotional Support and Suicide Prevention Helpline

Bangladesh's first suicide prevention helpline, Kaan Pete Roi, was set up in April 2013. Dr. Yeshim Iqbal started KPR, a non-profit volunteer-run organization (Iqbal et al., 2019). KPR employs a "befriending" approach, as opposed to typical counseling or psychotherapy. The core of the Befriending concept is active listening, in which a volunteer receives training on how to actively listen to someone with empathy and nonjudgmental support over the phone in order to de-escalate the risk of suicide. KPR is the forty-first member to join the globally recognized organization "Befrienders Worldwide" dedicated to suicide prevention (Befrienders Worldwide, 2012).

Dr. Yeshim established the helpline with a group of youthful volunteers, believing that their objective to establish such a helpline would be worthwhile and legitimate if they could save even one life. With a pool of 70 to 80 active volunteers on the weekly roster at present, KPR has trained over 400 helpline volunteers in the last 10 years. In the past decade, KPR has assisted over 50,000 vulnerable individuals grappling with suicidal thoughts or plans.

The precise suicide rate in Bangladesh remains a subject of debate due to the absence of a national suicide surveillance system, resulting in varying figures across different sources and studies. However, existing evidence points to a higher prevalence of suicides among the youth, particularly those under 30, with a notable gender disparity as females surpass males in mortality rates (Kabir et al., 2023). Despite of heightened need, Bangladesh lacks a national crisis hotline, and with limited resources, initiatives like Kaan Pete Roi become essential to address the burden of stigma, cost-effectiveness, and accessibility in suicide prevention. With KPR's nonstop service for more than a decade, it is needless to say that the organization has successfully established a volunteer-based model for suicide prevention in Bangladesh. During COVID-19, when a nationwide lockdown caused everything to stop and operations to be scaled back. Over the phone, KPR continued offering their services. During the COVID-19 pandemic, people from all walks of life realized how crucial it was to have such a helpline because there was clearly a mental health emergency at hand (Iqbal et al., 2021). Consequently, there was a greater need than ever for such helpline services. At that point, SAJIDA Foundation began sponsoring KPR's activities. This allowed KPR to increase the number of calls it received each day from 15 to 40 by extending its operating hours from 6 to 12, including night shifts. With the goal of expanding this service across the country, SF has been sponsoring KPR operations since 2020. It is evidence of KPR's innovation of a volunteer-run model so successful in Bangladesh that was lacking previously.

### *19.5.2 Humanitarian Play Lab (HPL) of BRAC*

BRAC pioneers in developing Humanitarian Play Lab (HPL) in Bangladesh which has been scaled up in Tanzania and Uganda since 2015. HPL helps children from 0 to 2 learn and heal through play in humanitarian emergency settings. It provides children with a safe and supportive space to express themselves, develop their skills, and build resilience. The program focuses on psychosocial support, early learning, and community engagement. HPL has been implemented in a variety of humanitarian emergency settings, including the Rohingya refugee camps in Cox's Bazar, Bangladesh, and the refugee settlements in Uganda. Based on a recent study, the program has been shown to have a positive impact on children's psychosocial well-being, early learning outcomes, and community engagement (BRAC, 2021).

In a world where one in six children live in a conflict zone, countless children find themselves grappling with the profound impacts of conflict, displacement, and adversity (Save The Children, n.d). The need for compassionate and specialized care such as HPL is paramount, as these young souls grapple with the scars of their experiences. BRAC Humanitarian Play Labs are staffed by trained Play Leaders who are sensitive to the needs of children in humanitarian emergency settings. The Play Leaders are responsible for creating a safe and supportive environment for children to play and learn. They also work with parents, caregivers, and community members to support children's learning and development at home and in the community.

This innovation of HPL by RAC is an effective model and sets an example for the world on how a culturally sensitive, participatory approach can be seamlessly integrated into humanitarian initiatives. By placing emphasis on the unique cultural contexts of each community, BRAC ensures that its programs resonate authentically with the people they aim to serve. This holistic approach not only addresses immediate needs but also fosters sustainable solutions that empower communities to navigate challenges and rebuild, showcasing the transformative impact of a community-led model on a global scale. More than 40,000 Rohingya children accessed 250 BRAC play labs since 2017 (BRAC, 2019).

### *19.5.3 SHOJON Tele Mental Health Service of SAJIDA Foundation*

People with untreated mental diseases are more likely to become impoverished, more likely to be marginalized, and more likely to become disabled. Because of stigma and discrimination, people with mental illnesses commonly suffer from infringement of their human rights, including the denial of their economic, social, and cultural rights. The expense of mental health treatments is one of the numerous barriers that the people of Bangladesh must overcome in order to obtain mental health treatment. Because service providers and services are mostly centralized in Dhaka, it was time the country needed to utilize digital mental health in order to tackle the gap.

Aligned with the organization's commitment to ensure health, happiness, and dignity for all and the emerging need of mental health, *SAJIDA Foundation,* a value-driven non-profit organization, designed and developed SHOJON tele-mental health service in 2021 to address the service gap especially in the lower socioeconomic strata. Shojon uses a tiered model where a range of mental health professionals work in different tiers based on a referral pathway, using an innovative tech platform. It includes para-counselors, psychologists, and psychiatrists. Anyone from any part of Bangladesh can call to get long-term counseling support and psychiatric consultation from SHOJON using their phone, with a minimum cost based on their affordability. Thus, SHOJON makes a difference by bridging the rural and low-income community into the access of quality MH services with minimum cost leveraging digital mental health.

While the effectiveness of digital mental health is well established in high-income countries, there has been limited evidence in the context of LMICs. A recent meta-analysis, encompassing nine LMICs and published in September 2023, revealed promising results. The study demonstrated that digital mental health interventions were more effective than controls in reducing symptoms of common mental disorders such as anxiety and depression at the post-test (Karyotaki et al., 2023). Additionally, there was a small but significant improvement in the quality of life at the post-test stage. These findings instill hope for interventions like SHOJON, suggesting that with proper operational and clinical planning, tele-mental health services can stand out in addressing the community's mental health needs, a critical requirement at this time.

Over the past 2 years, SHOJON has provided assistance to approximately 9000 individuals with mental health needs. This exemplifies the positive impact achievable through such initiatives. As SF advances to scale up its operations, there is a growing optimism that SHOJON, with its effective approach, will play a crucial role in meeting the psychological needs of the country. The journey from pilot phase to expansion signifies not only the success of SF's initiatives but also the increasing recognition of the importance of accessible and innovative digital solutions for mental health in LMICs. The road ahead holds promise for SHOJON as it continues to make strides in improving the mental health landscape in Bangladesh through digital mental health.

## 19.6 Challenges of NGOs in Bangladesh

NGOs working in this field of mental health in Bangladesh face an array of difficulties and challenges in their efforts to provide support, advocacy, and awareness. Mental health issues have gained prominence globally, yet the journey toward understanding, acceptance, and effective treatment remains an uphill battle for many NGOs. These organizations encounter several hurdles that often impede their noble intentions and impact. Some of the significant difficulties and challenges faced by NGOs are presented below:

### 19.6.1 Funding, Sustainability, and Long-Term Impact

A major roadblock for NGOs is securing sustainable funding. Mental health programs typically require long-term support, yet funding often comes in the form of short-term grants or donations. This makes it difficult for NGOs to plan for long-term sustainability and ensure the continuity of their services. Additionally, measuring the impact of mental health interventions can be complex, making it challenging to demonstrate the effectiveness of programs and secure long-term funding.

### 19.6.2 Dearth of Ethical Practice

The absence of a regulatory body and licensing system for psychologists in Bangladesh has resulted in significant challenges for mental health services. This gap often led NGOs to recruit underqualified staff at lower salaries, often without proper mechanism of clinical supervision. As a consequence, there is a notable deficiency in technical expertise within mental health services, heightening the risk of potential malpractice. This situation not only compromises the quality of care available to those seeking mental health support but also underscores the urgent need for regulatory frameworks to ensure the competence and ethical standards of mental health professionals in Bangladesh.

### 19.6.3 Regulatory Oversight

Some NGOs, particularly those providing institutional care, require stricter regulatory monitoring. Ensuring the safety, welfare, and ethical treatment of residents is a crucial responsibility. However, inadequate oversight can lead to abuse, neglect, and violations of human rights. Robust regulatory frameworks and consistent monitoring are essential to safeguard the well-being of individuals under NGO care.

### 19.6.4 Limited Resources and Personnel

Mental health services in Bangladesh are significantly under-resourced. The government allocates a minimal budget to mental health care, leading to a shortage of qualified professionals and inadequate infrastructure. Additionally, the shortage of trained mental health professionals exacerbates the challenges faced by NGOs. Bangladesh grapples with a scarcity of psychiatrists, psychologists, and counselors, creating an imbalance in service delivery. NGOs often struggle to recruit and retain qualified staff, constraining their ability to provide comprehensive care. These limitations can impact the quality and scope of NGOs programs, leaving many individuals without access to vital mental health support.

### 19.6.5 Burnout Among Staff

The demanding nature of working in mental health, coupled with limited resources and challenging work environments, can lead to burnout among NGO staff. This not only impacts individual well-being but also affects the quality-of-service delivery and the overall effectiveness of the organization.

## 19.7 Future Scope and Opportunities

In this section, we will delve into the potential avenues and opportunities that lie ahead, paving the way for further evolution and advancement of mental health services provided by NGOs.

### 19.7.1 Integration of Theory and Research

One notable deficiency in the current approaches employed by NGOs to deliver mental health services in the Bangladeshi context is the absence of interventions rooted in well-established theories and research evidence. This gap contributes to the challenge of sustaining and scaling up interventions designed and implemented by NGOs over the long term. In the evolving landscape of mental health opportunities and challenges in Bangladesh, the amalgamation of theory and research can be a crucial element for NGOs seeking sustainability and a positive impact on the community, society, and the nation. As the understanding of mental health continues to deepen, NGOs have a distinct opportunity to bridge the gap between theoretical frameworks and practical applications. Collaborations with academic institutions and research organizations, such as Department of Clinical or Counseling Psychology, University of Dhaka and ICDDR, B practices are not only endorsed but actively ingrained into the realm of mental health service initiatives. Such integration and collaboration can ensure the context-specificity and adaptability of interventions provided by NGOs to address the nuanced mental health challenges faced by the diverse population in Bangladesh.

### 19.7.2 Evidence-Based Practice and Quality of Care

To foster scientific credibility and enhance the sustainable impact of interventions provided by NGOs, there is no alternative to evidence-based practice. This approach is crucial because it ensures the quality of care by offering comprehensive and person-centered mental health services. To achieve this, a comprehensive approach involving continuous supervision, monitoring, and ongoing capacity-building initiatives is imperative. NGOs can establish robust supervision frameworks that involve regular and structured oversight of mental health interventions. This continuous supervision framework can be designed through collaboration with mental health professional bodies, such as Bangladesh Clinical Psychology Society and Bangladesh Psychiatric Association. These professional bodies can assist NGOs in developing monitoring tools to track staff adherence to evidence-based protocols, ensuring the competence of mental health service providers and addressing any emerging challenges promptly. Furthermore, ensuring the capacity development of staff through the implementation of continuous training and workshop programs in clinical skills, journal clubbing, literature review, research designs, data interpretations, and culturally sensitive practices can enhance their proficiency in delivering evidence-based care, thereby ensuring the quality of care.

### 19.7.3 Community-Based Mental Health Intervention

Future focus and investment of the NGOs should be implementing community-based mental health interventions. This approach has the potential to reduce the burden on tertiary care facilities by offering accessible mental health services at the community level enabling promotion, prevention, and early intervention. A significant contributor to the mental health burden is the stigma attached to mental health conditions and lack of primary care (Faruk et al, 2023). Hence, NGOs can play a crucial role in reducing this stigma through diverse approaches such as outreach programs, peer support networks, and culturally sensitive awareness campaigns. NGOs can provide primary mental health screening and care collaborating with educational institutions, community health clinics, and local government bodies.

### 19.7.4 Utilization of Digital Innovations in Mental Health

In an era characterized by rapid technological advancements, NGOs have the opportunity to leverage innovative solutions for enhancing mental health services. Telemedicine, mobile applications, and online platforms, for instance, can serve as accessible mediums for counseling, psychoeducation, awareness-raising, and support (Arafat et al., 2021). Social media platforms, blogs, and web portals are additional

**Table 19.1** List of NGOs working with vulnerable communities

| Sl | Vulnerable group | NGOs |
|---|---|---|
| 1 | Forcibly displaced myanmar national (Rohingya) | Action Aid Bangladesh (AAB), Agrajattra, Ain o Salish Kendra (ASK), Bandhu Social Welfare Society (Bandhu), Bangladesh Legal Aid and Services Trust (BLAST), Bangladesh Red Crescent Society (BDRCS), BRAC, Care Bangladesh, Center for Disability in Development (CDD), Dhaka Ahsania mission (DAM), Gonosasthaya Kendra (G.K.), International Centre for Diarrheal Disease Research, Bangladesh (ICDDR, B), Jago Foundation, Mukti Coxbazar, Prottyashi, Samaj Kalyan O Unnoyon Shangstha (SKUS), Partners in Health and Development (PHD), Care Bangladesh |
| 2 | Climate change | SAJIDA Foundation, BRAC, Friendship, Coastal Association for Social Transformation Trust (COAST) |
| 3 | Indigenous community | Supporting People and Rebuilding Communities (SPaRC), Manusher Jonno Foundation (MJF), Kapaeeng Foundation |
| 4 | LGBTQ community | Bandhu Social Welfare Society (Bandhu), ICDDR, B, Badhan Hijra Sangha (BHS), Dhaka Ahsania mission (DAM), TransEnd |

tools that can be employed to disseminate mental health literacy, teach self-help strategies, foster positive living, and develop resiliency. Other ICT-based platforms, such as text messaging, audio-visual animations, and email, can be utilized to deliver customized and targeted information to specific communities as interventions to enhance mental health awareness. Podcasts represent another potential medium for education, where mental health professionals can provide specific information related to mental health for the general population. Additionally, the integration of artificial intelligence (AI)-driven technologies, including chatbots, holds the potential to open new avenues for developing innovative mental health services for remotely accessible populations. Therefore, by embracing these technological innovations, NGOs can overcome geographical barriers, reaching individuals in remote areas where mental health resources are often scarce.

## 19.8 Conclusion

In the realm of Bangladesh's mental health, it is undeniable that NGOs have played a pioneering role in significantly alleviating the burden of the mental health treatment gap on a national scale. From addressing the unique needs of vulnerable communities to introducing innovative approaches, NGOs have become indispensable partners in mental health care. In synergy with government efforts, the collective impact of NGOs has been instrumental in expanding access to mental health services and fostering a more comprehensive and inclusive approach.

## References


ADD Internation Bangladesh. (2021). *Nationwide Mental Health Service Mapping. Community Based Mental Health Services for Children and Young People in Marginalized Communities* ($2^{nd}$ edition). ADD International Bangladesh.

Ambekar, A., Lewi, G., Rao, S., & Sethi, H. (2005). *South Asia: Regional Profile (Drugs and Crime)*. UNODC. Retrieved December 12, 2023 from https://www.unodc.org/documents/india/South%20Asia%20Regional%20Profile%20(Sept%202005).pdf.

Arafat, M. Y., Zaman, S., & Hawlader, M. D. H. (2021). Telemedicine improves mental health in COVID-19 pandemic. *Journal of Global Health, 11*,. https://doi.org/10.7189/jogh.11.03004

Bangladesh Bureau of Statistics. (2023). *Population and Housing Census 2022*. Bangladesh Bureau of Statistics. Retrieved December 12, 2023 from https://bbs.gov.bd/site/page/47856ad0-7e1c-4aab-bd78-892733bc06eb/Population-&-Housing.

Baser, S., & Abu Hasnath, S. (2023). The rise and fall of the NGOs in Bangladesh: What does the future hold? *IntechOpen*. https://doi.org/10.5772/intechopen.107855

Befienders Worlwide. (2012). *Find support now*. Retrieved December 12, 2023 from https://befrienders.org/.

BRAC. (2019). *Humanitarian Play Labs: Helping Rohingya children heal and learn through play*. Retrieved December 12, 2023 from https://www.brac.net/latest-news/item/1213-humanitarian-play-labs-helping-rohingya-children-heal-and-learn-through-play#:~:text=More%20than%2040%2C000%20Rohingya%20children,collaboration%20with%20the%20LEGO%20Foundation.

BRAC. (2021). *Play Lab Research Brief*. Retrieved December 13, 2023 from https://playlabs.bracusa.org/wp-content/uploads/2021/12/BRAC-Play-Labs-Research-Brief-Bangladesh-Final.pdf.

Department of Narcotics Control. (2023). *List of private treatment centre*. Department of Narcotics Control. Retrieved December 13, 2023 from https://dnc.gov.bd/site/page/efb131fc-a930-43b2-aaa5-41a1cd1817ca.

Diaz, M. L., & Rahaman, M. M. (2022). *Deep scars of climate change: The need for addressing mental health issues in Bangladesh*. The Business Standard. Retrieved December 13, 2023 from https://www.tbsnews.net/thoughts/deep-scars-climate-change-need-addressing-mental-health-issues-bangladesh-557758.

Faruk, M. O., Khan, A. H., Chowdhury, K. U. A., Jahan, S., Sarker, D. C., Colucci, E., & Hasan, M. T. (2023). Mental illness stigma in Bangladesh: Findings from a cross-sectional survey. *Cambridge Prisms: Global Mental Health, 10*, e59. https://doi.org/10.1017/gmh.2023.56

Faruk, M. O., Nijhum, R. P., Khatun, M. N., & Powell, G. E. (2021). Anxiety and depression in two indigenous communities in Bangladesh. *Global Mental Health, 8*, e34. https://doi.org/10.1017/gmh.2021.33

JRP. (2022). *Joint response plan: Rohingya humanitarian crisis*. Inter Sector Coordination Group (ISCG). Retrieved December 12, 2023 from https://www.humanitarianresponse.info/en/operations/bangladesh.

Iqbal, Y., Jahan, R., & Matin, M. R. (2019). Descriptive characteristics of callers to an emotional support and suicide prevention helpline in Bangladesh (first five years). *Asian Journal of Psychiatry, 45*, 63–65. https://doi.org/10.1016/j.ajp.2019.09.005

Iqbal, Y., Jahan, R., Yesmin, S., Selim, A., & Siddique, S. N. (2021). COVID-19-related issues on tele-counseling helpline in Bangladesh. *Asia-Pacific Psychiatry, 13*(2), e12407. https://doi.org/10.1111/appy.12407

Islam, A., & Biswas, T. (2015). Mental health and the health system in Bangladesh: situation analysis of a neglected domain. *Am J Psychiatry Neurosci, 3*(4), 57–62. https://doi.org/10.11648/j.ajpn.20150304.11.

Islam, M. S. (2016). The NGOs sector in Bangladesh: Emergence, contribution and current debate. *Advances in Asian Social Science, 7*(2), 1182–1188.

Kabir, R., Hasan, M. R., & Arafat, S. M. Y. (2023). Epidemiology of Suicide and Data Quality in Bangladesh. In: Arafat, S.M.Y., Khan, M.M. (eds) Suicide in Bangladesh. New Perspectives in Behavioral & Health Sciences. Springer, Singapore. https://doi.org/10.1007/978-981-99-0289-7_1.

Karim, M. E., & Shaikh, S. (2021). Newly enacted mental health law in Bangladesh. *Bjpsych International, 18*(4), 85–87. https://doi.org/10.1192/bji.2021.1

Karyotaki, E., Miguel, C., Panagiotopoulou, O. M., Harrer, M., Seward, N., Sijbrandij, M., Araya, R., Patel, V., & Cuijpers, P. (2023). Digital interventions for common mental disorders in low-and middle-income countries: A systematic review and meta-analysis. *Cambridge Prisms: Global Mental Health, 1–28,*. https://doi.org/10.1017/gmh.2023.50

MacMillan, S. (2022). *Hope Over Fate: Fazle Hasan Abed and the Science of Ending Global Poverty*. Rowman & Littlefield Publishers.

Mental Health Act. (2018). *Bangladesh [Online]*. Retrieved December 12, 2023 from http://bdlaws.minlaw.gov.bd/act-1273.html.

Ministry of Health & Family Welfare. (2021). *National Mental Health Survey 2019*. National Institute of Mental Health. Retrieved December 12, 2023 from http://nimh.gov.bd/wp-content/uploads/2021/11/Mental-Health-Survey-Report.pd.

Rukmana, D. (2014). Vulnerable Populations. In A. C. Michalos (Ed.), *Encyclopedia of Quality of Life and Well-Being Research* (pp. 6989–6992). Springer Netherlands. https://doi.org/10.1007/978-94-007-0753-5_3184.

Save The Children. (n.d.). *Every child deserves a childhood - no matter who they are and where they live*. Retrieved December 12, 2023 from https://www.savethechildren.org/us/what-we-do/global-policy-advocacy/humanitarian-crises#:~:text=Over%20150%20million%20children%20around,living%20outside%20of%20conflict%20settings.

Tay, A. K., Riley, A., Islam, R., Welton-Mitchell, C., Duchesne, B., Waters, V., Varner, A., Moussa, B., Alam, A. M., & Elshazly, M. (2019). The culture, mental health and psychosocial wellbeing of Rohingya refugees: A systematic review. *Epidemiology and Psychiatric Sciences, 28*(5), 489–494. https://doi.org/10.1017/S2045796019000192

UNHCR. (2023). *Rohingya Refugee Crisis Explained*. Retrieved December 12, 2023 from https://www.unrefugees.org/news/rohingya-refugee-crisis-explained/#:~:text=Now%2C%20more%20than%20960%2C000%20Rohingya,populated%20camps%20in%20the%20world.

Wahid, S. S., Raza, W. A., Mahmud, I., & Kohrt, B. A. (2023). Climate-related shocks and other stressors associated with depression and anxiety in Bangladesh: A nationally representative panel study. *The Lancet Planetary Health, 7*(2), e137–e146. https://doi.org/10.1016/S2542-5196(22)00315-1

Wei, D., Wang, X., You, X., Luo, X., Hao, C., Gu, J., Peng, S., Yang, X., Hao, Y., & Silenzio, V. M. (2020). Prevalence of depression, anxiety and suicide among men who have sex with men in China: A systematic review and meta-analysis. *Epidemiology and Psychiatric Sciences, 29*, e136. https://doi.org/10.1017/S2045796020000487

SPRINGER NATURE

# GPSR Compliance

*The European Union's (EU) General Product Safety Regulation (GPSR) is a set of rules that requires consumer products to be safe and our obligations to ensure this.*

*If you have any concerns about our products, you can contact us on ProductSafety@springernature.com*

In case Publisher is established outside the EU, the EU authorized representative is:

Springer Nature Customer Service Center GmbH
Europaplatz 3
69115 Heidelberg, Germany

The manufacturer's authorised representative in the EU is Springer Nature Customer Service Centre GmbH, Europaplatz 3, 69115 Heidelberg, Germany. If you have any concerns regarding our products, please contact ProductSafety@springernature.com

Printed and bound by CPI Group (UK) Ltd, Croydon, CR0 4YY
30/09/2026
02225314-0010